Recent Progress in

HORMONE RESEARCH

Proceedings of the Laurentian Hormone Conference

VOLUME 46

RECENT PROGRESS IN
HORMONE RESEARCH

Proceedings of the
1989 Laurentian Hormone Conference

Edited by
JAMES H. CLARK

VOLUME 46

PROGRAM COMMITTEE

C. W. Bardin
J. H. Clark
H. G. Friesen
D. K. Granner
P. A. Kelly
I. A. Kourides
S. McKnight

A. R. Means
D. Orth
J. E. Rall
G. Ringold
N. B. Schwartz
J. L. Vaitukaitis
W. Vale

ACADEMIC PRESS, INC.
Harcourt Brace Jovanovich, Publishers
San Diego   New York   Boston
London   Sydney   Tokyo   Toronto

This book is printed on acid-free paper. ∞

Copyright © 1990 By Academic Press, Inc.
All Rights Reserved.
No part of this publication may be reproduced or transmitted in any form or
by any means, electronic or mechanical, including photocopy, recording, or
any information storage and retrieval system, without permission in writing
from the publisher.

Academic Press, Inc.
San Diego, California 92101

United Kingdom Edition published by
Academic Press Limited
24-28 Oval Road, London NW1 7DX

Library of Congress Catalog Card Number: Med. 47-38

ISBN   0-12-571146-8   (alk. paper)

Printed in the United States of America
90 91 92 93   9 8 7 6 5 4 3 2 1

CONTENTS

LIST OF CONTRIBUTORS AND DISCUSSANTS

D. Accili

R. Arakaki

M. Ascoli

C. W. Bardin

L. Beitz

C. Bevins

S. P. Bottari

H. Brady

T. R. Brown

A. Cama

J.-L. Castrillo

G. C. Chamness

J. H. Clark

C. Conover

F. Courtney

W. F. Crowley

G. B. Cutler

D. D. De Leon

S. M. Donovan

B. A. J. Evans

C. M. Foster

C. Frapier

F. S. French

H. G. Friesen

D. L. Garbers

L. Giudice

P. J. Godowski

G. A. Gonzalez

P. Gorden

C. Grunfeld

R. G. Hammonds

I. A. Hughes

E. Imano

D. R. Joseph

N. Josso

H. Kadowaki

T. Kadowaki

A. Kakizuka

M. Karin

K. K. Kidd

J. Kirkland

G. Lamson

D. W. Leung

D. B. Lubahn

B. Marcus-Samuels

R. Margolis

A. McCormick

C. McKeon

A. R. Means

H. Meunier

C. J. Migeon

V. Moncada

M. R. Montminy

S. Najjar

M. New

S. Nakanishi

K. Nikolics

I. Ocrant

Y. Oh

H. Ohkubo

K. Ojamaa

N. Perrotti

H. Pham

C. Quigley

R. Rees-Jones

G. Ringold

C. Rivier

D. Rodbard

V. Roberts

R. G. Rosenfeld

S. M. Rosenthal

J. Roth

M. Rozakis

N. A. Samaan

M. Sar

Y. Sasai

N. B. Schwartz

D. L. Segaloff

R. Shigemoto

J. A. Simental

N. E. Simpson

S. A. Spencer

R. Sprengel

S. Shenolikar

vii

R. S. Swerdloff

T. Takumi

J.-an Tan

S. I. Taylor

L. Theill

J. L. Vaitukaitis

W. Vale

M. R. Walters

M. J. Waters

E. M. Wilson

W. I. Wood

K. K. Yamamoto

W. G. Yarbrough

Y. Yokota

PREFACE

This volume provides a superior summary of the most recent developments in the field of hormone research.

Giving a talk at the Laurentian Hormone Conference is an honor, and the presentations of those who participated were excellent. Each of the lectures was followed by an interesting discussion–question session. These were conducted by the session chairpersons: Gordon Ringold, Tony Means, Henry Friesen, Wylie Vale, Neena Schwartz, and Judy Vaitukatis. I thank them for a job well done. I also thank Robert Lacroix who recorded the sessions, Lucy Felicissimo and Linda Carsagnini who transcribed them, and Rose Copenhaver who made the final corrections.

James H. Clark

Molecular Basis of Androgen Insensitivity

FRANK S. FRENCH,* DENNIS B. LUBAHN,* TERRY R. BROWN,† JORGE
A. SIMENTAL,* CHARMIAN A. QUIGLEY,* WENDELL G.
YARBROUGH,* JIANN-AN TAN,* MADHABANANDA SAR,* DAVID R.
JOSEPH,* BRONWYN A. J. EVANS,‡ IEUAN A. HUGHES,‡ CLAUDE J.
MIGEON,† AND ELIZABETH M. WILSON*

*University of North Carolina School of Medicine, Chapel Hill, North Carolina 27599,
†Department of Pediatrics and Endocrinology, Johns Hopkins University School
of Medicine, Baltimore, Maryland 21205, and ‡University of Wales College
of Medicine, Cardiff CF4 4XN, Wales

The earliest sex phenotype of a human fetus is female, regardless of its genetic sex. Development of male external genitalia in the 46,XY embryo and virilization of the pubertal male are dependent on androgen binding to its receptor and subsequent activation of gene expression. Male sex differentiation fails to occur in the absence of androgen, as in the normal female fetus, or without a functioning androgen receptor (AR), as in the genetic male who develops female external genitalia because of androgen insensitivity. Thus, androgen, acting through its receptor, functions as a morphogen to direct formation of the male phenotype during a critical period of early fetal development. At puberty the AR complex functions as a growth and differentiation factor, acting in concert with other hormones and growth factors to stimulate reproductive functions that characterize the fully virilized male.

Studies of the androgen insensitivity syndrome (AIS) [also referred to as testicular feminization (Tfm)] in rats, mice, and humans have established that this disorder is linked to the X chromosome (Meyer *et al.*, 1975; B. R. Migeon *et al.*, 1981; Lyon and Hawkes, 1970). Androgen insensitivity is characterized by lack of a target cell response to androgen (testosterone and its 5-α-reduced metabolite, dihydrotestosterone) (Wilkins, 1950; French *et al.*, 1965, 1966; Strickland and French, 1969; Keenan *et al.*, 1974; Griffin *et al.*, 1976; Amrhein *et al.*, 1976).

To further localize the AR gene, C. J. Migeon *et al.* (1981) produced a series of Tfm mouse–human cell hybrids containing X:autosome translocation chromosomes lacking specific segments of the human X chromosome. Expression of AR

1

androgen binding indicated that either the AR locus or a factor controlling AR expression is located on the human X chromosome near the centromere between Xq13 and Xp11. Cloning the AR enabled Lubahn *et al.* (1988a) to demonstrate that it is the AR structural gene that occupies this locus on the X chromosome and enabled Brown *et al.* (1988) to establish that a mutation in the AR gene can result in AIS.

I.   Cloning of AR

AR belongs to the subfamily of steroid hormone receptors within a larger family of nuclear proteins that likely evolved from a common ancestral gene. Each contains an amino-terminal region, variable in length, that could have a role in transcriptional activation, a central cysteine-rich DNA-binding domain, and a carboxyl-terminal ligand-binding domain (Hollenberg *et al.*, 1985; Arriza *et al.*, 1987; Misrahi *et al.*, 1987; S. Green *et al.*, 1986; Weinberger *et al.*, 1986; Petkovich *et al.*, 1987). Highest sequence identity occurs in the DNA-binding domain, including the conserved positioning of cysteines resembling the zinc-binding motif (i.e., finger structure) of the *Xenopus laevis* 5 S RNA gene transcription factor IIIA (Miller *et al.*, 1985; Diakun *et al.*, 1986; Berg, 1986; Fairall *et al.*, 1986).

The strategy for isolating AR DNA was based on evidence that the AR gene is X chromosome linked and that no other steroid receptor gene is located on the X chromosome. In addition, it was assumed that AR would resemble other members of the steroid receptor family in the conserved DNA-binding domain. A consensus oligonucleotide probe was synthesized from homologous sequences within the DNA-binding domains of human progesterone, glucocorticoid, thyroid hormone, and estrogen receptors (Hollenberg *et al.*, 1985; Misrahi *et al.*, 1987; G. L. Green *et al.*, 1986; S. Green *et al.*, 1986). Screening an X chromosome library with the consensus oligonucleotide A resulted in several recombinants whose inserts were cloned into bacteriophage M13 DNA and sequenced. One recombinant clone contained a sequence similar to, yet distinct from, the cystine-rich DNA-binding domains of the other steroid hormone receptors.

This cloning strategy is shown in Fig. 1 (Lubahn *et al.*, 1988a). The genomic fragment was subsequently used to screen cDNA libraries derived from human fibroblasts and epididymides. Two overlapping cDNA clones were isolated which had identical sequences in the DNA-binding domain and shared sequence identity with the genomic fragment used in screening.

Isolation of the partial AR cDNA sequence led to the identification and sequencing of additional clones to obtain the full-length coding sequence of human (Lubahn *et al.*, 1988b) and rat (Tan *et al.*, 1988) ARs. The size of AR determined from the deduced amino acid sequences (i.e., rat AR, MW 98,227; human AR, MW 98,999) is in reasonable agreement with that determined from biochemical evidence (rat AR, MW 117,000) (Wilson and French, 1979).

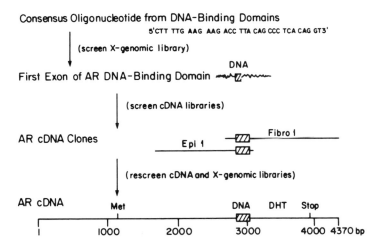

FIG. 1. Human AR cloning strategy. DHT, Dihydrotestosterone.

Transient expression in monkey kidney cells (COS M6) demonstrated that the human foreskin fibroblast cDNA encodes the steroid-binding domain of human AR. A DNA fragment extending 5′ to 3′ from the *Hin*dIII site within the putative DNA-binding domain through the stop codon (TGA) (Fig. 2A) was cloned into the plasmid vector (pCMV) containing the cytomegalovirus promoter (Fig. 2B). Expression was facilitated by adding to the 5′ end a consensus translation initiation sequence containing the methionine codon (ATG) in the reading frame. Transfection of the recombinant construct produced a protein with high affinity for [^{3}H]dihydrotestosterone, saturable at physiological levels of hormones (Fig. 3A). The binding constant [$K_d = 2.7$ ($\pm$ 1.4) $\times$ 10^{-10} M] (Fig. 3B) was nearly identical to that of native AR (Wilson and French, 1976). The level of expressed protein, 1.3 pmol/mg of protein, was 20–60 times greater than that in male reproductive tissues (Wilson and French, 1976, 1979). Mock transfections without plasmid or transfections with plasmid DNA lacking the AR insert yielded no specific binding of dihydrotestosterone. Steroid specificity was identical to that of native AR, with highest affinity for dihydrotestosterone and testosterone, intermediate affinity for progesterone and estradiol, and low affinity for cortisol (Fig. 3C).

Sublocalization of human AR was achieved with known fragments of the X chromosome in human–rodent hybrids (Willard and Riordan, 1985). A 900-bp *Hin*dIII DNA probe from the human AR genomic isolate (X05AR) hybridized to a 0.9-kb *Hin*dIII DNA fragment from hybrid cells that contained human Xcen–qter or Xp21–qter fragments, but not to DNA fragments from hybrid cells containing Xq21–qter or Xq13–qter (Fig. 4). Thus, the AR gene is located between the X centromere and Xq13. More recently, the AR gene locus has been further defined to Xq11–q12 (C. J. Brown *et al.*, 1989). This chromosome map position

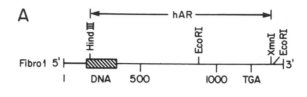

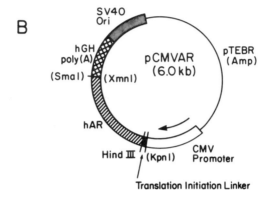

FIG. 2. (A) Partial AR cDNA cloned from human fibroblast cDNA library. hAR, Human androgen receptor. (B) Expression vector (pCMV) with the partial cDNA insert shown in (A). pCMV (constructed by David W. Russell) contains the cytomegalovirus promoter, CMV, the immediate early gene, the poly(A) addition–transcription terminator region of the human growth hormone gene [hGH poly(A)], the simian virus 40 origin of replication, and a polylinker region for the insertion of cDNAs. The plasmid pTEBR contains the ampicillin resistance gene (Amp). Restriction endonuclease sites in parentheses are lost during cloning. (From Lubahn et al., 1988a.)

is similar to that determined by expression of AR from X chromosome fragments in hybrid cells (C. J. Migeon et al., 1981) and is consistent with X chromosome linkage of AIS (Grumbach and Barr, 1958; Stanley et al., 1973; Lyon and Hawkes, 1970).

II. Antisera to AR

A peptide with a sequence derived from a 15-amino acid region common to rat and human AR was synthesized and used to raise antibodies in rabbits. The sequence shown in Fig. 5 is immediately 5′ to the DNA-binding domain and is unique to the AR, based on available steroid receptor sequence information. An additional criterion for peptide selection was hydrophilicity, as determined from a hydropathic plot of the AR sequence (Lubahn et al., 1988b). It was predicted that the region selected for peptide synthesis would extend to the hydrophilic exterior and that contiguous proline residues might contribute secondary struc-

STEROID BINDING PROPERTIES OF THE EXPRESSED ANDROGEN RECEPTOR

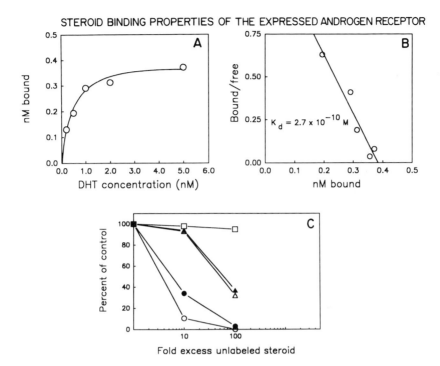

FIG. 3.   (A) Saturation analysis of [^{3}H]dihydrotestosterone (DHT) binding in extracts of pCMV AR-transfected COS M6 cells. Portions of cytosol (0.1 ml; 0.3 mg of protein per milliliter) were incubated overnight at 4°C with increasing concentrations of ^{3}H-labeled hormone and analyzed by charcoal adsorption. Nonspecific binding increased from 18% to 37% of the total bound radioactivity. (B) Scatchard plot of [^{3}H]DHT binding. Error estimation was based on linear regression analysis ($r = 0.966$). (C) Competition of unlabeled steroids for binding of 10- and 100-fold excess of labeled hormone. Specific binding was determined as previously described (Wilson and French, 1976). Unlabeled competitor steroids included DHT (○), testosterone (●), estradiol (△), progesterone (▲), and cortisol (□). (From Lubahn et al., 1988a.)

ture and thus increase peptide antigenicity. The 15-amino acid AR sequence and three linker amino acids, Gly–Gly–Cys, were synthesized (peptide 875) and covalently coupled to keyhole limpet hemocyanin for use in antibody production. The antisera demonstrated high titer reactivity toward peptide 875 in an enzyme-linked immunosorbent assay (ELISA), showing reactivity against peptide 875 at dilutions greater than 25,000.

Antiserum reactivity with native AR was investigated by sucrose gradient centrifugation. Antibodies obtained by antigen-affinity chromatography caused the 4.5 S [^{3}H]dihydrotestosterone-labeled AR to sediment at 10 S (Fig. 6). No peak of radioactivity was observed when cytosol was incubated with

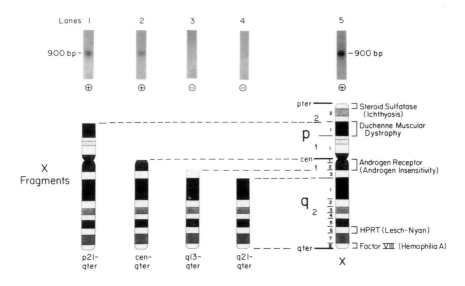

FIG. 4. Androgen localization on the human X chromosome by Southern blot analysis. A hybridization signal (900 bp) was detected only with gene fragments containing DNA from X centromere to Xq13 (Lubahn *et al.*, 1988a). At the top of the figure is a Southern blot of fragments shown schematically below. More recently, the AR gene locus has been further defined to Xq11–q12. HPRT, Hypoxanthine phosphoribosyltransferase.

[^{3}H]dihydrotestosterone and a 100-fold excess of unlabeled dihydrotestosterone. Preincubation of the antiserum preparations with peptide 875 prior to combining with [^{3}H]dihydrotestosterone-labeled receptor eliminated the reactive antibodies, as measured by ELISA, and abolished the increased sedimentation of the 4.5 S receptor.

The antibody is effective in immunocytochemical localization of AR in human prostate, shown in Fig. 7. Sections of human prostate tissue obtained by radical prostatectomy contained regions of benign prostatic hyperplasia. Strong nuclear

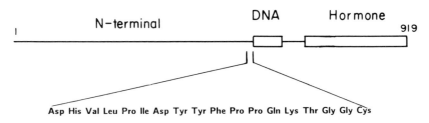

FIG. 5.   Synthetic peptide used as antigen for AR antibody.

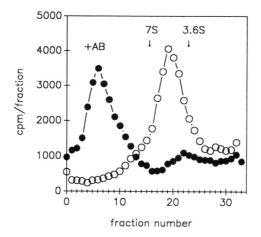

FIG. 6. Sucrose gradient analysis of the [³H]dihydrotestosterone-labeled AR after incubation with polyclonal antibody AR52 raised against peptide 875. Dunning tumor AR fraction was incubated for 3 hours at 0°C with (●) or without (○) an immunoglobulin fraction of immune serum purified on a peptide-affinity column (150 μg protein in 0.1 ml). Centrifugation was performed as described in a 2–20% (w/v) sucrose gradient containing 5 mM mercaptoethanol, 10% glycerol, 0.15 M KCl, and 50 mM Tris, pH 7.2. The migration positions of the molecular weight markers ovalbumin (3.6 S) and γ-globulin (7 S) were determined as previously described. (From Tan *et al.,* 1988.)

immunostaining was detected in acinar epithelial cells of glandular benign prostatic hyperplastic tissue, with weaker immunostaining in nuclei of stromal cells. This and other antibodies to synthetic peptides corresponding to amino-terminal AR sequences homologous in humans and rats have been effective in localizing AR in reproductive tissues and the brains of rats, mice, and guinea pigs. Staining of AR in cultured genital skin fibroblasts (Fig. 8) is especially valuable in analyses of mutant AR proteins causing androgen insensitivity syndrome.

III. Comparison of Human and Rat AR cDNAs

Rat androgen receptor cDNA was cloned from a λ-gt11 rat epididymal cDNA library (Tan *et al.,* 1988). Comparison of amino acid sequences revealed overall amino acid sequence homologies of 85% and 83% at the nucleotide level. Within the DNA- and hormone-binding domains amino acid sequences of the two receptors are identical (Fig. 9). The carboxyl-terminal halves of the human and rat ARs, including the DNA- and hormone-binding domains, differ by only seven amino acid residues. In contrast, the amino-terminal regions of human and rat ARs have significant sequence divergence. The overall amino-terminal homology is only 77%, primarily due to repeated single amino acid motifs, which,

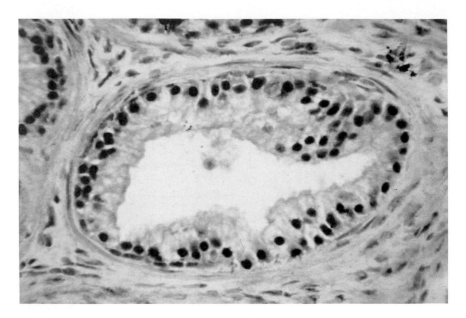

FIG. 7. Immunocytochemical localization of AR in epithelial cell nuclei of human benign hyperplastic prostate. Tissue was obtained by radical prostatectomy from a patient with both benign hyperplasia and adenocarcinoma. Frozen sections (10 μm) were fixed with 4% paraformaldehyde, pH 7.4, incubated with the immunoglobulin G (IgG) fraction of AR antiserum (10 μg/ml), and stained by the avidin–biotin–peroxidase method (Sar, 1985). Rabbit polyclonal antibody, AR52, was raised against a conjugate of the synthetic peptide shown in Fig. 5 and the IgG fraction was purified (Tan *et al.*, 1988). Magnification ×460.

though variable in length, generally occur at the same position. For example, there are 24 repeated glycines in human AR, but only five in rat AR at the same location. Similarly, five repeated glutamines in human AR correspond in position to 22 glutamines in rat AR, and eight prolines in human AR correspond to a broken sequence of seven prolines in rat AR. Additional repeats of glutamine and arginine occur in one receptor, but not in the other. Sequence homology between the repeats is 78–90%, and at one location five consecutive alanine residues in human AR correspond to an equal number in rat AR.

One group of repeated amino acids varied in length within the human species. The 21 glutamines in the human AR were observed in two cDNA clones, while there were 25 repeated glutamines at the same location in the genomic clone. These clones were isolated from independent libraries prepared from DNA of different individuals.

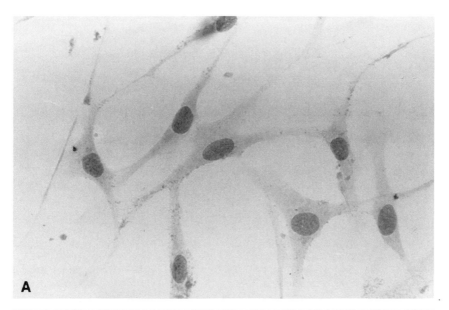

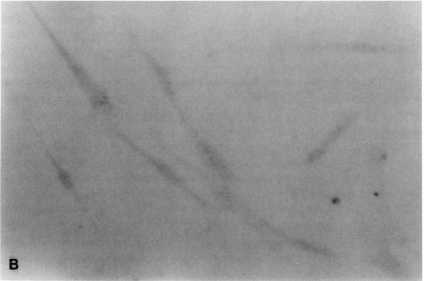

FIG. 8. Immunocytochemical localization of AR in normal human foreskin fibroblasts. A primary culture of human foreskin fibroblasts obtained from newborn circumcision was maintained in minimum essential medium containing antibiotics and 10% fetal calf serum. Twenty-four hours before harvest, the medium was replaced with serum-free medium containing 70 nM methyltrienolone (R1881). Cells were washed with phosphate-buffered saline, fixed with 2% paraformaldehyde overnight at 0°C, and incubated with an anti-AR peptide IgG fraction (AR32, 2 μg of IgG protein per milliliter), a polyclonal antibody raised against a sequence close to the amino terminus of the human AR. In preadsorption studies the immune IgG fraction was incubated with 5 μg peptide per milliliter for 48 hours at 0°C. The cells were stained by the avidin–biotin–peroxidase method (Sar, 1985). Magnification ×460. (A) AR staining in nuclei. (B) Absence of AR staining with peptide preabsorbed immune IgG.

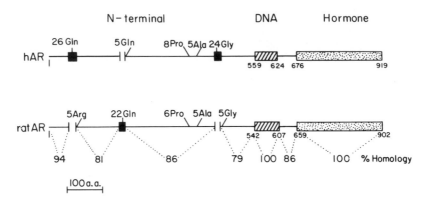

FIG. 9. Human (hAR) and rat AR amino acid (aa) alignment. The schematic drawing compares the percentage of amino acid homology (indicated at the bottom) of individual segments (dotted lines) between rat and human ARs. Amino acid residues are numbered immediately below the hatched and stippled boxes. Repeated amino acid motifs (more than four in length) within the amino-terminal region are indicated (some by solid boxes). (From Lubahn et al., 1988b.)

IV. Detection of an AR Gene Deletion by Southern Hybridization

In their initial study Brown et al. (1988) selected six unrelated 46,XY phenotypic females with negative receptor binding associated with complete AIS and 10 normal subjects for analysis of genomic DNA by Southern blotting with the human AR cDNA probes (Fig. 10). Using the cDNA probe hAR-1, the 10 normal subjects and five of the six AIS patients had identical restriction fragment patterns of EcoRI and BamHI digests. In one AIS patient a deletion was identi-

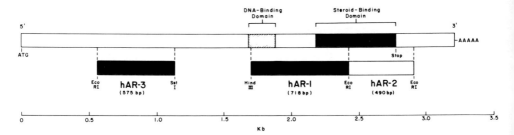

FIG. 10. Diagram of the human AR (hAR) cDNA and the three fragments used as radiolabeled hybridization probes on Southern blots of genomic DNA. The hAR from its 5′ initiation site (ATG) to its 3′ stop codon is encoded by 2757 nucleotides. The poly(A) tail indicates a poly(A)-rich region in the 3′-untranslated region, but not the true 3′ end of the mRNA, which is probably several kb farther 3′. The positions of the DNA (hatched bar)- and steroid (solid bar)-binding domains are shown. The three cDNA probes used for hybridization and their respective positions within the cDNA structure are designated as hAR-1, hAR-2, and hAR-3. (From Brown et al., 1988.)

fied (Fig. 11A) with probes hAR1 and hAR2. However, the deletion could not be detected with hAR3, indicating that it was located in the steroid-binding domain. Analysis of other members of the family (see pedigree in Fig. 11B) confirmed the deletion and its association with receptor binding-negative androgen insensitivity. In poly(A) RNA extracted from genital skin fibroblasts of this AIS patient neither 10-kb AR mRNA nor smaller hybridizing bands were detected by Northern hybridization, suggesting that the deleted AR mRNA is rapidly degraded. Deletion of the entire steroid-binding domain was confirmed by the amplification of genomic DNA using the polymerase chain reaction (PCR), as described in Section VI.

Brown *et al.* (1988) elected to perform this initial study in patients with complete AIS who had undetectable ARs by ligand binding assays, in the expectation that some of them might present a deletion of the AR gene. [About 5–10% of mutations found in genetic disorders are due to gene deletions (Monaco *et al.*, 1985; Antonarakis *et al.*, 1985; Hobbs *et al.*, 1987).] Assuming a 5% frequency, screening of 14 independent mutations of the AR gene should result in a greater than 50% chance of finding a gene deletion. This group of patients included one affected subject from each of six unrelated families. One of them showed a deletion when using two endonucleases, *Eco*RI and *Bam*HI. This finding demonstrated further the genetic heterogeneity in AIS; some patients with the complete receptor-negative form have a deletion of the AR gene, whereas others have no detectable deletion when assessed by identical techniques. In other AIS mutations the AR gene might not be expressed due to a point mutation, or a mutant gene might express a structurally modified receptor incapable of binding androgen. Thus far, several deletions and point mutations have been demonstrated by PCR and DNA sequencing, as shown below.

V.   Sequence of the Intron–Exon Junctions of the Coding Region of the AR Gene

Rapid analysis of the coding region of the AR gene using PCR required sequencing of the intron–exon junctions so that oligonucleotide primers bracketing each exon could be designed. Six genomic clones containing the eight exons of the amino acid coding regions of the human AR gene were isolated from a human X chromosome λ phage library using human AR cDNA and synthetic oligonucleotide probes (Lubahn *et al.*, 1989). Although the genomic clone inserts averaged 15 kb and the mRNA of human AR was 10–11 kb, only exons D and E and exons F–H were found in the same clones. Calculations based on five nonoverlapping clones averaging 15 kb yielded a size estimate of greater than 75 kb for the human AR gene. Sequences of the human AR coding exons and flanking intron regions are shown in Fig. 12. Cloned genomic exon and flanking intron sequences were confirmed by sequencing PCR-amplified fragments of

A

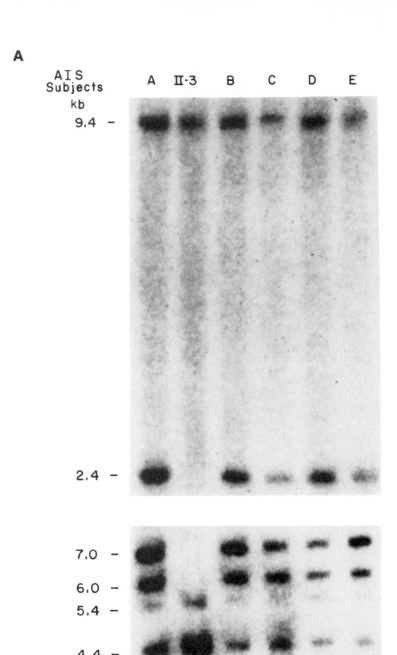

FIG. 11. (A) Southern blots of genomic DNA from genital skin fibroblasts of six unrelated subjects with the receptor-negative form of complete AIS. DNA (8 μg) was digested with *Eco*RI (top) or *Bam*HI (bottom) and analyzed for hybridization with ^{32}P-labeled hAR-1 cDNA. (B) Pedigree of a family with receptor-negative form of complete AIS. The father (I-1) is deceased; the mother (I-2) is an obligate heterozygote of this X chromosome-linked trait (solid circle inside open circle); and the three affected 46,XY subjects (solid symbols) and dizygotic twins, II-3 [AR gene deletion shown in (A)] and II-4, and a sibling II-7. (From Brown *et al.*, 1988.)

B

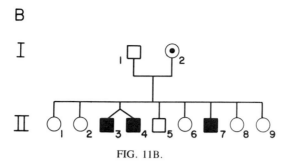

FIG. 11B.

genomic DNA. Development of a method utilizing PCR for rapid analysis of mutations in the coding regions of the AR gene required sequencing only far enough into the flanking introns to allow selection of suitable synthetic oligonucleotide primers to bracket each exon. Thus, the large central regions of each intron remain to be sequenced.

The intron–exon boundaries contain the canonical splice consensus sequences (double-underlined in Fig. 12) (Breathnach and Chambon, 1981). Splice sites of the human AR gene and those of human estrogen receptor (ER) (Ponglikit-mongkol et al., 1988) and the chicken progesterone receptor (PR) (Huckaby et al., 1987) genes are remarkably similar in location and flanking amino acid sequences. By comparison with other homologous steroid receptor cDNAs and cloned steroid receptor genes, the splice sites of the other as yet unreported steroid receptor gene sequences could be predicted. Comparisons of their exons reveal regions of evolutionary conservation of essential functions (Fig. 13). The most highly conserved exons, B and C, encode the first and second zinc finger motifs, respectively, and make up the DNA-binding domain (Evans, 1988; Green and Chambon, 1988; Beato, 1989). Within these and other exons sequence identity of human AR is closer to human PR, MR, and GR than to human ER. Only the second zinc finger exon of human ER, exon C, has a high degree of sequence similarity with human AR. The large amino-terminal domain contained within the A exon has little similarity to other receptors. This exon appears to contain a transcription-enhancing function and might also modulate DNA bind-ing (Hollenberg and Evans, 1988; Danielscn et al., 1987; Miesfeld et al., 1987; Tora et al., 1988a,b). Neither exon A nor exons B and C are known to have any influence on ligand binding. In the ER and GR, it was demonstrated that the steroid-binding domain encompasses exons E–G and portions of exons D and H (Giguere et al., 1986; Kumar et al., 1987). The human AR exons E–G exhibit a relatively high degree of similarity to human PR, MR, and GR. Although exon D is less homologous overall, a 23-amino acid region positioned near its 3' junc-tion is highly conserved among all nuclear receptors (Lubahn et al., 1988a).

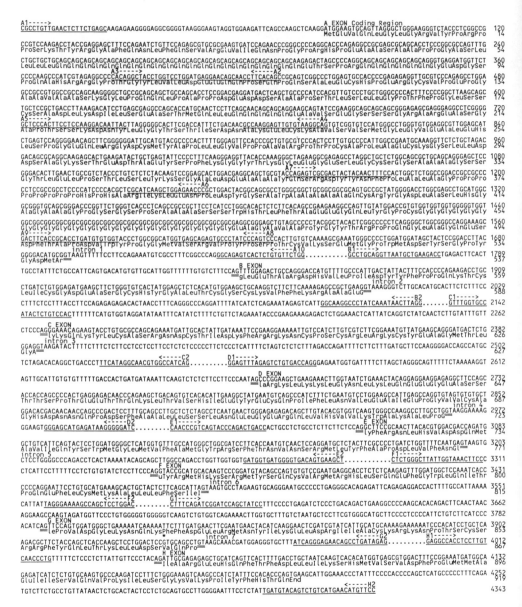

FIG. 12. Sequence of human AR gene intron–exon splice sites. Oligonucleotides used for PCR are underlined, with orientation indicated by arrows. Gaps in sequence (indicated by dots) represent an undetermined intron sequence. Canonical donor and acceptor splice sites are double-underlined. A point mutation found in the G exon is marked by an asterisk. (From Lubahn et al., 1989.)

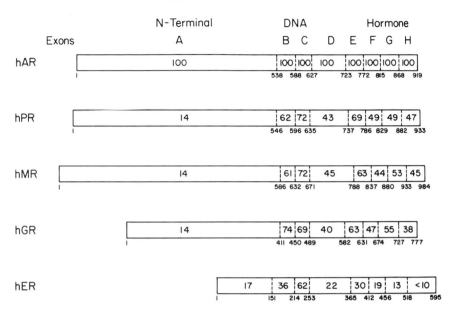

FIG. 13. Amino acid homology among steroid receptors compared by exons. The amino acid sequence of human AR is compared by exon with amino acid sequences of the human PR, MR, GR, and ER (Evans, 1988; Green and Chambon, 1988; Beato, 1989, Arriza *et al.*, 1987). Indicated are the percentages of homologies with human AR (boxed) and amino acid residue numbers (below boxes). Intron–exon splice sites are indicated by the vertical dashed lines. Amino acid residue numbers of the splice sites of human AR and ER (Ponglikitmongkol *et al.*, 1988) and the exon B splice sites of human MR (Arriza *et al.*, 1987) are known. Human PR splice sites were derived from sequence homology with the known splice sites of chicken PR (Huckaby *et al.*, 1987). The splice sites of human GR and the remaining splice sites of human MR were derived from sequence homology with human AR. Amino acid sequences of the predicted splice sites, with the exception of the exon A/B sites, were homologous (data not shown). The percentages of homologies among the same exons of different receptors were calculated by the GAP program of the GCG sequence analysis program (Devereux *et al.*, 1984). (From Lubahn *et al.*, 1989.)

Experimental mutations within this conserved region were found to interfere with ligand binding, suggesting that it is part of a hydrophobic ligand-binding pocket (Pratt *et al.*, 1988). Throughout exons D–G a variety of deletion and linker insertion mutations of the PR, GR, and ER result in decreased steroid binding and transcriptional activation (Kumar *et al.*, 1987; Giguere *et al.*, 1986; Dobson *et al.*, 1989).

VI. Detection of AR Receptor Gene Deletions Using PCR

With the oligonucleotide primers shown in Fig. 12, it was possible to amplify DNA fragments containing each of the AR gene coding exons for the detection of deletions. Amplified fragments can be analyzed by agarose gel electrophoresis and ethidium bromide staining. Using this approach, several additional AR gene deletions have been detected in individuals with AIS.

Two 46,XY children, ages 3 and 7 years, with complete AIS and their normal female relatives were studied using the PCR strategy diagrammed in Fig. 14. Both affected siblings demonstrated normal testosterone biosynthesis, as evidenced by increased serum testosterone in response to stimulation with human chorionic gonadotropin (Hughes *et al.*, 1986). Ratios of testosterone to dihydrotestosterone indicated normal 5α-reductase activity. The total cellular concentrations of AR in genital skin fibroblasts were increased about 2-fold above the normal. AR ligand binding at 40°C was stable, and the nuclear retention of [^{3}H]dihydrotestosterone was similar to that of human foreskin fibroblasts obtained from normal prepubertal males.

All amplified exon DNA fragments were of the correct size, with the exception of exon C, which codes for the second zinc finger (Fig. 15). Southern blot analysis using a C exon-specific PCR-generated probe confirmed the deletion of exon C. In addition, PCR of cDNA [reverse transcribed from poly(A) RNA] derived from cultured genital skin fibroblasts produced an amplified fragment approximately 117 bp smaller in the exon C-deleted patients than the 664-bp fragment found in controls. Dideoxy sequencing of the amplified cDNA revealed continuity of sequence between the B and D exons; the deletion of the C exon did not disturb the translational reading frame. This naturally occurring mutation demonstrates the functional importance of the second zinc finger of this steroid receptor and suggests that androgen insensitivity in these patients results from a failure of transactivation of androgen-dependent genes due to defective interaction of the mutant receptor with its androgen response elements. Interestingly, nuclear retention of the AR was not disturbed, as shown by immunocytochemical analysis of cultured genital skin fibroblasts.

Additional AR gene deletions detected by PCR and confirmed by Southern blot hybridization using ^{32}P-labeled AR cDNA or exon-specific probes are

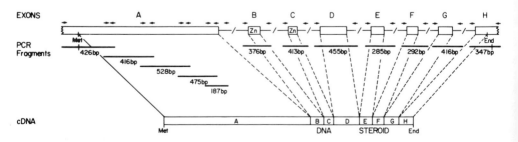

FIG. 14.   Amplification by PCR of the coding region in the human AR gene.

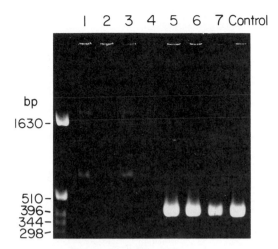

FIG. 15. Detection of AR gene C exon deletion using PCR. Genomic DNA (1.0 μg) was amplified through 30 cycles of PCR using the C exon primers shown in Fig. 12. Amplified DNAs were fractionated by electrophoresis on a 1.4% agarose gel and stained with ethidium bromide. Lanes 1–4 are duplicates for each of the two affected siblings showing absence of the expected 413-bp fragment present in female siblings (lanes 5 and 6), the mother (lane 7), and a normal control male.

shown in Fig. 16. All of these individuals have complete AIS. The lower three types of AR gene deletions were associated with the absence of AR steroid binding activity and were familial. The family with the total AR gene deletion harbored a HindIII polymorphism (C. J. Brown et al., 1989) (Fig. 17) that could be used for carrier detection in female siblings of affected males (Quigley et al.,

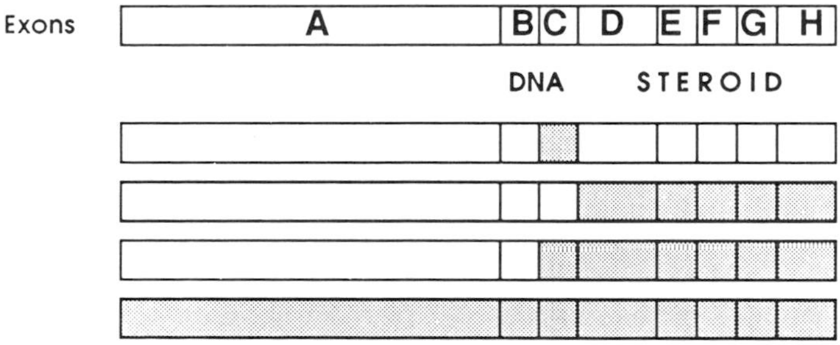

FIG. 16. Complete androgen insensitivity with deletions in the AR gene. Horizontal bars are divided to indicate the splice junctions separating exons A–H. The amino-terminal domain is contained within exon A, the DNA-binding domain is in exons B (first zinc finger) and C (second zinc finger), exon D contains the "hinge" region and a portion of the steroid-binding domain, which includes exons E–H. AR gene deletions are indicated by the stippled areas.

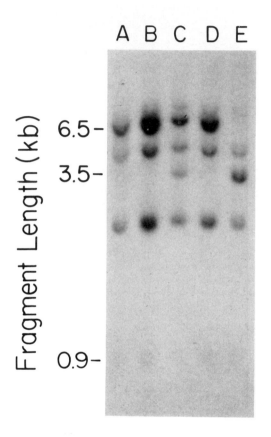

FIG. 17. *Hin*dIII restriction fragment-length polymorphism in the human AR gene. Genomic DNA was digested with *Hin*dIII and analyzed by Southern blot hybridization. Polymorphic bands are observed at 7.0 kbp (absent in lane E) or 3.5 kbp (absent in lanes A, B, and D). The frequency of the *Hin*dIII polymorphism is such that it should be informative in 20% of carrier females.

1990). Another large deletion of the AR gene was detected (Pinsky *et al.*, 1989) in a patient with complete AIS associated with mental retardation. PCR of genomic DNA from this patient in our laboratories suggested a total AR gene deletion. The association with mental retardation in this patient suggests the possible deletion of a contiguous gene on the X chromosome.

VII. Detection of Point Mutations in the AR Gene Causing Androgen Insensitivity

As a first step in understanding further the structure–function relationships of AR at the molecular level, we analyzed a family with complete AIS first described by Brown et al. (1982). For a prototypical study we chose a family in which three 46,XY siblings expressed AR proteins with abnormal ligand-binding properties. Affected individuals had the external female phenotype of complete AIS, except that there was a sparse to moderate amount of pubic hair. Levels of circulating testosterone were in the normal adult male range, and normal 5α-reductase activity was assayed in genital skin fibroblasts. Saturation binding analysis with [³H]dihydrotestosterone indicated normal amounts of AR in genital skin fibroblasts, and the AR protein had a normal 8 S sedimentation rate by sucrose density gradient centrifugation. However, AR binding affinity for [³H]di-hydrotestosterone in affected 46,XY siblings was 3-fold lower than normal (K_d, 1.5 nM; normal, 0.5 nM) (Fig. 18), and the binding activity exhibited increased thermolability (Brown et al., 1982). Moreover, the mutant AR affinity for progesterone was relatively higher than normal (2.5-fold) in binding displacement assays with [³H]dihydrotestosterone. These findings suggested the presence of a mutation in the AR steroid-binding domain.

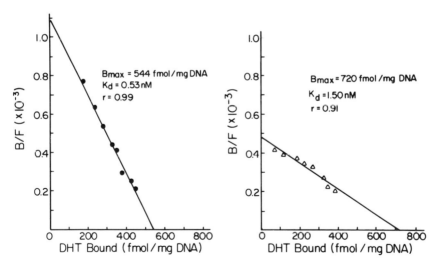

FIG. 18. Scatchard analysis of androgen binding in genital skin fibroblasts. Replicate cell monolayers were incubated for 45 minutes at 37°C with 0.2–2.5 nM [³H]dihydrotestosterone (DHT) and assayed for specific DHT binding in total cell sonicates. The B_{max} and K_d were calculated from the Scatchard plots for fibroblasts from a normal newborn foreskin (left) and the labia majora of a patient with complete androgen insensitivity (right). B/F, Bound-to-free ratio. (From Brown et al., 1982.)

Southern blot analysis of genomic DNA with human AR cDNA probes spanning the coding region revealed no major deletion in the human AR gene of any member of this family. Northern blot analysis of mRNA from one of the 46,XY siblings with AIS revealed the 10- to 11-kb and 7-kb mRNA species characteristic of human AR. With no indication of a gross gene deletion or defect involving mRNA transcription in the three affected siblings of this study, sequence analysis was performed for a small deletion or point mutation.

Oligonucleotides (underlined in Fig. 12) bracketing each of the amino acid coding exons were used as primers for PCR amplification of genomic DNA from one 46,XY sibling with complete AIS (II-1). All amplified exons produced fragments of predicted size (Fig. 14), verifying the Southern and Northern analyses that indicated the absence of a major human AR gene deletion. Sequence analysis of amplified exon DNA revealed a point mutation in exon G of the steroid-binding domain (Fig. 19). A guanine residue in the normal sequence was replaced by adenine, changing amino acid 866 from valine to methionine. No other amino acid sequence difference from normal was found in the entire 2757-bp AR coding region or in the flanking intron sequences, except within repeated glutamine and glycine regions of the A exon, where the numbers of glutamines (22) and glycines (15) differ from normal. However, variation in the numbers of these repeated amino acids has been found in all published sequences of the normal human AR receptor (Chang *et al.*, 1988b; Tilley *et al.*, 1989; Faber *et al.*, 1989).

To confirm the human AR gene mutation, genomic DNA of exon G from the affected individual was reamplified and sequenced. In addition, genomic DNAs

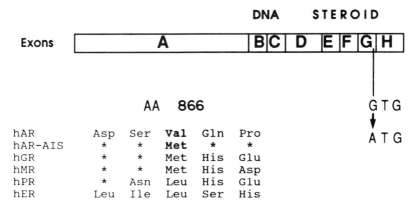

FIG. 19.   Complete androgen insensitivity with point mutation in the AR gene. Point mutation in amino acid (AA) 866 of the human AR (hAR). Amino acid sequences in the same region of other human steroid receptors are shown. hGR, Glucocorticoid; hMR, mineralocorticoid; hPR, progesterone; hER, estrogen receptor. Identity with hAR is indicated by an asterisk.

from the two other affected siblings (II-2 and II-3) and their mother (I-1) were analyzed. Each contained the AR allele with a guanine replaced by an adenine, while their carrier mother contained, in addition, the normal allele (Fig. 20). The valine-to-methionine alteration is therefore linked to AIS in this family.

Cytidine–guanine dinucleotides, such as those found at the locus mutated in this family with AIS, are sometimes methylated on the cytidine. Methylated cytidine can deaminate spontaneously to form thymidine. Methylation can result in relative "hot spots" for the formation of mutations such as those in the X chromosome-linked factor VIII gene, which causes hemophilia A (Youssoufian et al., 1986).

AR protein was expressed in normal amounts in the siblings described above with complete AIS, as evidenced by the number of [^{3}H]dihydrotestosterone-binding sites (Fig. 18); however, binding affinity for androgen was decreased. There was also a relative increase in affinity for progesterone. Although human PR has a leucine at the position corresponding to the AR point mutation, chicken PR does contain a methionine, as do human GR and MR (Fig. 19). It is interesting to speculate that this region of the G exon could be important in determining the steroid-binding specificity of AR. Estradiol has no increase in affinity for the mutated AR, and its receptor has little homology with AR in exon G (Fig. 19).

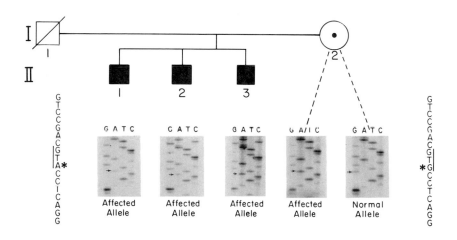

FIG. 20.   Partial pedigree of a family with complete AIS (Brown et al., 1982) and nucleotide sequence of the AR gene mutation. The solid squares indicate 46,XY genetic males with the complete androgen insensitivity syndrome phenotype, the slashed open square indicates the deceased father, and the circle with the dot indicates the heterozygous mother. The abnormal AR sequence is shown on the left, and the normal sequence is shown on the right. A single-base mutation (asterisk and arrows) of guanine to adenine resulted in the only identified amino acid sequence change in this kindred. The mutation was found in all amplified G exon clones from individuals II-1, -2, and -3 and in two of the six clones sequenced from I-2. I-2, a heterozygous carrier, displayed the normal allele in the other four sequenced clones. (From Lubahn et al., 1989.)

Confirmation was obtained by site-directed mutagenesis that the change in amino acid 866 from valine to methionine altered the binding properties of the AR. Site-directed mutagenesis was performed using PCR in a procedure similar to that described by Higuchi *et al.* (1988) (Fig. 21). Human AR cDNA containing the entire coding region was inserted into the vector pCMV5 (Lubahn *et al.*, 1988a), which was modified by insertion of an f1 origin of replication and a polylinker region. Mutated and wild-type human AR cDNAs were expressed in COS cells as described previously (Lubahn *et al.*, 1988a). Binding affinity of the mutated AR for [³H]R1881 (a synthetic androgen) was 4-fold lower than that of the wild-type AR. This difference in androgen-binding affinities is similar to that demonstrated earlier in cultured genital skin fibroblasts from normal males and siblings with AIS in this family (Fig. 22; see also Fig. 18).

The exon G mutation has the potential of affecting both the steroid-binding and transcription-activating functions of the AR protein. Ligand binding to AR and other steroid hormone receptors initiates a transformation process that results in

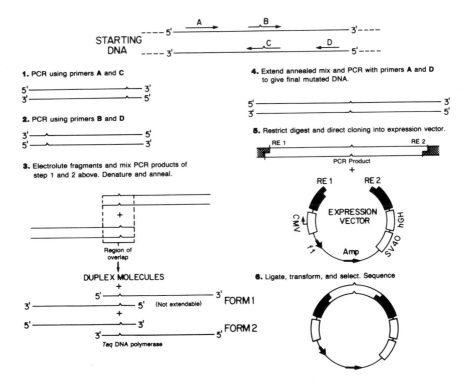

FIG. 21.   The method for site-directed mutagenesis using the PCR modified from Higuchi *et al.* (1988). SV40, Simian virus 40; hGH, human growth hormone; Amp, ampicillin resistance gene; RE, restriction enzyme.

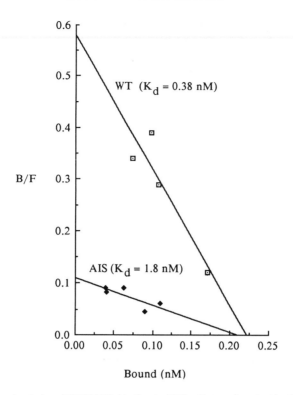

FIG. 22. Scatchard plot of [³H]R1881 binding in COS cells transfected with pCMV expression vectors containing mutant (AIS) and wild-type AR cDNAs. COS-7 cells at 80% confluence were transfected with 1 μg of DNA per 6-cm dish, using the diethylaminoethyl–dextran method (Lopata *et al.*, 1984). Cells were cleared of serum 20 hours after transfection and 18 hours later were incubated with increasing concentrations of [³H]methyltrienolone (R1881) in duplicate dishes in the presence and absence of 100-fold excess unlabeled R1881 for 2 hours at 37°C. [³H]R1881 was used rather than [³H]dihydrotestosterone to minimize steroid metabolism during the incubation. Cells were washed twice in cold phosphate-buffered saline and harvested in 2% sodium dodecyl sulfate, 10% glycerol, and 10 m*M* Tris, pH 6.8. Aliquots were taken for the determination of radioactivity and for Western blot analysis using an antibody specific for AR. Specific binding was estimated from the difference in radioactivity determined in the presence and absence of unlabeled hormone.

enhanced binding of receptors to their hormone response elements. This process could involve a conformational change in the receptor protein or separation from a nonsteroid-binding component that unmasks the DNA-binding domain and a nuclear transfer sequence located in the carboxyl-terminal region downstream from the DNA-binding domain. The process might also activate within the steroid-binding domain a dimerization sequence shown to be required for strong interaction of the steroid receptor with its response element and for transactivation of gene expression (Tsai *et al.*, 1988; Kumar and Chambon, 1988).

The mechanism by which this point mutation, resulting in only a modest change in steroid-binding properties of the AR, could cause complete loss of AR functional activity is not clear; however, it appears that complete transformation of the receptor subsequent to steroid binding requires precise structural interaction between receptor and ligand. Steroid antagonists, for example, have recently been shown to bind ERs and GRs and to promote specific binding to hormone response elements without enhancing gene transcription, as would a normal agonist (Green and Chambon, 1988). Hormone-binding domains of nuclear receptors are now recognized to have transcriptional enhancer effects (Kumar *et al.*, 1987; Webster *et al.*, 1988). A point mutation might abolish this function without greatly affecting steroid binding. Expression of this mutated human AR *in vitro* will allow further studies to determine whether it is capable of binding to its response element and enhancing transcription of a reporter gene.

VIII. AR Gene Point Mutation in the Androgen-Insensitive (Stanley–Gumbreck) Rat

Androgen insensitivity in a strain of King/Holtzman rats was discovered by Stanley and Gumbreck and propagated as a substrain. Affected genetic male rats retain the female phenotype, although abdominal testes produce normal to elevated male levels of testosterone and there is a normal rate of conversion of testosterone to dihydrotestosterone. In affected genetic males Müllerian ducts are absent due to testicular Müllerian inhibiting substance, but androgen-dependent male accessory sex glands fail to develop.

The molecular defect in the androgen-insensitive *Tfm* rat was investigated at the levels of AR gene and mRNA expression, subcellular localization of the AR protein, androgen binding to AR, and functional properties of the AR recreated by site directed mutagenesis (Yarbrough *et al.*, 1990).

Southern hybridization analysis of genomic DNA showed no indication of a major deletion or rearrangement of the AR gene in the *Tfm* rat, and Northern blot analysis of poly(A) RNA revealed the characteristic 10-kb AR mRNA band in *Tfm* rat kidney, which was indistinguishable in size and intensity from the wild type (Fig. 23). Thus, AR mRNA abundance and size were consistent with normal AR gene transcription and RNA processing in the *Tfm* rat. AR binding of [^{3}H]dihydrotestosterone in kidney cytosol fractions of the *Tfm* rat using a charcoal adsorption assay (Wilson and French, 1976) was only 10–15% of that observed in wild-type siblings and too low to determine apparent binding affinity, indicating a major reduction in androgen binding activity in the *Tfm* rat AR.

To identify a possible single-base mutation or small gene deletion, synthetic oligonucleotides homologous to rat AR cDNA (Tan *et al.*, 1988) were used in the PCR to prime the amplification of wild-type and *Tfm* rat AR DNA and to generate overlapping fragments within the coding region. Genomic DNA was

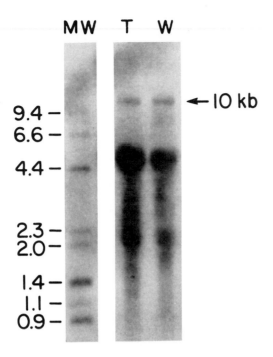

FIG. 23.   Poly(A) RNA was isolated from the kidneys of *Tfm* (T) and wild-type (W) sibling rats, and 10-μg aliquots were denatured and analyzed by Northern blot hybridization. Not shown is actin cDNA hybridization, which indicated nearly equivalent loading of RNA in the two lanes. Molecular weight markers (MW) were ^{32}P-labeled *Hin*dIII-digested λ DNA and *Hae*III-digested φX174 DNA. (From Yarbrough *et al.*, 1990.)

used as template to amplify four fragments from exon A; the remaining coding sequence was amplified from single-stranded cDNA obtained by reverse transcription of poly(A) RNA. These fragments were cloned into M13 bacteriophage and sequenced (Sanger *et al.*, 1977).

A single-base change in the *Tfm* rat AR cDNA, compared with the wild-type King/Holtzman, was observed at nucleotide residue 2201, approximately one-third the distance (5′–3′) into the steroid-binding domain. The guanine-to-adenine mutation resulted in conversion of basic arginine (codon CGG) to neutral glutamine (codon CAG) at amino acid residue 734 (Fig. 24). The single-base mutation occurs within exon E of the AR gene, based on sequence homology and exon position of the human AR gene (see Fig. 13). Arginine 734, which is replaced by glutamine in the *Tfm* rat AR, is positionally conserved throughout the nuclear receptor family (Fig. 25) and therefore appears to be critical for the function of this group of nuclear proteins. Interestingly, it is adjacent to an almost equally

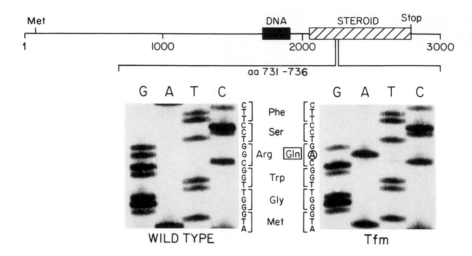

FIG. 24. Single-base mutation in *Tfm* rat AR. (Top) The AR functional domains. (Bottom) Autoradiograms of DNA sequencing gels from coding strands of normal male sibling (wild-type) and *Tfm* male animals with the sequencing reactions guanine (G), adenine (A), thymine (T), and cytosine (C). The DNA sequence shown codes for amino acid (aa) residues 731–736 of rat AR, starting from the lower portion of the gel. A single-base change from G in wild-type DNA to A (circled) in *Tfm* rat DNA changes arginine at position 734 in wild-type rat AR to glutamine (boxed) in the *Tfm* rat AR. (From Yarbrough *et al.*, 1990.)

RECEPTOR	CONSERVED REGION OF THE LIGAND-BINDING DOMAIN						
Androgen (rat)	Met	Gly	Trp	Arg	Ser	Phe	Thr
Androgen (human)	*	*	*	*	*	*	*
Androgen (rat Tfm)	*	*	*	Gln	*	*	*
Progesterone	Leu	*	*	*	*	Tyr	Lys
Glucocorticoid	Leu	*	*	*	*	Tyr	Arg
Mineralocorticoid	Leu	Ser	*	*	*	Tyr	Lys
Estrogen	Leu	Val	*	*	*	Met	Glu
Retinoic acid	Ile	Cys	Thr	*	−	Tyr	*
Thyroid	Ala	Ala	Val	*	−	Tyr	Asp

FIG. 25. Partial amino acid sequence comparisons of nuclear receptors within the region of the single-base mutation in the *Tfm* AR steroid-binding domain. The amino acid (aa) sequence of rat AR (aa 731–737) is compared to the corresponding sequence of human AR (aa 749–755), *Tfm* rat AR (aa 730–737), and receptors for human progesterone (aa 763–769), glucocorticoid (aa 608–614), mineralocorticoid (aa 814–820), estrogen (aa 391–397), retinoic acid (aa 243–249), and thyroid hormone (aa 263–269). Identical (*) and missing (−) amino acids are indicated relative to wild-type rat AR. (From Yarbrough *et al.*, 1990.)

conserved serine residue, which, together, might form a recognition sequence for phosphorylation. The conserved arginine is probably not a determinant of ligand-binding specificity, since it occurs among receptors that bind diverse ligands. However, the low level of androgen binding by the *Tfm* rat AR suggests that the arginine is essential for normal steroid-binding capacity.

Proof that the guanine-to-adenine transition mutation at nucleotide 2201 caused the functional defect in AR was obtained by site-directed mutagenesis in M13 bacteriophage using wild-type rat AR cDNA as template for DNA synthesis, and as primer, a single-stranded oligonucleotide containing the mutant sequence. Mutant and wild-type AR cDNAs were cloned into pCMV and expressed in COS-7 cells. A 10-fold reduction in binding capacity was observed with the mutant AR (Fig. 26A and B). Mutant AR protein expressed in COS cells was equivalent to wild type, as determined by immunoblot analysis (see inset, Fig. 26A). Interestingly, the mutant AR had an apparent affinity for [³H]methyl-trienolone (R1881, a synthetic androgen) equivalent to that of the wild-type receptor (Fig. 26B), despite its low binding capacity. No specific binding was measured in mock-transfected COS cells. The reduced binding capacity of the recreated *Tfm* rat AR was similar to the low or undetectable binding reported previously for endogenous *Tfm* male rat AR (Bardin *et al.*, 1973; Naess *et al.*, 1976; Smith *et al.*, 1975; Fox and Wieland, 1981). The rat pituitary gland AR of the *Tfm* rat had low binding capacity, but retained normal binding affinity for [³H]testosterone (Naess *et al.*, 1976). Thus, both the *Tfm* rat AR and the recreated mutant AR have reduced androgen binding capacity with affinity equivalent to that of wild-type AR.

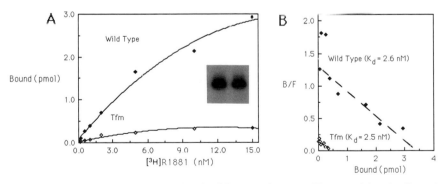

FIG. 26. Saturation binding analysis of wild-type and mutant ARs created by site-directed mutagenesis in M13. (A) Saturation binding curves for wild-type (♦) and *Tfm* (◇) rat AR; binding of [³H]R1881 was determined as described in Fig. 22. (Inset) Immunoblot of equivalent aliquots of cells transfected with wild-type (left) and *Tfm* (right) rat AR DNA expression vectors. (B) Scatchard plot of wild-type (♦) and *Tfm* (◇) rat AR binding. Standard deviation of the binding constants was ± 1.3 n*M*. (From Yarbrough *et al.*, 1990.)

Subcellular localization of the *Tfm* rat AR in the pituitary gland revealed intense nuclear immunostaining indistinguishable from wild-type littermate males (Fig. 27). The finding of nuclear AR protein in the *Tfm* rat would appear to contradict previous biochemical evidence that [^{3}H]testosterone does not accumulate in nuclei of the *Tfm* male rat *in vivo*; (Ritzen *et al.*, 1972; Max, 1981; Wieland and Fox, 1981) however, the results can be explained by a mutant AR with low androgen binding capacity.

Transcriptional activity of the *Tfm* rat AR was tested by cotransfection into CV1 cells of expression vectors containing either mutant or wild-type AR cDNA together with a reporter plasmid (Fig. 28). In CV1 cells expressing the mutant AR, androgen in high concentration induced a low level of chloramphenicol acetyltransferase activity relative to wild type. It was shown previously in cell lines containing endogenous AR that androgen stimulates transcriptional activity of the enhancer/promoter of the mouse mammary tumor virus (Darbe *et al.*, 1986; Cato *et al.*, 1987; Otten *et al.*, 1988). *Tfm* male rats are unresponsive to physiological concentrations of androgen (Bardin *et al.*, 1973), and hence the androgen insensitivity syndrome develops. However, pharmacological doses of testosterone and dihydrotestosterone can induce detectable biological effects. For example, serum

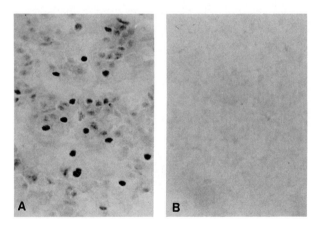

FIG. 27.   Immunocytochemical localization of AR in the *Tfm* male rat pituitary gland. Adult *Tfm* rats received a 15-mg injection of testosterone propionate in sesame oil intramuscularly 16 hours prior to tissue removal and rapid freezing. Treatment with the high dose of testosterone propionate was to enhance AR occupancy and recognition by the antibody. Frozen sections (6 μm) of pituitary gland were incubated with the IgG fraction of AR antibody (A) or preimmune serum (B) and stained by the avidin–biotin–peroxidase method (Sar, 1985). The antibody, AR-52, was raised against a synthetic peptide with a sequence just 5' of the AR DNA-binding domain (Fig. 5). The IgG fraction was prepared (Tan·et al., 1988) and used at a dilution of 5 μg/ml of protein. Magnification ×690. (From Yarbrough *et al.*, 1990.)

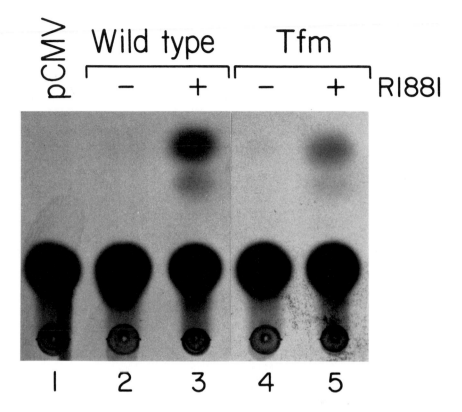

FIG. 28. A functional assay for AR by cotransfection with the mouse mammary tumor virus–chloramphenicol acetyltransferase (MMTV–CAT) reporter plasmid. CV1 cells were transfected with wild type and the recreated mutant AR expression vectors in pCMV together with the MMTV–CAT reporter plasmid, using the calcium phosphate method. After transfection cells were maintained in 0.2% fetal calf serum in Dulbecco's modified Eagle's medium with or without the addition of 50 nM R1881. Shown is the fluorogram of CAT activity separated into its acetylated forms by silica plate chromatography for (1) pCMV parent plasmid lacking the AR sequence, (2) wild-type AR without androgen, (3) wild-type AR with androgen treatment, (4) *Tfm* mutant AR without androgen, and (5) *Tfm* mutant AR with androgen treatment. The results are representative of four independent experiments. (From Yarbrough *et al.*, 1990.)

luteinizing hormone levels were decreased in *Tfm* males in response to high doses of androgen in a manner similar to the normal feedback effect in the wild-type rat at physiological androgen levels (Naess *et al.*, 1976). Similarly, high doses of androgen induced preputial gland growth in the *Tfm* rat (Sherins and Bardin, 1971). An AR with reduced androgen-binding capacity might be insufficient to elicit androgen responses at physiological hormone concentrations, while a high concentration of androgen might stabilize nuclear interactions of the defective

AR, perhaps including that fraction of AR with binding activity below the level of detection in our assay. Thus, even with their reduced binding capacity, the *Tfm* rat AR and the recreated mutant AR are functionally active in the presence of pharmacological levels of androgen.

It is not understood, at present, why a single-base mutation results in a major loss of binding activity, with retention of a small amount of high-affinity androgen binding. As noted above, however, adjacent to arginine 734 in AR are potential phosphorylation sites (Blackshear *et al.*, 1988) on serine or threonine. In addition, a partially conserved tyrosine occurs in the region in other members of the nuclear receptor family (see Fig. 25). Arginine 734 might be a necessary amino acid in a phosphorylation recognition sequence. Other possible consequences of the single-base mutation include distortion of protein folding and/or loss of dimer formation or interactions with other proteins (Bresnick *et al.*, 1989; Pratt *et al.*, 1988; Colvard and Wilson, 1984).

IX.   Screening for Point Mutations in the Human AR Gene

Two methods can be readily applied to the detection of point mutations in exon fragments generated by PCR, as described above. One is the chemical mismatch cleavage method described by Cotton *et al.* (1988) and Cotton and Campbell (1989) and later applied by Grompe *et al.* (1989) to map mutation sites in patients with ornithine transcarbamylase deficiency. When applied to screening AR gene mutations, wild-type exon fragments prepared as described above (Figs. 12 and 14) are labeled with [^{32}P]ATP and hybridized with an excess of the corresponding exon DNA from a mutant AR gene to form a labeled heteroduplex. Two reagents, osmium tetroxide and hydroxylamine, can potentially recognize all variants and, together with piperidine, cleave DNA at mismatched thymine and cytosine, respectively. Cleavage products are identified by electrophoresis on a sequencing gel.

A second method, denaturing gradient gel electrophoresis (Fischer and Lerman, 1983), has been modified by attachment of a G+C-rich sequence (G–C clamp) to genomic DNA fragments using PCR (Myers *et al.*, 1985a; Sheffield *et al.*, 1989). This method is based on the melting property of DNA under denaturing conditions. As DNA fragments move through polyacrylamide gels containing an ascending gradient of denaturant (e.g., formamide plus urea), regions called melting domains undergo a strand separation to produce partially denatured molecules with decreased electrophoretic mobility. As these DNA molecules continue to move slowly into higher concentrations of denaturant, additional melting domains undergo strand separation. Single-base changes in any of these domains alter their melting temperature and lead to differences in the pattern of electrophoresis in the denaturing gradient gel. However, when the final, or most stable, domain melts, the fragment undergoes complete strand

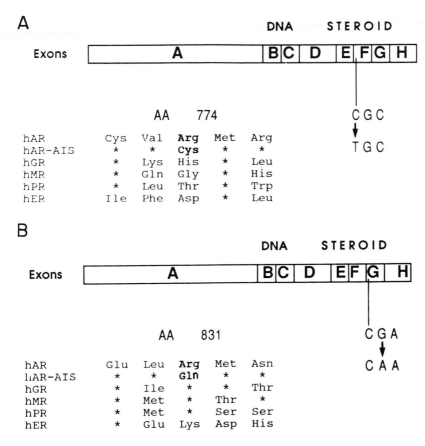

FIG. 29. Point mutations associated with complete androgen insensitivity and absence of AR binding activity. (A) Mutation of amino acid (AA) 774 in F exon. (B) Mutation of amino acid 831 exon G. Both mutations were identified by PCR amplification of genomic DNA as in Fig. 14, but using G+C-tailed oligonucleotide primers. Amplified exon DNA was screened by denaturing gradient gel electrophoresis, and exons containing the mutations were sequenced. Amino acid sequences within the same regions of other steroid hormone receptors are shown as in Fig. 19. An asterisk indicates identity with human AR. (From T. R. Brown *et al.*, 1989.)

separation and the resolving power of the gel is lost. Therefore, base substitutions in the highest temperature melting domain of the DNA molecule cannot be detected by denaturing gradient gel electrophoresis. Myers *et al.* (1985b) found that addition of a G+C-rich sequence (80% G+C), because of its resistance to melting, held the DNA strands together through a higher concentration of denaturant, thus allowing a more complete comparison of melting domains.

T. R. Brown *et al.* (1989) have added G+C sequences to the oligonucleotide primers (Fig. 12) and have used these G+C-tailed primers to amplify and compare exons B–H from several 46,XY individuals with complete androgen insensitivity. Four suspected mutations were identified by denaturing gradient gel electrophoresis and confirmed by sequencing, site-directed mutagenesis, and expression of the mutated coding DNA. The AR mutations in two of these individuals are shown in Fig. 29A and B. While this method might not detect all mutations, its simplicity makes it attractive for an initial screen. Its power is increased by making a heteroduplex and thus creating a base mismatch between labeled wild-type and mutant AR gene exons (Theophilus *et al.*, 1989).

X. Conclusion

Cloning of the human (Lubahn *et al.*, 1988a,b; Chang *et al.*, 1988a,b; Trapman *et al.*, 1988; Tilley *et al.*, 1989) and rat (Tan *et al.*, 1988; Chang *et al.*, 1988b) ARs has made it possible to localize the AR gene to the X chromosome and to establish that AIS is caused by mutations of the AR gene, both point mutations and deletions. In studies of complete androgen insensitivity reported thus far, single-base transition mutations have been identified in a variety of positions within the steroid-binding domain (Fig. 30), and it appears that the

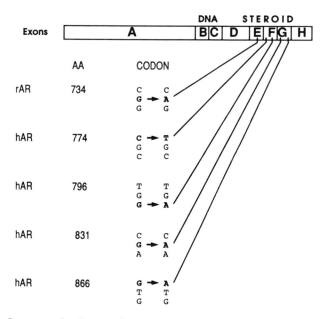

FIG. 30.   Summary of point mutations in the AR gene of human (hAR) and rat AR (rAR) associated with androgen insensitivity.

number of different mutations will become very large as studies of both the complete and partial forms of the syndrome continue. Thus, AIS in humans provides an opportunity to relate sex phenotype with AR genotype within what now appears to be a large spectrum of different natural mutations. Recreation of these natural mutations and *in vitro* expression of the mutated receptors in cell lines should enable much to be learned about the structure–function relationships of the AR. Knowledge of the sex phenotype associated with the mutation and comparisons of natural and recreated mutant androgen receptor functions will be enormously helpful in validating these *in vitro* studies.

REFERENCES

Ainman, J., Griffin, J. E., Gazak, J. M., Wilson, J. D., and MacDonald, P. C. (1979). *N. Engl. J. Med.* **300,** 223–227.

Amrhein, J. A., Meyer, W. J., III, Jones, H. W., Jr., and Migeon, C. J. (1976). *Proc. Natl. Acad. Sci. U.S.A.* **73,** 891–894.

Andersson, S., Davis, D. N., Dahlback, H., Jornvall, H., and Russell, D. W. (1989). *J. Biol. Chem.* **264,** 8222–8229.

Antonarakis, S. E., Waber, P. G., Kittur, S. D., Patel, A. S., Kazazian, H. H., Jr., Mellis, M. A., Counts, R. B., Stamatoyannopoulos, G., Bowie, E. J. W., Fass, D. N., Pittman, D. D., Wozney, J. M., and Toole, J. J. (1985). *N. Engl. J. Med.* **313,** 842–848.

Arriza, J. L., Weinberger, C., Cerelli, G., Glaser, T. M., Handelin, B. L., Housman, D. E., and Evans, R. M. (1987). *Science* **237,** 268–275.

Baker, A. R., McDonnell, D. P., Hughes, M., Crisp, T. M., Mangelsdorf, D. J., Haussler, M. R., Pike, J. W., Shine, J., and O'Malley, B. W. (1988). *Proc. Natl. Acad. Sci. U.S.A.* **85,** 3294–3298.

Bardin, C. W., and Wright, W. (1980). *Ann. Clin. Res.* **12,** 236–242.

Bardin, C. W., Bullock, L. P., Sherins, R. J., Mowszowicz, I., and Blackburn, W. R. (1973). *Recent Prog. Horm. Res.* **29,** 65–109.

Beato, M. (1989). *Cell (Cambridge, Mass.)* **56,** 335–344.

Benbrook, D., and Pfahl, M. (1987). *Science* **238,** 788–791.

Benbrook, D., Lernhardt, E., and Pfahl, M. (1988). *Nature (London)* **333,** 669–672.

Berg, J. M. (1986). *Science* **232,** 485.

Bigsby, R. M., and Cunha, G. R. (1986). *Endocrinology (Baltimore)* **119,** 390–396.

Blackshear, P. J., Nairn, A. C., and Kuo, J. F. (1988). *FASEB J.* **2,** 2957–2969.

Brand, N., Petkovich, M., Krust, A., Chambon, P., de Thé, H., Marchio, A., Tiollais, P., and Dejean, A. (1988). *Nature (London)* **332,** 850–853.

Breathnach, R., and Chambon, P. (1981). *Annu. Rev. Biochem.* **50,** 349–383.

Bresnick, E. H., Dalman, F. C., Sanchez, E. R., and Pratt, W. B. (1989). *J. Biol. Chem.* **264,** 4992–4997.

Brown, T. R. (1987). *Semin. Reprod. Biol.* **5,** 243–258.

Brown, T. R., and Migeon, C. J. (1981). *Mol. Cell. Biochem.* **36,** 3–22.

Brown, T. R., and Migeon, C. J. (1987). *In* "Hormone Resistance and Other Endocrine Paradoxes" (M. P. Cohen and P. P. Foa, eds.), pp. 157–203. Springer-Verlag, New York.

Brown, C. J., Goss, S. J., Lubahn, D. B., Joseph, D. R., Wilson, E. M., French, F. S., and Willard, H. F. (1989). *Am. J. Hum. Genet.* **44,** 264–269.

Brown, T. R., Maes, M., Rothwell, S. W., and Migeon, C. J. (1982). *J. Clin. Endocrinol. Metab.* **55,** 61–69.

Brown, T. R., Lubahn, D. B., Wilson, E. M., Joseph, D. R., French, F. S., and Migeon, C. J. (1988). *Proc. Natl. Acad. Sci. U.S.A.* **85,** 8151–8155.

Brown, T. R., Lubahn, D. B., Kruter, R., and Migeon, C. J. (1989). *Endocrinology (Baltimore)* **124,** 178 (abstr.).

Bruchovsky, N., and Wilson, J. D. (1968). *J. Biol. Chem.* **243,** 5953–5960.

Catelli, M. G., Binart, N., Jung-Testas, I., Renoir, J. M., Baulieu, E. E., Feramisco, J. R., and Welch, W. J. (1985). *EMBO J.* **4,** 3131–3135.

Cato, A. C. B., Henderson, D., and Ponta, H. (1987). *EMBO J.* **6,** 363–368.

Chang, C., Kokontis, J., and Liao, S. (1988a). *Science* **240,** 324–326.

Chang, C., Kokontis, J., and Liao, S. (1988b). *Proc. Natl. Acad. Sci. U.S.A.* **85,** 7211–7215.

Colvard, D. S., and Wilson, E. M. (1981). *Endocrinology (Baltimore)* **109,** 496–504.

Colvard, D. S., and Wilson, E. M. (1984). *Biochemistry* **23,** 3479–3486.

Conneely, O. M., Dobson, A. D. W., Tsai, M. J., Beattie, W. G., Toft, D. O., Huckaby, C. S., Zarucki, T., Schrader, W. T., and O'Malley, B. W. (1987a). *Mol. Endocrinol.* **1,** 517–525.

Conneely, O. M., Dobson, A. D. W., Tsai, M., Beattie, W. G., Toft, D. O., Huckaby, C. S., Zarucki, T., Schrader, W. T., and O'Malley, B. W. (1987b). *Mol. Endocrinol.* **1,** 517–525.

Cotton, R. G. H., and Campbell, R. D. (1989). *Nucleic Acids Res.* **17,** 4223–4232.

Cotton, R. G. H., Rodrigues, N. R., and Campbell, R. D. (1988). *Proc. Natl. Acad. Sci. U.S.A.* **85,** 4397–4401.

Cunha, G. R., and Lung, B. (1979). *In Vitro* **15,** 50–71.

Danielsen, M., Northrop, J., and Ringold, G. (1986). *EMBO J.* **5,** 2513–2522.

Danielsen, M., Northrop, J. P., Jonklass, J., and Ringold, G. M. (1987). *Mol. Endocrinol.* **1,** 816–822.

Darbe, P. D., Moriarty, A., Curtis, S. A., and King, R. J. B. (1985). *J. Steroid Biochem.* **23,** 379–384.

Darbe, P., Page, M., and King, R. J. B. (1986). *Mol. Cell. Biol.* **6,** 2847–2854.

Davies, P., Roach, A., and Hew, C.-L. (1982). *Proc. Natl. Acad. Sci. U.S.A.* **79,** 335–339.

Devereux, J., Haeberli, P., and Smithies, O. (1984). *Nucleic Acids Res.* **12,** 387.

Diakun, G. P., Fairall, L., and Klug, A. (1986). *Nature (London)* **324,** 698.

Dobson, A. D. W., Conneely, O. M., Beattie, W., Maxwell, B. L., Mak, P., Tsai, M.-J., Schrader, W. T., and O'Malley, B. W. (1989). *J. Biol. Chem.* **264,** 4207–4211.

Evans, R. M. (1988). *Science* **240,** 889–899.

Evans, R. M., and Hollenberg, S. M. (1988). *Cell (Cambridge, Mass.)* **52,** 1–3.

Faber, P. W., Kuiper, G. G. J. M., van Rooij, H. C. J., van der Korput, J. A. G. M., Brinkman, A. O., and Trapman, J. (1989). *Mol. Cell. Endocrinol.* **61,** 257–262.

Fairall, L., Rhodes, D., and Klug, A. (1986). *J. Mol. Biol.* **192,** 577.

Fichman, K., Migeon, B., and Migeon, C. J. (1980). *Adv. Hum. Genet.* **10,** 331–377.

Fischer, S., and Lerman, L. (1983). *Proc. Natl. Acad. Sci. U.S.A.* **80,** 1579.

Fox, T. O., and Wieland, S. J. (1981). *Endocrinology (Baltimore)* **109,** 790.

French, F. S., Van Wyk, J. J., Baggett, B., Easterling, W. E., Talbert, L. M., Johnston, F. R., Forchielli, E., and Dey, A. C. (1966). *J. Clin. Endocrinol. Metab.* **26,** 493–503.

French, F. S., Baggett, B., Van Wyk, J. J., Talbert, L. M., Hubbard, W. R., Johnston, F. R., Weaver, R. P., Forchielli, E., Rao, G. S., and Sarda, I. R. (1965). *J. Clin. Endocrinol. Metab.* **25,** 661–677.

Giannelli, F., Choo, K. H., Rees, D. J. G., Boyd, Y., Rizza, C. R., and Brownlee, G. G. (1983). *Nature (London)* **303,** 181–182.

Giguere, V., Hollenberg, S. M., Rosenfeld, M. G., and Evans, R. (1986). *Cell (Cambridge, Mass.)* **46,** 645–652.

Giguere, V., Ong, E. S., Segui, P., and Evans, R. M. (1987). *Nature (London)* **330,** 624–629.

Giguere, V., Yang, N., Segui, P., and Evans, R. (1988). *Nature (London)* **331,** 91–94.

Gottleib, B., Kaufman, M., Pinsky, L., Leboeue, G., and Sotos, J. F. (1987). *J. Steroid Biochem.* **28**, 279–284.

Green, S., and Chambon, P. (1988). *Trends Genet.* **4**, 309–313.

Green, G. L., Gilna, P., Waterfield, M., Baker, A., Hort, Y., and Shine, J. (1986). *Science* **231**, 1150–1154.

Green, S., Walter, P., Kumar, V., Krust, A., Bornert, J., Argos, P., and Chambon, P. (1986). *Nature (London)* **320**, 134–139.

Griffin, J. E., and Wilson, J. D. (1986). *In* "Steroid Hormone Resistance: Mechanisms and Clinical Aspects" (G. P. Chrousos, D. L. Loriaux, and M. B. Lipsett, eds.), pp. 257–268. Plenum, New York.

Griffin, J. E., Punyashthiti, K., and Wilson, J. D. (1976). *J. Clin. Invest.* **57**, 1342–1351.

Grima, B., Lamouroux, A., Blanot, F., Biguet, N. F., and Mallet, J. (1985). *Proc. Natl. Acad. Sci. U.S.A.* **82**, 617–621.

Grompe, M., Muzny, D. M., and Caskey, C. T. (1989). *Proc. Natl. Acad. Sci. U.S.A.* **86**, 5888–5892.

Grumbach, M. M., and Barr, M. L. (1985). *Recent Prog. Horm. Res.* **14**, 255–335.

Hansson, V., Ritzen, E. M., French, F. S., and Nayfeh, S. N. (1975). *Handb. Physiol., Sect. 7: Endocrinol. 1972–1976* pp. 173–201.

Higuchi, R., Krummel, B., and Jaiki, R. K. (1988). *Nucleic Acids Res.* **16**, 7351.

Hobbs, H. H., Brown, M. S., Russell, D. W., Davignon, J., and Goldstein, J. L. (1987). *N. Engl. J. Med.* **317**, 734–737.

Hollenberg, S. M., and Evans, R. M. (1988). *Cell (Cambridge, Mass.)* **55**, 899–906.

Hollenberg, S. M., Weinberger, C., Ong, E. S., Cerelli, G., Oro, A., Lebo, R., Thompson, E. B., Rosenfeld, M. G., and Evans, R. M. (1985). *Nature (London)* **318**, 635–641.

Huckaby, C., Conneely, O. M., Beattie, W. G., Dobson, A. D. W., Tsai, M., and O'Malley, B. (1987). *Proc. Natl. Acad. Sci. U.S.A.* **84**, 8380–8384.

Hughes, I. A., and Evans, B. A. J. (1987). *Horm. Res.* **28**, 25–29.

Hughes, I. A., Evans, B. A. J., Ismail, R., and Mathews, J. (1986). *J. Clin. Endocrinol. Metab.* **63**, 309–315.

Hughes, M. R., Malloy, P. J., Kieback, D. G., Kesterson, R. A., Pike, J. W., Feldman, D., and O'Malley, B. W. (1988). *Science* **242**, 1702–1705.

Joab, I., Radanyi, C., Renoir, M., Buchou, T., Catelli, M.-G., Binart, N., Mester, J., and Baulieu, E.-E. (1984). *Nature (London)* **308**, 850–853.

Kaufman, M., Straisfeld, C., and Pinsky, L. (1976). *J. Clin. Invest.* **58**, 345–350.

Kaufman, M., Pinsky, L., Baird, P. A., and McGillivray, B. C. (1979). *Am. J. Med. Genet.* **4**, 402–411.

Keenan, B. S., Meyer, W. J., III, Hadjian, A. J., Jones, H. W., Jr., and Migeon, C. J. (1974). *J. Clin. Endocrinol. Metab.* **38**, 1143–1146.

Klug, A., and Rhodes, D. (1987). *Trends Biol. Sci.* **12**, 464–469.

Koike, S., Sakai, M., and Muramatsu, M. (1987). *Nucleic Acids Res.* **15**, 2499–2513.

Korach, K. S., Horigome, T., Tomooka, Y., Yamashita, S., Newbold, R., and McLachlan, J. A. (1988). *Proc. Natl. Acad. Sci. U.S.A.* **85**, 3334–3337.

Kozak, M. (1986). *Cell (Cambridge, Mass.)* **44**, 283–292.

Krust, A., Green, S., Argos, P., Kumar, V., Walter, P., Bornert, J.-M., and Chambon, P. (1986). *EMBO J.* **5**, 891–897.

Kuiper, G. G. J. M., Faber, P. W., van Rooij, H. C. J., van der Korput, J. A. G. M., Ris-Stalpers, C., Klaassen, P., Trapman, J., and Brinkmann, A. O. (1989). *J. Mol. Endocrinol.* **2**, R1–R4.

Kumar, V., and Chambon, P. (1988). *Cell (Cambridge, Mass.)* **55**, 145–146.

Kumar, V., Green, S., Stack, G., Berry, M., Jin, J.-R., and Chambon, P. (1987). *Cell (Cambridge, Mass.)* **51**, 941–951.

Loosfelt, H., Atger, M., Misrahi, M., Guiochon-Mantel, A., Meriel, C., Logeat, F., Benarous, R., and Milgrom, E. (1986). *Proc. Natl. Acad. Sci. U.S.A.* **83,** 9045–9049.

Lopata, M. A., Cleveland, D. W., and Sollner-Webb, B. (1984). *Nucleic Acids Res.* **12,** 5707.

Lubahn, D. B., Joseph, D. R., Sullivan, P. M., Willard, H. F., French, F. S., and Wilson, E. M. (1988a). *Science* **240,** 327–330.

Lubahn, D. B., Joseph, D. R., Sar, M., Tan, J., Higgs, H. N., Larson, R., French, F. S., and Wilson, E. M. (1988b). *Mol. Endocrinol.* **2,** 1265–1275.

Lubahn, D. B., Brown, T. R., Simental, J. A., Higgs, H. N., Migeon, C. J., Wilson, E. M., and French, F. S. (1989). *Proc. Natl. Acad. Sci. U.S.A.* **86,** 9534–9538.

Lyon, M. F., and Hawkes, S. G. (1970). *Nature (London)* **227,** 1217–1219.

Max, S. R. (1981). *Biochem. Biophys. Res. Commun.* **101,** 792–799.

Maxwell, B. L., McDonnell, D. P., Conneely, O. M., Schulz, T. Z., Greene, G. L., and O'Malley, B. W. (1987). *Mol. Endocrinol.* **1,** 25–35.

Meyer, W. J., III, Migeon, B. R., and Migeon, C. J. (1975). *Proc. Natl. Acad. Sci. U.S.A.* **72,** 1469–1472.

Miesfeld, R., Rusconi, S., Godowski, P. J., Maler, B. A., Okret, S., Wikstrom, A.-C., Gustafsson, J.-A., and Yamamoto, K. R. (1986). *Cell (Cambridge, Mass.)* **46,** 389–399.

Miesfeld, R., Godowski, P. J., Maler, B. A., and Yamamoto, K. R. (1987). *Science* **236,** 423.

Migeon, B. R., Brown, T. R., Azelman, J., and Migeon, C. J. (1981). *Proc. Natl. Acad. Sci. U.S.A.* **78,** 1469–1472.

Migeon, C. J., Brown, T. R., and Fichman, K. (1981). *In* "The Intersex Child" (N. Josso, ed.), Vol. 8, pp. 171–202. Karger, Basel, Switzerland.

Migeon, C. J., Brown, T. R., Lanes, R., Palacios, A., Amrhein, J. A., and Schoen, E. J. (1984). *J. Clin. Endocrinol. Metab.* **59,** 672–678.

Migliaccio, A., Di Domenico, M., Green, S., de Falco, A., Kajtaniak, E. L., Blasi, F., Chambon, P., and Auricchio, F. (1988). *Mol. Endocrinol.* **3,** 1061–1069.

Miller, J., McLachlan, A. D., and Klug, A. (1985). *EMBO J.* **4,** 1609.

Misrahi, M., Atger, M., d'Auriol, L., Loosfelt, H., Megrier, C., Fridlansky, F., Guiochon-Mantel, A., Galibert, F., and Milgrom, E. (1987). *Biochem. Biophys. Res. Commun.* **143,** 740–748.

Monaco, A. P., Bertlsen, C. J., Middlesworth, W., Colletti, C. A., Aldridge, J., Fishbeck, K. H., Bartlett, R., Pericak-Vance, M. A., Roses, A. D., and Kunkel, I. M. (1985). *Nature (London)* **316,** 842–845.

Mullis, K., Faloona, F., Scharf, S., Saiki, R., Horn, G., and Erhlich, H. (1986). *Cold Spring Harbor Symp. Quant. Biol.* **51,** 263–273.

Myers, R. M., Fischer, S. G., Lerman, L. S., and Maniatis, T. (1985a). *Nucleic Acids Res.* **13,** 3131–3145.

Myers, R. M., Larin, Z., and Maniatis, T. (1985b). *Science* **230,** 1242–1246.

Naess, O., Haug, E., Attramadal, A., Aakvaag, A., Hansson, V., and French, F. S. (1976). *Endocrinology (Baltimore)* **99,** 1295–1303.

Ohno, S., and Lyon, M. F. (1970). *Clin. Genet.* **1,** 121–129.

Olsen, K. L. (1979). *Horm. Behav.* **13,** 66–84.

Olsen, K. L. (1989). *In* "Handbook of Behavioral Neurobiology. Sexual Differentiation: A Lifespan Approach" (A. A. Gerall, H. Mottz, and I. C. Ward, eds.). Plenum, New York.

Otten, A. D., Sanders, M. M., and McKnight, G. S. (1988). *Mol. Endocrinol.* **2,** 143–147.

Peters, C. A., and Barrack, E. R. (1985). *Program Annu. Meet. Endocr. Soc., 67th* p. 108 (abstr.).

Peters, C. A., and Barrack, E. R. (1987a). *J. Histochem. Cytochem.* **35,** 755–762.

Peters, C. A., and Barrack, E. R. (1987b). *Cytochemistry* **35,** 755–762.

Petkovich, M., Brand, N., Krust, A., and Chambon, P. (1987). *Nature (London)* **330,** 444–450.

Pinsky, L., Kaufman, M., Gil-Esteban, C., and Sumbulian, D. (1983). *Can. J. Biochem. Cell Biol.* **71,** 770–778.

Pinsky, L., Trifiro, M., Sebbaghian, N., Kaufman, M., Chang, C., Trapman, J., Brinkman, A. O., Kuiper, G. G. J. M., Ris, C., Brown, C. J., Willard, H. F., and Sergovich, F. (1989). *Am. J. Hum. Genet.* **45,** A212.

Ponglikitmongkol, M., Green, S., and Chambon, P. (1988). *EMBO J.* **7,** 3385–3388.

Pratt, W. B., Jolly, D. J., Pratt, D. V., Hollenberg, S. M., Giguere, V., Cadepond, F. M., Schweizer-Groyer, G., Catelli, M. G., Evans, R. M., and Baulieu, E. E. (1988). *J. Biol. Chem.* **263,** 267–273.

Quigley, C. A., Simental, J. A., Evans, B. A., Lubahn, D. B., Hughes, I. A., and French, F. S. (1990). *Endocrinology (Baltimore)* 72nd Meeting, p. 223.

Ritzen, E. M., Nayfeh, S. N., French, F. S., and Aronin, P. A. (1972). *Endocrinology (Baltimore)* **91,** 116–124.

Rivarola, M. A., Saez, J. M., Meyer, W. J., III, Kenny, F. M., and Migeon, C. J. (1967). *J. Clin. Endocrinol. Metab.* **27,** 371–378.

Sanger, F., Nicklen, S., and Coulson, A. R. (1977). *Proc. Natl. Acad. Sci. U.S.A.* **64,** 5463–5467.

Sar, M. (1985). *Tech. Immunocytochem.* **3,** 43–54.

Sar, M., Liao, S., and Stumpf, W. E. (1970). *Endocrinology (Baltimore)* **86,** 1008–1011.

Shannon, J. M., and Cunha, G. R. (1983). *Prostate* **4,** 367–373.

Sheffield, V., Cox, D. R., Lerman, L. S., and Myers, R. M. (1989). *Proc. Natl. Acad. Sci. U.S.A.* **86,** 232–236.

Sherins, R. J., and Bardin, C. W. (1971). *Endocrinology (Baltimore)* **89,** 835–841.

Smith, A. A., McLean, W. S., Nayfeh, S. N., French, F. S., Hansson, V., and Ritzen, E. M. (1975). *Curr. Top. Mol. Endocrinol.* **2,** 257–280.

Stanley, A. J., and Gumbreck, L. G. (1964). *Proc. Endocr. Soc.* **46,** 40 (abstr.).

Stanley, A. J., Gumbreck, L. G., Allison, J. E., and Easley, R. B. (1973). *Recent Prog. Horm. Res.* **29,** 43–64.

Strickland, A. L., and French, F. S. (1969). *J. Clin. Endocrinol. Metab.* **29,** 1284–1286.

Tan, J. A., Joseph, D. R., Quarmby, V. E., Lubahn, D. B., Sar, M., French, F. S., and Wilson, F. M. (1988). *Mol. Endocrinol.* **2,** 1276–1285.

Theophilus, B. D. M., Latham, T., Gabrowski, G. A., and Smith, F. I. (1989). *Nucleic Acids Res.* **13,** 3131–3145.

Tilley, W. D., Marcelli, M., Wilson, J. D., and McPhaul, M. (1989). *Proc. Natl. Acad. Sci. U.S.A.* **86,** 327–331.

Tora, L., Gronemeyer, H., Turcotte, B., Gaub, M. P., and Chambon, P. (1988a). *Nature (London)* **333,** 185–188.

Tora, L., Gaub, M. P., Mader, S., Dierich, A., Bellard, M., and Chambon, P. (1988b). *EMBO J.* **7,** 3771–3778.

Trapman, J., Klaassen, P., Kuiper, G. G. J. M., van der Korput, J. A. G. M., Faber, P. W., van Rooij, H. C. J., Geurts van Kessel, A., Voorhorst, M. M., Mulder, E., and Brinkmann, A. O. (1988). *Biochem. Biophys. Res. Commun.* **153,** 241–248.

Tremblay, R. R., Foley, T. P., Jr., Corvol, P., Park, I.-J., Kowarski, A., Blizzard, R. M., Jones, H. W., Jr., and Migeon, C. J. (1972). *Acta Endocrinol. (Copenhagen)* **70,** 331–341.

Tsai, S. Y., Carlstedt-Duke, J., Weigel, N. L., Dahlman, K., Gustafsson, J.-A., Tsai, M.-J., and O'Malley, B. W. (1988). *Cell (Cambridge, Mass.)* **55,** 361–369.

Webster, N. J. G., Green, S., Jin, J. R., and Chambon, P. (1988). *Cell (Cambridge, Mass.)* **54,** 199–207.

Wei, L. L., Krett, N. L., Francis, M. D., Gordon, D. F., Wood, W. M., and O'Malley, B. W. (1988). *Mol. Endocrinol.* **2,** 62–72.

Weiler, I. J., Lew, D., and Shapiro, D. J. (1987). *Mol. Endocrinol.* **1,** 355–362.

Weinberger, C., Thompson, C. C., Ong, E. S., Lebo, R., Gruol, D. J., and Evans, R. M. (1986). *Nature (London)* **324,** 641–646.

Wharton, K. A., Yedvobnick, B., Finnerty, V. G., and Artavanis-Tsa-Konas, S. A. (1985). *Cell (Cambridge, Mass.)* **40,** 55–62.

White, R., Lees, J. A., Needham, M., Ham, J., and Parker, M. (1987). *Mol. Endocrinol.* **1,** 735–744.

Wieacker, P., Griffin, J. E., Wienker, T., Lopez, J. M., Wilson, J. D., and Breckwoldt, M. (1987). *Hum. Genet.* **76,** 248–252.

Wieland, S. J., and Fox, T. O. (1981). *J. Steroid Biochem.* **14,** 409–414.

Wilkins, L. (1950). "The Diagnosis and Treatment of Endocrine Disorders in Childhood and Adolescence." Thomas, Springfield, Illinois.

Willard, H. F., and Riordan, J. R. (1985). *Science* **230,** 940.

Wilson, E. M. (1985). *J. Biol. Chem.* **260,** 8683–8689.

Wilson, E. M., and Colvard, D. S. (1984). *Ann. N.Y. Acad. Sci.* **438,** 85–100.

Wilson, E. M., and French, F. S. (1976). *J. Biol. Chem.* **251,** 5620–5629.

Wilson, E. M., and French, F. S. (1979). *J. Biol. Chem.* **254,** 6310–6319.

Wilson, E. M., Lubahn, D. B., French, F. S., Jewell, C. M., and Cidlowski, J. A. (1988). *Mol. Endocrinol.* **2,** 1018–1026.

Wilson, J. D., Griffin, J. E., Leshin, M., and MacDonald, P. C. (1983). *In* "The Metabolic Basis of Inherited Disease" (J. B. Stanbury, J. B. Wyngaarden, D. S. Fredrickson, J. L. Goldstein, and M. S. Brown, eds.), pp. 1001–1026. McGraw-Hill, New York.

Yarbrough, W. G., Quarmby, V. E., Simental, J. A., Joseph, D. R., Sar, M., Lubahn, D. B., Olsen, K. L., French, F. S., and Wilson, E. M. (1990). *J. Biol. Chem.* **265,** 8893–8900.

Young, C. Y. F., Murthy, L. R., Prescott, J. L., Johnson, M. P., Rowley, D. R., Cunningham, G. R., Killian, C. S., Scardino, P. T., Von Eschenbach, A., and Tindall, D. J. (1988). *Endocrinology (Baltimore)* **123,** 601–610.

Youssoufian, H., Kazazian, H. H., Jr., Phillips, D. G., Aronis, S., Tsiftis, G., Brown, V. A., and Antonarakis, S. E. (1986). *Nature (London)* **324,** 380–382.

Zahraoui, A., and Cuny, G. (1987). *Eur. J. Biochem.* **166,** 63–69.

DISCUSSION

W. F. Crowley. On the Western blot of your expressed protein, in addition to the 114 kDa protein, there were two smaller bands of 80 Kd and 64 Kd. You also had in a Northern blot some smaller 6.4 and 4.4 kb sizes. What is the significance of these? Does this have anything to do with the differential between testosterone (T) and dihydrotestosterone (DHT) binding and the absolute requirement of certain tissues to have DHT?

F. S. French. All we can say now is that these smaller bands on the Western blot are either proteolytic fragments of the receptor or protein products from alternate translation initiation sites.

W. F. Crowley. What do you think about T versus DHT binding in tissue specificity? Does it reside in the receptor? Certain tissues, such as hair follicles, prostate, and seminal vesicles, have testosterone converted to DHT.

F. S. French. I believe the requirement for DHT is related to its formation of a more stable complex with the androgen receptor. Where the concentration of T is high, T can probably do everything that DHT does. However, where concentrations of T and DHT are lower, DHT is likely to be the functional androgen simply because it dissociates from the receptor more slowly than T.

J. H. Clark. Were you able to see any androgen receptor message or protein in skeletal muscle?

F. S. French. Yes, we have been able to detect low levels of androgen receptor mRNA in skeletal muscle.

J. H. Clark. It is easily discernible?

F. S. French. The bands are weaker, but it can be detected in skeletal muscle.

J. H. Clark.   It is very difficult for us to even detect binding of androgen receptor in skeletal muscle.

F. S. French.   We have trouble with that too. There is a low level of message there. I agree that it is difficult to measure binding.

C. Grunfeld.   The point mutation at 831 with the substitution of glutamine for arginine is an interesting one. Has anyone done site-directed mutagenesis in a steroid hormone receptor other than the androgen receptor to see what the effects might be?

F. S. French.   I do not think so, but it would be interesting to do so.

J. H. Clark.   In *Tfm* and wild-type rats there are similar affinities, but decreased binding in a large number of sites not binding in *Tfm*. Isn't this a paradox? There are many sites by Western in the *Tfm* rat.

F. S. French.   When we express *Tfm* and wild-type AR cDNAs in COS cells, there are equal amounts of the AR proteins, as measured by Western blotting; however, the *Tfm* rat AR has a lower binding capacity for [^{3}H]R1881, even though the binding affinities of *Tfm* and wild type for [^{3}H]R1881 are similar.

J. H. Clark.   Do you know whether there is anything in the cell extracts of these animals which will inhibit the binding of normal androgen receptors? Is something else involved?

F. S. French.   We have not done that experiment. The evidence we have would suggest that there is a defect in the receptor itself, rather than an inhibitor of androgen binding to the receptor.

J. H. Clark.   It is a fairly common problem, even with the hi-tech expression of receptors in bacterial cells in which one can detect a lot of receptor by Westerns, but the binding is much reduced, as though something were blocking it or maybe aggregating the receptor.

F. S. French.   The *Tfm* rat will respond to high doses of testosterone. Sherins and Bardin reported this many years ago, and later Naess and co-workers demonstrated that serum LH is suppressed by DHT in the *Tfm* rat, but only at very high doses.

J. H. Clark.   This is strictly for the rat, not for the *Tfm* mouse.

F. S. French.   The *Tfm* mouse is different in that it has a low level of mRNA for the receptor and also has a low level of androgen binding activity. In fact, Barbara Attardi and others who have studied binding in brain have found that the androgen receptor binding activity of the *Tfm* mouse is about 10% of normal. More recently, Don Tindall's laboratory reported that the mutant androgen receptor of the *Tfm* mouse is smaller than the wild type. The *Tfm* mouse is totally unresponsive to androgen.

M. R. Walters.   I always thought, prior to cloning information, that androgen and estrogen receptors would be very closely related evolutionarily. Does the difference surprise you as much as it does me? Do you understand why they might not be so similar?

F. S. French.   I did not have a preconceived notion about this, so I was not that surprised.

M. R. Walters.   My surprise was based on the cross-affinity of the steroids.

F. S. French.   Estradiol binds to the androgen receptor reasonably well, about like progesterone, but testosterone and dihydrotestosterone do not bind very well to the estrogen receptor. Bonita Katzenellenbogen and co-workers did studies on the uterus showing there is a response to high doses of dihydrotestosterone and suggested that it might be acting, in part, through the estrogen receptor system. However, the antiestrogenic effects of androgen may be mediated largely through the androgen receptor, rather than by inhibition of the estrogen receptor.

J. H. Clark.   I think that this is what most people believe.

D. Rodbard.   I would like to comment on the interpretation of the Scatchard plots for the wild-type and mutant androgen receptors. The present results do not allow one to conclude whether there has been a change in maximal binding capacity B_{max} or affinity or both. One needs additional data at higher ligand concentrations, spanning a 10- to 100-fold higher range of concentrations, to obtain more precise estimates of B_{max} and to search for curvature. The presence of curvature, possibly due to two states or two sites, or dimerization or negative cooperativity, could conceivably account for the present results and still have a B_{max} consistent with the wild type, as you indicated was suggested by your immunohistochemical data. Also, the uncertainty in the estimate of nonspecific binding can have a major effect on the estimate of B_{max}, especially in the case of a curvilinear Scatchard plot.

G. C. Chamness.   In response to Dr. Walters' comment on the cross-talk or interaction of estrogen on androgen receptors and vice versa, there are, in fact, both types of evidence. A long time ago we did some work with MCF 7 cells which showed a definite growth response to DHT which was inhibited by antiestrogen and thus presumably involved the estrogen receptor. The levels required were such that binding of the DHT to the estrogen receptor could have caused this. This was a highly hyperphysiological response. In another study of brain receptors, where I do not think there was any actual physiological response, estradiol, but not other estrogens, did bind to the DHT receptor reasonably specifically, though, again, not too strongly.

The questions I have deal with some of the deletion mutants. It has been stated that if you get rid of the hormone-binding region, you might actually have a constitutively activating receptor, since there would not be anything in the way of its binding to the response elements. Dr. French, you discussed one in which I think the entire hormone-binding region was deleted. Is all of the DNA-binding region still there? What is the phenotype of that deletion?

F. S. French.   All of the genomic DNA-binding domain was there in one of those deletions. That patient was completely androgen insensitive.

S. I. Taylor.   I have a question about the same deletion mutation. It is not always possible to predict from the sequence of the genomic DNA at what level the protein will be expressed. For example, nonsense mutations and other types of mutations which cause premature chain termination will often lead to low levels of mRNA. Alternatively, because this deletion removes the normal stop codon, this type of mutation has the potential of causing the synthesis of a fusion protein with the C-terminal portion encoded by DNA sequences downstream from the deletion break point. Such a fusion protein might be unstable or it might not be targeted to the nucleus. Have you measured the levels of androgen receptor mRNA by Northern blotting or have you detected the presence of a fusion protein by Western blotting?

F. S. French.   I am glad you brought that up since I meant to go on to say, in answer to the previous question, that in the patient with a deletion of the entire steroid binding domain, Terry Brown could not detect a 10-kb mRNA nor a smaller AR mRNA. It seems likely that a truncated AR message is transcribed, but is unstable and rapidly degraded.

S. I. Taylor.   That would certainly explain the observation.

F. S. French.   We have not done Western blot analysis for AR protein in genital skin fibroblasts and therefore this patient cannot be used to test the hypothesis that an AR missing its steroid-binding domain would be constitutively active.

R. S. Swerdloff.   Have you found in families with partial androgen insensitivity any examples of varying degrees of defect—one family member having a more severe degree of the defect than another affected family member? If so, have you had an opportunity to study in more detail the specific type of defect?

F. S. French.   This is a study we would like to pursue. In fact, we have one such patient we are working with now. She is a partially androgen-insensitive 46,XY phenotypic female with an enlarged clitoris and some posterior labial fusion. When she entered puberty at age 13, her serum testosterone increased and she became further virilized. Genital skin fibroblasts were found to have normal androgen binding affinity and binding capacity. This child has a maternal uncle with hypospadius deformity, suggesting that he has the same AR gene defect, but with less resistance to androgen. This type of variation is not likely to occur in the complete form of androgen insensitivty syndrome and will probably be observed more often in the incomplete form among siblings with different fathers.

J. H. Clark.   Couldn't some of these simply be developmentally mistimed expression of the androgen receptor—that the fetus did not have androgen receptors present during the development and differentiation of the Wolffian and Müllerian ducts, but later did have them? Are there examples of differential timing in the developmental expression of receptors? I do not know that there are.

F. S. French. I do not know either.

N. Josso. I do not know of any examples of variation in the timing of the expression of the androgen receptor, but we have observed a family with anorchia in which the atrophy of the fetal testes took place at different times in the different children. One of the children was a phenotypic male, only he had no testes. Another one, in which the abnormality had occurred earlier, had had no virilization of the genital tract and was declared a female at birth. Thus, I think that this is important. We have had a bit of the same problem in patients with persistent Müllerian duct syndrome in whom we found normal expression of the hormone but do not know whether this means that this family has the receptor defect or simply that the anti-Müllerian hormone was expressed too late—at a time when the Müllerian ducts themselves had become unresponsive.

W. F. Crowley. Have you found examples of alterations in receptor that seemed to be localized in certain tissues, or of tissues that seemed to retain their receptor function?

F. S. French. A kind of mosaic pattern in androgen insensitivity? No. However, this possibility has been suggested in children with hypospadius deformity. Some patients with partial androgen insensitivty have been described wherein the genital skin fibroblasts do not show any binding activity. In fact, I think Natalie Josso reported such a case. The question in such a case is: "Might androgen receptor binding be detected in skin fibroblasts from a different area?" Of course, another possibility is that this was a case with a constitutively active receptor without androgen binding activity.

R. S. Swerdloff. Or, as Dr. Clark suggested, there could be situations in which there is some other type of substance which interferes with binding.

F. S. French. That is an interesting possibility.

W. F. Crowley. We studied a patient with Klinefelter's syndrome and complete androgen insensitivity. This really should not happen, since Klinefelter's patients have two X chromosomes, and androgen sensitivity is an X-linked disorder. Hence, at least 50% of the receptors should be normal. However, this patient's androgen receptors exhibited no binding at all. There have been two cases reported in the literature of an identical occurrence of Klinefelter's syndrome with testicular feminization or complete androgen sensitivity. The possibility of an inhibitor being present is probably another potential explanation. Do you have any idea of what the mechanism of this might be genetically?

F. S. French. I am afraid not.

G. B. Cutler. That Klinefelter's patient could likely have had nondisjunction at the second meiotic division in the mother. If the same maternal X chromosome was duplicated, the androgen receptor mutation would be present on both the Xs.

Most women with androgen insensitivity seem to have a moderate amount of pubic hair, even the ones considered "completely insensitive." Has this also been your experience? If these two families had a deletion of the androgen receptor, did they have absolutely no pubic hair?

F. S. French. The presence of pubic hair indicates some androgen response, even though the phenotype is female without other signs of virilization. These individuals are said to have complete androgen insensitivity because they are essentially like the normal female. Within the complete androgen insensitivity group, pubic hair may be present, though sparse. These individuals with pubic hair are probably not completely androgen insensitive. However, there are affected individuals with no sexual hair, and these must be totally unresponsive to androgens. I would assume a deletion of the entire androgen receptor would result in that phenotype.

G. B. Cutler. One interesting thing about androgens is that there are major differences in androgen sensitivity of the hair follicle, depending on where it is placed regionally (pubis versus axilla versus mustache, beard, abdomen, upper back, etc., in decreasing order of sensitivity). Have you any thoughts on the mechanism for this difference in sensitivity, which may not be at the receptor level?

F. S. French. No, I do not have any thoughts on this, but I think it is something that might be possible to study in greater detail with the new probes that are available. Dr. L. L. Hsia and co-workers [Sawaya *et al., J. Invest. Dermatol.* **92,** 91–95 (1989)] have demonstrated androgen receptor binding in sebaceous glands and hair follicles. They found androgen receptors from areas of male-type balding as well as in hairy scalp. I do not know of other studies of androgen receptors in hair follicles. Regional differences in androgen metabolism might explain why androgen-stimulated hair growth occurs in some areas more than others.

D. Rodbard. One of the factors contributing to the distribution of androgen sensitivity in hair follicles on the body surface may be local temperature. We should recall that skin temperature is often 27–32°C, not 37°C, and there are characteristic temperature gradients (i.e., in the face). Certain areas (e.g., axilla and pubis) are much closer to 37°C. The equilibrium between testosterone and di-hydrotestosterone with TeBG is also temperature sensitive, so free testosterone concentrations may vary throughout the body. The genital fibroblasts from foreskin are not at their physiological temperature when cultured at 37°C. Since many known receptor mutants are temperature sensitive, it is conceivable that their activation depends, in part, on average local body temperature. This might account for some aspects of hirsutism in both normal males (e.g., beard growth, trunk versus extremities) and in some pathophysiological states, and might account for some disparities between clinical phenotype and androgen receptors at 37°C *in vitro.*

R. S. Swerdloff. There are differences in the amount of hair growth in different races, with the American Indian as the prototype of the markedly diminished response. Is this a postreceptor alteration?

J. H. Clark. No, it is a temperature response.

F. S. French. This would be interesting to study with an androgen receptor antibody using immunohistochemistry.

R. S. Swerdloff. Have there ever been any reports of estrogen receptor defects? If not, is this a lethal type of defect?

F. S. French. To my knowledge there has been no such report.

J. H. Clark. There are no such studies that I know of. We have tried to produce a transgenic strain of mice that would be receptorless, but have been unable to do so as yet; possibly because it is lethal, but I do not know for sure.

F. S. French. Could the estrogen receptor be required for normal placental function and essential for implantation?

J. H. Clark. Yes, I think it could be in many different places. I think estrogen is very important developmentally.

Tissue-Specific Expression of the Growth Hormone Gene and Its Control by Growth Hormone Factor-1

MICHAEL KARIN, LARS THEILL, JOSE-LUIS CASTRILLO,
ALISON MCCORMICK, AND HELEN BRADY

*Department of Pharmacology, School of Medicine, University
of California–San Diego, La Jolla, California 92093*

I. Introduction

One of the major challenges in molecular genetics is to decipher the mechanisms that control the utilization of genetic information in time- and space-dependent manners. Differential gene activation is the basis for the processes of cellular differentiation and specialization. Through genetic analysis a great deal has been learned about the general mechanisms that govern these processes in organisms such as *Drosophila melanogaster* and *Ceanorhabditis elegans.* Although mammals, on the other hand, are refractory to genetic analysis, significant progress has been made in understanding the mechanisms that control tissue-specific gene expression in these organisms. This can be attributed mostly to a biochemical approach based on the development of *in vitro* systems in which differential promoter utilization could be observed, resulting in identification of transcription factors mediating cell-type-specific gene expression (Schcidcrcit *et al.*, 1987; Lichtsteiner *et al.*, 1989; Bodner and Karin, 1987). Several of these factors were purified to homogeneity and their cDNAs were cloned (Bodner *et al.*, 1988; Ingraham *et al.*, 1988; Muller *et al.*, 1988; Scheidereit *et al.*, 1988).

In this review we describe our studies on the control of growth hormone (GH) gene expression. Emphasis is placed on the mechanisms responsible for the cell-type-specific expression of this gene. The GH gene family represents an excellent system for studying the mechanisms responsible for cell-type-specific gene expression (Karin, 1989). In addition to GH, this family includes several other genes coding for hormones of physiological and clinical importance, such as prolactin (PRL) and the various placental lactogens (PLs) (Miller and Eberhart, 1983). GH is specifically expressed in specialized cells, the somatotropes, of the anterior pituitary. It is required for postnatal growth and maintenance of nitrogen, mineral, lipid, and carbohydrate metabolism (Martin, 1973). Its most important

43

function is probably the stimulation of protein synthesis, especially collagen in cartilage (Jubiz, 1985). PRL, which is expressed in a different group of specialized cells in the anterior pituitary—the lactotropes—is responsible for the initiation and maintenance of lactation (Bern and Nicoll, 1968).

II. GH Gene Family

The GH and PRL genes arose by duplication of a common precursor more than 350 million years ago (Miller and Eberhardt, 1983), an estimate consistent with the presence of both genes in all vertebrates and the divergence of amphibians from fish some 400 million years ago. While rodents contain a single GH gene, primates contain five tandemly linked GH genes. However, only one of these genes codes for the physiological form of GH, while the other four encode variant GH polypeptides and PLs. Only the authentic GH gene, present at the 5' end of the gene cluster, is expressed in the anterior pituitary. Expression of the four other genes is restricted to the placenta during late pregnancy (Miller and Eberhardt, 1983). The function of the various PLs is not clear, but they are thought to have a role in lactogenesis, fetal growth, and stimulation of the corpus luteum and to affect carbohydrate and lipid metabolism (Chard, 1979).

It is evident that all of these hormones function mostly in the control of growth and development through fetal and adult life. Insufficient production of GH leads to growth retardation or dwarfism, while its overproduction before puberty leads to gigantism and to acromegaly after puberty (Jubiz, 1985). Insufficient production of PRL causes a failure in lactation. In contrast, overproduction of PRL leads to amenorrhea or impotence (Jubiz, 1985). Low levels of PLs seem to correlate with fetal growth retardation (Lee et al., 1980).

Studying the mechanism responsible for the tissue- and cell-type-specific expression of these genes is therefore of immediate importance for understanding the physiology and pathology of this group of hormones. Also, as mentioned above, due to recent progress, the GH gene family and its regulation represent an excellent paradigm for understanding the general mechanisms involved in cell-type-specific gene expression and differentiation in mammals and its regulation by hormones (Karin, 1989; Karin et al., 1990).

III. Promoter Structure and Regulation

To date, the individual members of both the human and rat GH gene family have been isolated and their complete nucleotide sequences have been determined (Miller and Eberhardt, 1983; Truong et al., 1984; Ogren and Talamantes, 1987). Most importantly, the promoter regions of the two genes expressed in the anterior pituitary, GH and PRL, were subjected to detailed scrutiny (Karin et al., 1990; Nelson et al., 1988). Comparison of the 5'-flanking regions of the rat and human GH genes reveals five blocks of extensive sequence similarity within the first 500 bp of DNA. The first two blocks encompass the TATA box and the binding sites for the pituitary-specific transcription factor, GH factor-1 (GHF-1). Similar comparison between the human and rat PRL 5'-flanking regions reveals four blocks of extensive similarity (80–90%) within the first 400 bp. On the other hand, only two short blocks of limited sequence similarity (60–70%) are revealed by comparison of the first 400 bp of the 5'-flanking regions of the human GH and PRL genes (Karin et al., 1990).

In addition to mediating pituitary-specific expression, the GH promoter region also contains several other cis elements responsible for the modulation of GH transcription in response to hormonal signals. Transcription of both human and rat GH genes is induced by GH-releasing factor via a mechanism involving cAMP. A region mediating induction by cAMP has been mapped (Brent et al., 1988; Dana and Karin, 1989; Copp and Samuels, 1989). Two elements within the 5'-flanking region and the first intron were found to mediate the induction of human GH by glucocorticoids, by serving as binding sites for the glucocorticoid receptor (Slater et al., 1985). The location of such elements in the rat GH gene has not been determined, however the 5' site is evolutionarily conserved. In contrast to GH-releasing factor and glucocorticoids, the response to thyroid hormone is species specific: The rat GH gene is induced, while its human counterpart is not. A thyroid hormone response element was mapped within the 5'-flanking region of the rat GH gene. In this case it appears that binding of the thyroid hormone receptor to DNA might not be sufficient and could require an interaction with an adjacently bound factor (Wright et al., 1988; Brent et al., 1989).

IV. Pituitary Development and Differentiation

GH is specifically expressed in the somatotropic cells of the anterior pituitary, and no other site of GH synthesis has been detected. The anterior pituitary originates from Rathke's pouch, a structure that first appears at embryonic day (e.d.) 8.5 of the mouse (timing is different in other mammals), as an invagination of the oral endoderm. By e.d. 12 Rathke's pouch detaches from the oral epithelium and becomes an individual structure, initiating a program of rapid cell proliferation (Rugh, 1968). Its ventral epithelium serves as the anterior pituitary anlagen, while the dorsal epithelium generates the intermediate lobe of the pituitary. Cytodifferentiation gives rise to different hormone-producing cells first detected during e.d. 15–16. Two more committed precursors, acidophils and basophils, are formed from the primordial stem cell. The acidophils are the progenitors for both the somatotropes (GH producing) and lactotropes (PRL producing), while the basophils give rise to cells that specialize to produce adrenocorticotropic hormone, thyroid-stimulating hormone, follicle-stimulating hormone, or luteinizing hormone (Chatelain *et al.*, 1979). The intermediate pituitary, on the other hand, specializes to synthesize various peptide hormones derived from the proopiomelanocortin gene.

The majority of PRL-expressing cells appear to be derived from GH-producing precursors. Complete ablation of somatotropes by expression of GH–diphtheria toxin and GH–thymidine kinase fusion genes inserted into the germ line of transgenic mice also resulted in elimination of most of the lactotropes (Behringer *et al.*, 1988; Borrelli *et al.*, 1989). However, a small portion of the lactotropes escaped ablation (Behringer *et al.*, 1988). These observations support the lineal relationship between somatotropes and lactotropes outlined in Fig. 1. Despite the common precursor, no PRL expression can be detected until about 1–12 days

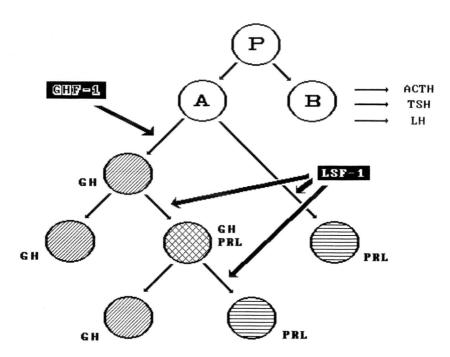

FIG. 1.   The lineal relationships between GH- and PRL-expressing cells. The primordial anterior pituitary stem cell (P) gives rise to the basophilic (B) and acidophilic (A) cells that serve as precursors for the various hormone-expressing cells. GH-expressing cells are first detected on e.d. 16, while a stable population of PRL-expressing cells is detected only 10–12 days after birth. Ablation experiments indicate that the majority (i.e., 80–90%) of PRL-expressing cells are derived from GH-expressing cells by direct descent; however, a small proportion of PRL expressors are derived from precursors that never contain GHF-1 or express GH. The stages at which GHF-1 and LSF-1 act are indicated. ACTH, Adrenocorticotropic hormone; TSH, thyroid-stimulating hormone; LH, luteinizing hormone.

postnatally in the mouse, while GH expression is first detected on e.d. 16 (Slabaugh *et al.*, 1982). Thus, the two genes are unlikely to be coordinately activated by a single common factor.

V. Identification of a Somatotrope-Specific Transcription Factor

Comparison of the 5'-flanking regions of the human and rat GH genes revealed extensive similarity over the first 500 bp of DNA, suggesting the importance of these sequences in controlling GH expression (Miller and Eberhardt, 1983). Indeed, by transfection of appropriate constructs, we found that the 300-bp evolutionarily conserved 5' region of the GH gene is sufficient for conferring somatotrope-specific expression in cultured cells (Lefevre *et al.*, 1987). These results were confirmed by others, using both transgenic mice (Behringer *et al.*, 1988; Borrelli *et al.*, 1989) and pituitary cell lines (West *et al.*, 1987). The location of protein-binding sites within this region was determined by DNase I "footprinting." Although several different protein factors binding to the GH promoter were detected, only one was unique to GH-expressing cells. The restricted distribution of this protein, named GHF-1, immediately suggested that it plays a major role in the pituitary-specific expression of the GH gene (Lefevre *et al.*, 1987).

This possibility was tested by constructing linker-scanning and internal deletion mutants affecting the GHF-1-binding sites and examining their activity by *in vivo* transfection and *in vitro* transcription. GHF-1 binds to two adjacent sites, one centered around position -80 and the other around position -120 upstream of the start of GH gene transcription. Both of these sites are important promoter elements *in vivo* (Lefevre *et al.*, 1987) and *in vitro* (Bodner and Karin, 1987). On the other hand, deletion of these elements has no effect on the low basal activity of the GH promoter in transfected HeLa cells or HeLa cell extracts (Bodner and Karin, 1987; Dana and Karin, 1989).

GHF-1 was purified to near-homogeneity from extracts of GC cells, a GH-expressing cell line derived from a rat pituitary tumor, and positively identified by elution from sodium dodecyl sulfate–polyacrylamide gels and renaturation as a 33-kDa polypeptide (Castrillo *et al.*, 1989). Most importantly, purified GHF-1 stimulates transcription from the GH promoter when added to extracts of cells such as HeLa, which do not express GH or GHF-1 (Bodner and Karin, 1987; Castrillo *et al.*, 1989). These findings indicate that, although GHF-1 is a pituitary-specific transcription factor, it is capable of interacting with the basic transcriptional machinery in both GH-expressing and nonexpressing cells. In fact, this was the first demonstration that a cell-type-specific transcription factor isolated from one cell type can be added to an extract of heterologous cell type and activate transcription. These results demonstrated that cell type specificity lies within factors recognizing upstream promoter elements and is not determined by the general transcription machinery. It is possible, therefore, that the mere presence or absence of GHF-1 is sufficient to determine whether the GH gene will be expressed.

Because of the close evolutionary and developmental relationships between GH and PRL, GHF-1 was examined for its ability to bind to the PRL promoter. Concentrations of GHF-1 which fully protect the low-affinity site of the GH promoter did not result in obvious protection of the PRL promoter (Castrillo *et al.*, 1989). However, at least one other factor present within the partially purified GC extract, which does not bind to the GHF-1-specific affinity column, was found to protect five sites within the PRL promoter (Castrillo *et al.*, 1989). These sites overlap with the sequences that are conserved between the human and rat PRL genes (Karin *et al.*, 1990; Truong *et al.*, 1984), some of which are essential promoter elements (Nelson *et al.*, 1988). This PRL-specific factor, lactotrope specific factor-1 (LSF-1), was purified to homogeneity using a PRL promoter-derived binding site as an affinity ligand and is clearly different from GHF-1 by both its molecular mass (38 versus 33 kDa) and its failure to cross-react with anti-GHF-1 antibodies (A. Guttierez-Hartman, personal communication).

Different results were obtained by Nelson *et al.* (1988), who claimed that a single factor, which they have named Pit-1, binds to both the GH and PRL promoters. After isolation of corresponding cDNA clones, it was found that Pit-1 is identical to GHF-1 (Bodner *et al.*, 1988; Ingraham *et al.*, 1988). Since, at concentrations sufficient to protect the GH promoter, no significant binding of GHF-1 to the PRL promoter can be detected (Castrillo *et al.*, 1989), it is possible that GHF-1 has much lower affinity toward the Prl promoter in comparison to the GH promoter. Only when present in very high and probably nonphysiological concentrations can it bind and activate the PRL promoter (Ingraham *et al.*, 1988; Theill *et al.*, 1989). This explanation is consistent with the noncoordinate activation of the two genes during development. In the mouse GH expression is first detected on e.d. 16, while PRL expression is first detected 10–12 days after birth (Slabaugh *et al.*, 1982). We have confirmed these results with the sole exception that, using more sensitive methods, we detected transient expression of PRL in a small number of cells during e.d. 16, but not on e.d. 17 (Dollé *et al.*, 1990). The mechanism of PRL gene activation should become more clear after isolation of the LSF-1 gene.

VI.   Structure of GHF-1

A partial amino acid sequence of GHF-1 was obtained and used for the construction of oligodeoxynucleotide hybridization probes. Screening of rat and bovine pituitary cDNA libraries with these probes resulted in the isolation of GHF-1 cDNA clones (Bodner *et al.*, 1988). Antipeptide antibodies generated against this peptide reacted specifically with GHF-1 and confirmed that the sequence of the isolated peptide was correct and that it was indeed derived from GHF-1. Other investigators isolated the same cDNA clone, Pit-1, by screening of an expression library prepared from rat pituitary with a labeled GHF-1-binding site (Ingraham et al., 1988). Deduction of the GHF-1 amino acid sequence from these cDNAs has identified it as a member of the ever-growing family of homeodomain proteins and confirmed its identity with Pit-1. In its carboxy-terminal region, GHF-1 contains a stretch of 60 amino acids which exhibit 73% sequence identity to a consensus homeodomain. The homeodomain is a 60-amino-acid DNA-binding domain first detected by its conservation among the products of genes involved in determining the morphogenesis of the fruit fly, *Drosophila* (Gehring, 1987).

At first, the closest relatives of GHF-1 were thought to be the *Drosophila* proteins encoded by the *eve*, *prd*, and *iab-7* genes and the yeast MAT-a1 protein (Bodner et al., 1988). However, within a short while the primary structures of three other transcriptional activators which also contain homeodomains had become available. The homeodomains of these proteins are much more similar (>90%) to the GHF-1 homeodomain. In addition to the homeodomain, these proteins, Oct-1, Oct-2, and unc-86, contain a second highly conserved sequence motif, termed the POU-specific domain, composed of 75 amino acids (Herr et al., 1988). The identification of two well-established mammalian transcription factors, GHF-1 and Oct-2, as homeodomain proteins was an important breakthrough that served to bridge the gap between two separate fields: transcriptional regulation and developmental biology. It provided the first conclusive proof that homeodomain proteins already known to be involved in developmental decisions do indeed function as transcription factors (Robertson, 1988).

The homeodomain serves as the minimal DNA-binding domain of several *Drosophila* proteins (Muller et al., 1988; Hoey and Levine, 1988; Desplan et al., 1988). It plays the same role in GHF-1. Bacterial fusion proteins containing this portion of GHF-1 bind to both sites on the GH promoter (Bodner et al., 1988). Fusion of the heterologous activation domain of cJun and cFos to the homeobox region of GHF-1 generates potent GH-specific chimeric transactivators (Angel et al., 1989). Deletion of sequences within the homeodomain interferes with the ability of GHF-1 to activate GH transcription. In addition, it appears that the homeodomain also contains the nuclear transfer signal of GHF-1 (Theill et al., 1989).

While the involvement of the homeodomain in DNA binding is well established, the role of the POU-specific domain is not very clear. Mutations within the POU-specific domain of Oct-1 were shown to interfere with DNA binding (Sturm and Herr, 1988). Thus, it was suggested that the POU-specific domain participates in DNA binding and that the DNA might actually be contacted by both the POU domain and the homeodomain. However, it was difficult to reconcile these results, suggesting that the mode of DNA binding could be different for the POU proteins than for other homeodomain proteins, with the demonstrations that the homeodomain alone is sufficient for DNA binding (Gehring, 1987; Muller *et al.*, 1988). The POU-specific domain also appears to contribute to DNA binding of GHF-1. However, fusion of the strong activation domain of cJun to GHF-1 sequences either containing both the homeodomain and the POU domain or only the homeodomain revealed that the protein lacking the POU domain was only 20% as active as the one containing this motif. Similar results were obtained by examining the binding activity of bacterial fusion proteins. A protein containing the intact POU-specific domain is only 3-fold more active than a protein missing one-half of this sequence. Furthermore, both proteins generate essentially identical DNase I footprints on the GH promoter (Theill *et al.*, 1989). Therefore, the POU-specific domain is unlikely to participate in direct contact with the DNA, although it does augment DNA binding by the homeodomain. It is possible that the POU-specific domain stabilizes the GHF-1–DNA complex by participating in protein–protein interactions.

While the carboxy-terminal half of GHF-1 is involved in DNA binding, its amino-terminal half is responsible for transcriptional activation. This activity is destroyed by the deletion of sequences residing within the first 72 amino acids. In addition, this part of GHF-1 can be fused to a heterologous DNA-binding domain derived from cJun to construct a chimeric protein capable of activating transcription from activator protein-dependent promoters (Theill *et al.*, 1989). Interestingly, this part of GHF-1 contains only a few negatively charged amino acids or glutamines, the residues shown to be associated with other known activation domains (Ptsashne, 1988; Courey and Tjian, 1988). Competition experiments indicate that an excess of a Jun·GHF-1 chimeric protein, which contains the DNA-binding domain of GHF-1 and the negatively charged activation domain of cJun, prevents activation by wild-type cJun binding to the collagenase promoter (L. E. Theill, unpublished observations). This is essentially the same phenomenon described as "squelching" by Gill and Ptashne (1988). On the other hand, wild-type GHF-1 does not compete against cJun. These results suggest that GHF-1 has a novel type of activation domain that could interact with components of the transcriptional machinery different from those contacted by other types of activation domains. The various features of GHF-1 are summarized in Fig. 2.

VII.   Extinction of GH Expression in Somatic Cell Hybrids

The results described above are consistent with a model according to which GH expression is positively regulated by GHF-1. If GHF-1 is present, GH is expressed; if GHF-1 is absent, no GH expression can be detected. So far, no substantial evidence for negative regulation of GH expression could be found. However, this relatively simple picture seemed to be contradicted by the finding that, like many other cell-type-specific genes, expression of GH is extinguished

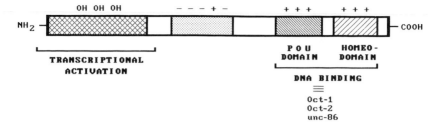

FIG. 2.   The architecture of GHF-1. GHF-1 is 291 amino acids long. Near its carboxy terminus, it contains a 60-amino-acid homeodomain (hatched box), which is preceded by a 75-amino-acid POU-specific domain (hatched box). The two are separated by a putative hinge region. The transactivation domain is located near the amino terminus and contains a 72-amino-acid serine-, threonine-rich region (cross-hatched box). The stippled box indicates a region rich in negatively charged amino acids.

in somatic cell hybrids (Thompson *et al.*, 1980; Sonnenschein *et al.*, 1971). Fusion of GH3 rat pituitary cells, which express GH to mouse L cell fibroblasts, results in first-generation hybrids which cease to express GH. However, these hybrids are metastable and, upon prolonged culturing, loose parts of the mouse genome contributed by the L cell parent. Second-generation hybrids containing different fractions of the mouse genome were isolated by subcloning. A small number of these subclones have begun to reexpress GH, which correlates with loss of the majority of the mouse genome (McCormick *et al.*, 1988). These experiments therefore suggest that the L cell parent contributes a specific extinguisher of GH expression, whose loss leads to reexpression of the GH gene. The chromosomal location of this extinguisher is yet to be determined.

We used these subclones to determine the mechanism of extinction. We found that extinction was extended to transiently transfected GH·chloramphenicol acetyltransferase (CAT) constructs and even observed in cell-free extracts with naked DNA templates. Therefore, altered chromatin structure or methylation of the GH gene was unlikely to be directly involved. Examination of proteins which bind to the GH promoter in extracts of the two parental cell lines and several secondary hybrids, one of which reexpresses GH, has ruled out the involvement of a repressor that binds directly to the GH promoter. In fact, all of the proteins that bind to the GH promoter in nonexpressing cells are also present in the expressing cell lines. Likewise, mixing experiments have ruled out the presence of a factor which inactivates GHF-1. Finally, analysis of GHF-1 expression in the various cell lines indicated that GHF-1 is present only in GH-expressing cells. Therefore, extinction of GH is mediated by an indirect mechanism controlling expression of the positive activator, GHF-1 (McCormick *et al.*, 1988). These experiments provided the first established molecular mechanism accounting for the extinction of cell-type-specific genes in somatic cell hybrids. This indirect mechanism is, in fact, economical. Instead of using several different repressors for direct extinction of individual pituitary-specific genes, a single fibroblast factor can be sufficient for extinguishing the entire repertoire of pituitary-specific gene expression by preventing expression of one or a few specific transactivators.

Although the mechanism responsible for extinction of GHF-1 itself is not known, preliminary results indicate that it occurs at the transcriptional level. The GHF-1 promoter has been identified and fused to the CAT reporter gene. Transfection of this GHF-1·CAT construct into the various hybrid and parental cell lines reveals expression only in GH-expressing cells. Thus, whatever mechanisms are responsible for extinction, they affect the activity of the GHF-1 promoter. Similar results were obtained *in vitro* using extracts of the various cell lines: The GHF-1 promoter is active only in extracts of GH-expressing cells (A. McCormick, unpublished observations). Analysis of the factors that recognize the GHF-1 promoter in expressing and nonexpressing hybrids should reveal the mechanism of extinction. It could be due to direct repression of the GHF-1 promoter, or it might be mediated by extinction of a positive-acting factor required for GHF-1 expression.

VIII. Developmental Regulation of GHF-1 Expression

The role of GHF-1 in maintaining GH expression in already differentiated cells seems unequivocal. However, none of the experiments described above provided strong support for participation of GHF-1 in activation of the GH gene during the development of the anterior pituitary. Therefore, we analyzed GHF-1 expression during mouse embryogenesis by *in situ* hybridization and immunohistochemical analyses. GHF-1 transcripts were first detected during e.d. 13, 24 hours after the individualization of Rathke's pouch. Expression is specific to the anterior pituitary anlagen and even morphologically similar cells that line the dorsal side of Rathke's pouch and give rise to the intermediate lobe do not express GHF-1. Expression of GHF-1 RNA increased during the next 48 hours and peaked between days 14 and 15, after which it declined. GH transcripts, on the other hand, first appeared during e.d. 16. Thus, there is a gap of approximately 3 days between the onset of GHF-1 transcription and the activation of GH gene expression. Immunohistochemical analysis of GHF-1 protein expression indicated that this lag period is probably due to delayed accumulation of the GHF-1 protein. Using anti-GHF-1 antibodies, no GHF-1 could be detected until e.d. 16. On this and the following day, the appearance of GHF-1 protein showed excellent temporal and spatial correlation with GH expression (Dollé *et al.*, 1990).

Although the mechanism responsible for the delayed accumulation of GHF-1 is not clear, these experiments provide strong support for the involvement of GHF-1 in the activation of GH expression during pituitary development. It appears that GHF-1 expression itself is controlled both transcriptionally and post-transcriptionally. The posttranscriptional regulation is likely to involve translational control, an unusual situation because delayed translation has been observed mostly for maternally inherited mRNAs (McDonald and Struhl, 1986; Steward *et al.*, 1988). This posttranscriptional event plays an important role in the regulation of GH gene activation, because the appearance of GHF-1 protein most likely represents the last step in the specialization pathway leading to formation of fully determined somatotropes.

While the appearance and accumulation of GHF-1 protein show excellent correlation with the onset of GH gene transcription, the correlation with PRL gene expression is more nebulous. PRL transcripts were detected in only a small number of cells during e.d. 16. No such cells could be found on day 17, while the number of cells expressing high levels of GH transcripts has dramatically increased (Dollé *et al.*, 1990). These results suggest that high levels of GHF-1 present during e.d. 16 lead to transient activation of the PRL gene. However, full expression of these genes probably requires the PRL-specific factor LSF-1, which might not appear until later. This interpretation of the results is consistent with the finding that GHF-1 has much lower affinity to the PRL promoter in comparison to the GH promoter (Castrillo *et al.*, 1989).

IX. Model for GH Gene Activation

The large body of experimental evidence described above indicates that GHF-1 is probably the only cell-type-specific factor responsible for activation of the GH gene in the anterior pituitary. Thus, the tissue specificity of GH expression appears to be controlled in a relatively simple manner in comparison to the albumin, immunoglobulin, or interleukin-2 genes, whose promoters are recognized by multiple cell-type-specific factors (Scheidereit *et al.*, 1987; Lichsteiner and Schibler, 1989; Serfling *et al.*, 1989). To understand how a single factor can be responsible for the highly specific expression of the GH gene, we constructed derivatives of the HeLa cell line in which GHF-1 expression is Cd^{2+} inducible by introducing into their genome a metallothionein–GHF-1 fusion gene. In these cells, expression of a transiently transfected GH·CAT reporter gene is Cd^{2+} dependent. In the absence of Cd^{2+} (and GHF-1), no significant GH promoter activity can be detected (Theill *et al.*, 1989).

Furthermore, in agreement with our previous results (Dana and Karin, 1989) in the absence of GHF-1, GH·CAT expression is also refractory to forskolin (cAMP) and glucocorticoids, even though the level of glucocorticoid receptor has been increased by cotransfection with a specific expression vector. Likewise, in the absence of GHF-1, GH·CAT shows little response to a cotransfected cJun expression vector. However, after induction of GHF-1, GH·CAT expression increases by at least two orders of magnitude and can now be further activated by glucocorticoids, forskolin, or a cotransfected cJun expression vector. The glucocorticoid effect is mediated via the glucocorticoid response element in the GH promoter, while the cJun effect is mediated by binding of this protein to AP-1 sites within the vector (L. E. Theill, unpublished observations).

Collectively, these findings suggest the following mechanism for explaining cell-type-specific GH gene activation (Fig. 3). In the absence of GHF-1, the inactive GH promoter is refractory to ubiquitous factors such as the glucocorticoid and thyroid hormone receptors. While even a transient transfected GH·CAT construct is refractory to these factors, the complete nonresponsiveness of the endogenous GH gene might be further secured by formation of a nucleosome covering its promoter region. Appearance of GHF-1 at a specific stage during development leads to occupancy of the promoter of the newly replicated GH gene, thereby preventing reformation of the nucleosome. GHF-1 binding alone only leads to partial activation of the promoter; however, synergistic in-

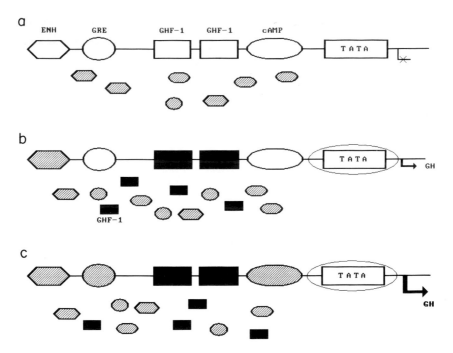

FIG. 3.   A model illustrating the role of GHF-1 in cell-type-specific activation of the GH gene. (a) Prior to e.d. 16 the precursors for the somatotropes contain most of the factors that can bind to the GH promoter, except GHF-1. In the absence of GHF-1, none of these factors is capable of activating the GH promoter (b). Together with ubiquitous factors that bind to an upstream enhancer element, it activates the GH promoter. (c) The rate of GH transcription can be further increased in response to GH-releasing factor, which acts via cAMP and a cAMP response factor, and glucocorticoids acting via the glucocorticoid receptor. ENH, enhancer; GRE, glucocorticoid response element.

teractions between GHF-1 and the ubiquitous activators already present within the pituitary cell are responsible for a much larger increase in GH transcription than the effect of GHF-1 alone. This cooperative activation could be brought about by GHF-1 interacting with one component of the basic transcriptional machinery and ubiquitous activators, such as the glucocorticoid receptor, which contain negatively charged activation domains (Ptashne, 1988), interacting with a different component. Together, the two factors stimulate the assembly of the initiation complex. Similar cooperativity between GHF-1 and enhancer factors can also be seen in transient cotransfection experiments performed in F9 cells. In these cells cotransfection of a suboptimal level of GHF-1 and cJun expression vectors leads to a large synergistic effect on GH·CAT expression. We found that mutations within the 72-amino-acid activation domain of GHF-1 interfere with its ability to cooperate with cJun. Thus, this serine-, threonine-rich domain is also required for synergistic interaction between GHF-1 and other transcription factors (L. E. Theill, unpublished observations). In the future it will be important to determine the mechanism by which this cooperativity is exerted.

The mechanism described above allows a single transcription factor whose abundance is itself regulated in a cell-type-specific manner to orchestrate the action of a number of more ubiquitous transcription factors, leading to precise activation of the GH gene only in the appropriate cell type. In addition to having a large synergistic effect on GH transcription, the ubiquitous activators are responsible for modulating its expression in response to various hormonal signals.

Due to the central role played by GHF-1, complete understanding of the pathway specifying the development of GH-expressing cells and the entire anterior pituitary will entail analysis of the mechanisms regulating GHF-1 expression.

ACKNOWLEDGMENTS

Work described here was supported by U.S. Public Health Service Grant DK-38527. L. Theill, J.-L. Castrillo, and H. Brady were supported by postdoctoral fellowships from the Danish Medical Research Council, the American Cancer Society–California Division, and the U.S. Public Health Service, respectively.

REFERENCES

Angel, P., Smeal, T., Meek, J., and Karin, M. (1989). *New Biol.* **1**, 35–43.
Behringer, R. R., Mathews, L. S., Palmiter, R. D., and Brinster, R. L. (1988). *Genes Dev.* **2**, 453–461.
Bern, H. A., and Nicoll, C. S. (1968). *Recent Prog. Horm. Res.* **24**, 681–705.
Bodner, M., and Karin, M. (1987). *Cell (Cambridge, Mass.)* **50**, 267–275.
Bodner, M., Castrillo, J.-L., Theill, L. E., Deerinck, T., Ellisman, M., and Karin, M. (1988). *Cell (Cambridge, Mass.)* **55**, 505–518.

Borrelli, E., Heyman, R. A., Arias, C., Sawchenko, P. E., and Evans, R. M. (1989). *Nature (London)* **339,** 538–541.

Brent, G. A., Harney, J. W., Moore, D. D., and Larsen, P. R. (1988). *Mol. Endocrinol.* **2,** 792–798.

Brent, G. A., Larsen, P. R., Harney, J. W., Koenig, R. J., and Moore, D. D. (1989). *J. Biol. Chem.* **264,** 178–182.

Castrillo, J.-L., Bodner, M., and Karin, M. (1989). *Science* **243,** 814–817.

Chard, T. (1979). *In* "Hormones in Blood" (C. H. Gray and V. H. T. Jones, eds.), pp. 333–409. Academic Press, New York.

Chatelain, A., Dupouy, J. P., and Dubois, M. P. (1979). *Cell Tissue Res.* **196,** 409–427.

Copp, R. P., and Samuels, H. H. (1989). *Mol. Endocrinol.* **3,** 790–796.

Courey, A. J., and Tjian, R. (1988). *Cell (Cambridge, Mass.)* **55,** 887–898.

Dana, S., and Karin, M. (1989). *Mol. Endocrinol.* **3,** 815–821.

Desplan, C., Theis, J., and O'Farrel, P. H. (1988). *Cell (Cambridge, Mass.)* **54,** 1081–1090.

Dollé, P., Castrillo, J.-L., Theill, L. E., Deerinck, T., Ellisman, M., and Karin, M. (1990). *Cell (Cambridge, Mass.)* **60,** 809–820.

Gehring, W. J. (1987). *Science* **236,** 1245–1252.

Gill, G., and Ptashne, M. (1988). *Nature (London)* **334,** 721–724.

Herr, W., Sturm, R. A., Clerc, R. G., Corcoran, L. M., Baltimore, D., Sharp, P. A., Ingraham, H. A., Rosenfeld, M. G., Finney, M., Ruvkun, G., and Horvitz, R. (1988). *Genes Dev.* **2,** 1513–1516.

Hoey, T., and Levine, M. (1988). *Nature (London)* **332,** 858–861.

Ingraham, H. A., Chen, R., Mangalam, H. J., Elsholtz, H. P., Flynn, S. E., Lin, C. R., Simmons, D. M., Swanson, L., and Rosenfeld, M. G. (1988). *Cell (Cambridge, Mass.)* **55,** 519–529.

Jubiz, W. (1985). "Endocrinology: A Logical Approach for Clinicians," 2nd ed. McGraw-Hill, New York.

Karin, M. (1989). *In* "Tissue Specific Gene Expression" (R. Renkawitz, ed.). VCH Publ., Weinheim, Federal Republic of Germany.

Karin, M., Castrillo, J.-L., and Theill, L. E. (1990). *Trend. Genet.* **6,** 92–96.

Lee, J. N., Grudzinskias, J. G., and Chard, T. J. (1980). *Obstet. Gynecol.* **1,** 87–92.

Lefevre, C., Imagawa, M., Dana, S., Grinlay, J., Bodner, M., and Karin, M. (1987). *EMBO J.* **6,** 971–981.

Lichtsteiner, S., and Schibler, U. (1989). *Cell (Cambridge, Mass.)* **57,** 1179–1187.

Lichtsteiner, S., Wuarin, J., and Schibler, U. (1989). *Cell (Cambridge, Mass.)* **57,** 963–973.

Martin, J. B. (1973). *N. Engl. J. Med.* **288,** 1384–1389.

McCormick, A., Wu, D., Castrillo, J.-L., Dana, S., Strobl, J., Thompson, E. B., and Karin, M. (1988). *Cell (Cambridge, Mass.)* **55,** 379–389.

McDonald, P. M., and Struhl, G. (1986). *Nature (London)* **324,** 537–545.

Miller, W. L., and Eberhardt, N. L. (1983). *Endocr. Rev.* **4,** 97–130.

Muller, M., Affolter, M., Leupin, W., Otting, G., Wüthrich, K., and Gehring, W. J. (1988). *EMBO J.* **7,** 4299–4304.

Nelson, C., Albert, V. R., Elsholtz, H. R., Lu, L. T. W., and Rosenfeld, M. G. (1988). *Science* **239,** 1400–1405.

Ogren, L., and Talamantes, F. (1987). *Int. Rev. Cytol.* **112,** 1–65.

Ptashne, M. (1988). *Nature (London)* **335,** 683–689.

Robertson, M. R. (1988). *Nature (London)* **336,** 522–524.

Rugh, R. (1968). "The Mouse: Its Reproduction and Development." Burgess.

Scheidereit, C., Heguy, A., and Roeder, R. D. (1987). *Cell (Cambridge, Mass.)* **51,** 783–793.

Scheidereit, C., Cromlish, J. A., Gerster, T., Kawakami, K., Balmaceda, C.-G., Alexander, R., and Roeder, R. G. (1988). *Nature (London)* **335,** 551–557.

Serfling, E. A., Barthelmaes, R., Pfeuffer, I., Schenk, B., Zarius, S., Swoboda, R., Mercurio, F., and Karin, M. (1989). *EMBO J.* **8**, 465–473.

Slabaugh, M. B., Lieberman, M. E., Rutledge, J. J., and Gorski, J. (1982). *Endocrinology (Baltimore)* **110**, 1489–1497.

Slater, E. P., Rabenau, O., Karin, M., Baxter, J. D., and Beato, M. (1985). *Mol. Cell. Biol.* **5**, 2984–2992.

Sonnenschein, C., Richardson, I., and Tashjian, A. H., Jr. (1971). *Exp. Cell Res.* **69**, 336–344.

Steward, R., Zushman, S. B., Huang, L. H., and Schedl, P. (1988). *Cell (Cambridge, Mass.)* **55**, 487–495.

Sturm, R. A., and Herr, W. (1988). *Nature (London)* **336**, 601–604.

Theill, L. E., Castrillo, J.-L., Wu, D., and Karin, M. (1989). *Nature (London)* **342**, 945–948.

Thompson, E. B., Dannies, P. S., Buckler, C. E., and Tashjian, A. H. (1980). *J. Steroid Biochem.* **12**, 193–210.

Truong, A. T., Duez, C., Belayew, A., Renard, A., Pictet, R., Bell, G. I., and Martial, J. A. (1984). *EMBO J.* **3**, 429–437.

West, B. L., Catanzaro, D. F., Mellon, S. H., Cattini, P. A., Baxter, J. D., and Rendelhuber, T. L. (1987). *Mol. Cell. Biol.* **7**, 1193–1197.

Wright, P. A., Crew, P. D., and Spindler, S. R. (1988). *Mol. Endocrinol.* **2**, 536–542.

DISCUSSION

G. Ringold. Do you have any idea whether activation of transcription by GHF-1 or the cooperativity between GHF-1 and the glucocorticoid receptor means that in the absence of GHF-1 the glucocorticoid receptor is incapable of binding to a GRE on that promoter? Alternatively, is the glucocorticoid receptor capable of binding, but not activating transcription in the absence of GHF-1?

M. Karin. We have no evidence, because the binding assays must be done *in vivo*. The 5' region of the gene binds the receptor very weakly *in vitro*, and even a footprint cannot be seen. I do not think there is cooperativity between the receptor and GHF-1 at the level of binding.

J. H. Clark. Do you think steroid receptor complexes might be interacting at the translational, rather than the transcriptional, level?

M. Karin. Maybe, but it is not likely.

J. H. Clark. Do you think that alterations of glucose blood levels in an adult animal change the level of the transcription factor?

M. Karin. GHF-1 has a rather long half-life. It is a rather stable protein and I think its role is just to open up the promoter. The transcription is then modulated by all the other factors that seem to be common to many different genes.

S. Nakanishi. Have you studied activation of the endogenous GH gene by transfection?

M. Karin. Yes, we have. So far, the results are negative, but I do not think they are conclusive. We examined HeLa cells that are not even from the same lineage as the pituitary. We have not eliminated the possibility that the endogenous growth hormone gene is so heavily methylated that it would be refractory to everything.

G. Ringold. Do you have any insight into what factors during development might influence the transcription activation of GHF-1? The generic issue to consider regarding organismal development is whether, in contrast to the activation of a transcription factor such as GHF-1, which is very tissue specific, the signals that activate other transcription factors will be more generalized. For example, the localized production of factors such as FGF or TGF-β might generate the signal(s) activating the expression of GHF-1.

M. Karin. I hope this will prove true, because I do not feel like purifying factors for the rest of my life! It is like an endless cascade of one specific factor activating another specific factor. We found at least two pituitary-specific footprints in this promoter, so for one of the levels of regulation we can actually see the influence of these sites *in vitro*. It will be another pituitary-specific factor that binds to the promoter, but I hope that at some point we will find some signal that comes from the outside so that we can end our search.

H. G. Friesen. Is GHF-1 expressed in the placenta? If not, do you have any thoughts on what regulates the expression of hGH-V in the placenta?

M. Karin. I cannot answer that question. We are just beginning to study the placenta now. We did some experiments with human placenta about 2 years ago. We failed to see any GHF-1-like activity in extracts of human placenta using footprinting, but this does not mean much, because placenta is essentially 50% necrotic tissue by the time it is used in experiments, so maybe the factor is very labile.

Molecular Characterization of Mammalian Tachykinin Receptors and a Possible Epithelial Potassium Channel

SHIGETADA NAKANISHI, HIROAKI OHKUBO, AKIRA KAKIZUKA,
YOSHIFUMI YOKOTA, RYUICHI SHIGEMOTO, YOSHIKI SASAI, AND
TORU TAKUMI

Institute for Immunology, Kyoto University Faculty of Medicine, Sakyo-ku, Kyoto 606, Japan

I. Introduction

Biologically active peptides of the neuroendocrine system exhibit a high degree of functional diversity not only through the regulation of peptide production, but also through peptide reception. Although mechanisms of peptide production in the neuroendocrine system have been widely explored for the past decade, the molecular basis for peptide reception largely remains to be elucidated. This is due to difficulty in the application of conventional biochemical approaches for investigating the membrane proteins involved in peptide reception and transmembrane signaling.

For the past few years we have been working on the mammalian tachykinin peptide system to study regulation of the expression of the peptide precursor genes and the molecular nature of peptide receptors. To explore the tachykinin receptors, we developed a new approach which combined molecular cloning and electrophysiology. Because ion channels also play an important role in controlling transmembrane signaling, our approach was extended to the characterization of ion channel proteins, and this enabled the identification of a possible novel potassium ion channel protein. This article deals with our recent studies of the molecular nature of multiple forms of tachykinin receptors and a possible epithelial potassium ion channel protein.

II. Mammalian Tachykinin Receptors

A. MAMMALIAN TACHYKININ PEPTIDES AND THEIR PRECURSOR GENES

The mammalian tachykinin system consists of three distinct peptides: substance P, substance K, and neuromedin K (Nakanishi, 1986, 1987) (Fig. 1). Substance P is one of the best-characterized neuropeptides and is believed to act

Substance P	Arg	Pro	Lys	Pro	Gln	Gln	Phe	Phe	Gly	Leu	Met-NH$_2$
Substance K		His	Lys	Thr	Asp	Ser	Phe	Val	Gly	Leu	Met-NH$_2$
Neuromedin K		Asp	Met	His	Asp	Phe	Phe	Val	Gly	Leu	Met-NH$_2$

FIG. 1.   Mammalian tachykinin peptides.

as a peptidergic neuromediator involved in the transmission of pain impulses by primary sensory neurons (Ohtsuka and Konishi, 1975). In addition to substance P, our molecular studies of the tachykinin precursors (Nawa *et al.*, 1983) as well as the peptide studies by Kimura *et al.* (1983) and by Kangawa *et al.* (1983) established that the mammalian tachykinin system comprises two more peptides: substance K and neuromedin K. The three peptides possess a common carboxy-terminal sequence, Phe–X–Gly–Leu–Met–NH$_2$, which accounts for the fundamental properties of the tachykinins. We elucidated the polypeptide sequences, mRNA sequences, and gene organizations of the tachykinin precursors (pre-protachykinins) by molecular cloning and sequence analyses of their cDNAs and genomic DNAs (Nawa *et al.*, 1983, 1984a; Kotani *et al.*, 1986; Kawaguchi *et al.*, 1986).

Figure 2 shows the structures and expressions of the preprotachykinin genes. The three mammalian tachykinins are derived from the two peptide precursor genes, designated the preprotachykinin A and B (PPT-A and PPT-B) genes. The PPT-A gene encodes the precursors common to substance P and substance K, while the PPT-B gene specifies the precursor for neuromedin K. These two genes possess a similar structural organization in terms of exon–intron arrangements, suggesting that they evolved from a common ancestor gene by duplication events

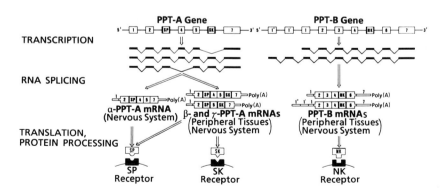

FIG. 2.   Expression of preprotachykinin A and B genes. Numbered boxes and boxes labeled as SP, SK, and NK represent corresponding exons and exons encoding substance P (SP; exon 3), substance K (SK; exon 6), and neuromedin K (NK; exon 5), respectively.

(Kotani *et al.*, 1986). The expressions of the two preprotachykinin genes differ in tissues and in regions of the nervous system. The PPT-A mRNAs are mainly expressed in the trigeminal ganglion and the striatum (Nawa *et al.*, 1984a), while the PPT-B mRNAs are synthesized in the hypothalamus and the intestines (Kotani *et al.*, 1986).

In both genes alternative RNA processing plays an important role in the regulation of tachykinin production. Substance K is specified by a discrete genomic segment, and alternative RNA splicing is involved in inclusion and exclusion of the substance K-coding region and results in the generation of multiple forms of the PPT-A mRNA (Nawa *et al.*, 1984a). This alternative splicing is regulated in a tissue-specific manner. The mRNA encoding substance P alone is mainly produced in the central nervous system, while the mRNAs encoding both substance P and substance K are generated in peripheral tissues as well as the nervous system (Nawa *et al.*, 1984a). Expression of the PPT-B gene also involves alternative RNA splicing combined with differential usage of different promoters and results in the generation of two forms of the mRNA (Kotani *et al.*, 1986). The mammalian tachykinin system thus exhibits its diversity at the level of peptide production by using a variety of cellular mechanisms characteristic of eukaryotic cells, including gene duplication, differential expression of the duplicated genes, and alternative RNA processing.

B. PHARMACOLOGY OF TACHYKININS

Since a new tachykinin sequence, substance K, was found to be contained in PPT-A, we chemically synthesized substance K and examined its biological potencies in parallel with those of substance P and an amphibian tachykinin, kassinin, in various pharmacological tests (Nawa *et al.*, 1984b). The results of this examination are presented in Fig. 3. The three tachykinins show a common spectrum of biological activities, but substance K is tens to hundreds of times more potent than substance P in some pharmacological tests, whereas substance P is as active as or more active than substance K in the others. The differing patterns of the biological activities of the two mammalian tachykinins strongly suggested the presence of multiple tachykinin receptors in mammalian tissues.

A large number of pharmacological experiments of three mammalian tachykinins as well as ligand-binding studies of these peptides were also conducted by different laboratories (Quirion, 1985; Buck and Burcher, 1986; Regoli *et al.*, 1988), and these studies led to the concept that there are at least three distinct tachykinin receptors in mammalian tissues, each specific for the respective tachykinin peptide. Furthermore, Matsuto *et al.* (1984) reported that both substance K and neuromedin K, like substance P, display a potent activity in the depolarization of the spinal motoneurons, suggesting that the three tachykinins function as neurotransmitters/neuromediators in the nervous system. Thus, the

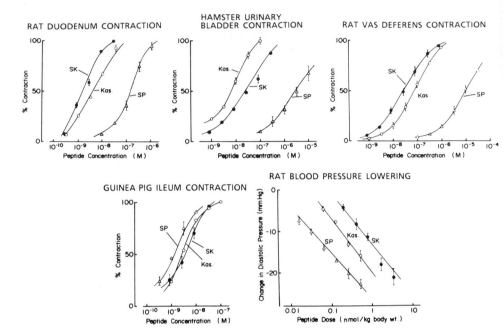

FIG. 3.   Dose–response curves of substance K (SK), substance P (SP), and kassinin (Kas.) in various pharmacological tests. (Data from Nawa *et al.*, 1984b.)

mammalian tachykinins should play different physiological roles in peripheral tissues as well as in the nervous system.

C.   ELECTROPHYSIOLOGY OF TACHYKININ RECEPTORS

Although substantial evidence indicating the presence of multiple tachykinin receptors has been accumulated, the molecular nature of the multiple tachykinin receptors remains to be clarified. This is because the tachykinin receptors, like other peptide receptors, are tightly embedded in the plasma membrane and are present only in small amounts as cellular components; thus, the characterization of the receptors at the biochemical and molecular levels was prevented. We therefore investigated tachykinin receptors by adopting a different approach, originally developed by Barnard *et al.* (1982). Figure 4 shows the principle of the method we used. When a *Xenopus* oocyte is injected with an appropriate exogenous mRNA, it is capable of producing a functional foreign receptor in the plasma membrane, and the expressed receptor can often be coupled to oocyte ion channels through the secondary messenger system. Therefore, the expression of the receptor can be measured electrophysiologically by application of a specific

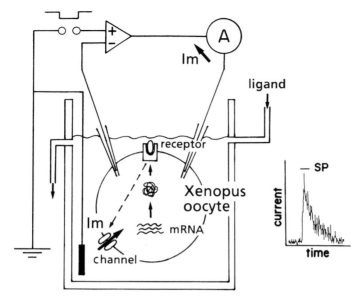

FIG. 4. Method for identification of a receptor mRNA in an oocyte through electrophysiological measurement. SP, Substance P; Im, current through cell membrane; A, current monitor.

receptor ligand. We adopted this system to characterize the mammalian tachykinin receptors.

Figure 5 shows electrophysiological responses to the application of different tachykinins in oocytes injected with brain and stomach mRNAs. The oocyte injected with brain mRNA showed a clear electrophysiological response to the application of substance P, while the oocyte injected with stomach mRNA produced a potent response to substance K (Harada *et al.*, 1987). When various tachykinins, including nonmammalian peptides, were tested for their potencies to induce electrophysiological responses of these receptors, the rank order of potencies for the substance P receptor was physalaemin > substance P > substance K > eledoisin ≥ kassinin > neuromedin K, while the order for the substance K receptor was substance K > kassinin > eledoisin > physalaemin > substance P.

Thus, there are at least two distinct types of mRNAs encoding the substance P and substance K receptors, and these two mRNAs are synthesized differentially between the brain and the peripheral tissue. It is noteworthy here that these two receptors were distinguished from each other in their desensitization (or tachyphylactic) behaviors. The substance P receptor was strongly desensitized by application of an agonist, while no such desensitization was observed for the substance K receptor. The different desensitization behaviors of the three tachykinin receptors are discussed in detail in section E.

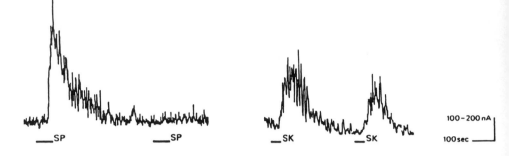

Brain mRNA   **Stomach mRNA**

FIG. 5. Responses of oocytes injected with brain and stomach mRNAs to different tachykinins. Upward deflections correspond to outward currents recorded at a holding potential of 0 mV. SP, Substance P; SK, substance K. (Data from Harada *et al.*, 1987.)

D. MOLECULAR CLONING OF TACHYKININ RECEPTORS

The experiment described above indicated that the oocyte expression system, in combination with electrophysiological measurements, serves as a useful tool for identifying the tachykinin receptor mRNAs. We therefore extended this observation and developed a new cloning strategy to isolate a cDNA clone for the bovine substance K receptor (Masu *et al.*, 1987). Figure 6 shows the principle of this strategy. We synthesized a cDNA mixture from an mRNA fraction, giving a potent substance K receptor expression in *Xenopus* oocytes after sucrose density gradient centrifugation of bovine stomach poly(A)$^+$ RNA. The double-stranded cDNAs were then synthesized and inserted immediately downstream of the SP6 promoter in the vector DNA. A stomach cDNA library was constructed, and a clonal cDNA mixture was extracted and subjected to *in vitro* transcription by specific SP6 RNA polymerase in the presence of the capping nucleotide. The mRNA mixture thus synthesized was injected into oocytes, which were tested for the expression of the receptor by measuring the electrophysiological response to application of substance K.

Since a clear electrophysiological response was observed, we purified a receptor cDNA clone by repeating the *in vitro* mRNA synthesis and electrophysiological measurements after stepwise fractionation of the response-evoking cDNA mixture. We began by examining the substance K receptor expression of the cDNA mixture comprising ~3×10^5 cDNA clones and obtained a single cDNA clone that encodes the substance K receptor.

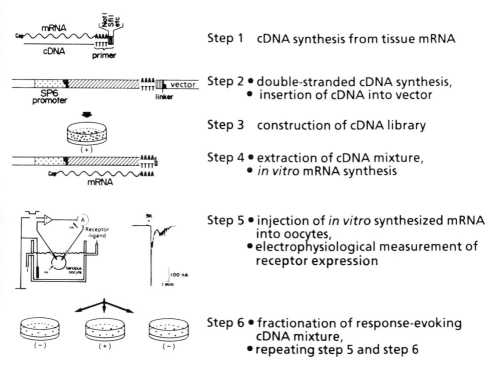

Step 1   cDNA synthesis from tissue mRNA

Step 2 • double-stranded cDNA synthesis,
       • insertion of cDNA into vector

Step 3   construction of cDNA library

Step 4 • extraction of cDNA mixture,
       • *in vitro* mRNA synthesis

Step 5 • injection of *in vitro* synthesized mRNA
         into oocytes,
       • electrophysiological measurement of
         receptor expression

Step 6 • fractionation of response-evoking
         cDNA mixture,
       • repeating step 5 and step 6

FIG. 6.   Strategy for isolating a receptor cDNA clone. Not1, Sfi1, etc., restriction sites; SK, substance K. (Data from Masu *et al.*, 1987.)

The sequence analysis of the cloned cDNA indicated that the bovine substance K receptor is a polypeptide consisting of 384 amino acid residues. The hydropathicity profile and the sequence homology analyses revealed that the substance K receptor has seven hydrophobic segments and shares significant sequence similarity with G protein-coupled receptors, including adrenergic and muscarinic receptors (Masu *et al.*, 1987). By using the same functional assay in *Xenopus* oocytes combined with cross-hybridization to the cloned substance K receptor cDNA or simply by using cross-hybridization to the same cDNA, we subsequently obtained functional cDNA clones for the substance P receptor and for the neuromedin K receptor from rat brain cDNA libraries (Yokota *et al.*, 1989; Shigemoto *et al.*, 1990). In addition, we also isolated a functional cDNA clone for the rat substance K receptor from a rat stomach cDNA library (Sasai and Nakanishi, 1989). The sequence analyses of these cloned cDNAs indicated that the rat substance P, substance K, and neuromedin K receptors consist of 407, 390, and 452 amino acid residues, respectively.

E.   CHARACTERIZATION OF TACHYKININ RECEPTORS

Because we succeeded in isolating a single functional cDNA clone for each of the three tachykinin receptors of the same species, we decided to characterize some properties of these receptors. We examined ionic mechanisms underlying activation of the tachykinin receptors expressed in oocytes (Harada *et al.*, 1987). When a tachykinin receptor was expressed in an oocyte, the reversal potential of the response to tachykinin was about -27 mV, which is close to the chloride equilibrium potential in the oocyte (Kusano *et al.*, 1982). Furthermore, when the concentration of external chloride was reduced, the shifted reversal potential agreed well with the value predicted by the Nernst equation for Cl^-. We thus conclude that Cl^- are the major ions involved in activation of the tachykinin receptor. Based on these experiments as well as others, Fig. 7 shows a scheme of the signal transduction coupled with the tachykinin receptors. The tachykinin receptor expressed in an oocyte acts through a G protein to cause production of inositol 1,4,5-triphosphate, which in turn elevates cytoplasmic Ca^{2+}. This Ca^{2+} then activates a Ca^{2+}-dependent chloride channel in the oocyte plasma membrane.

We examined the ligand specificity of each tachykinin receptor by characterizing not only electrophysiological responses of the receptors expressed in oocytes but also ligand-binding properties of the receptors expressed in mammalian cells.

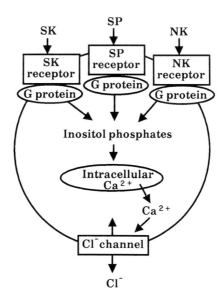

FIG. 7.   Scheme of the signal transduction coupled to tachykinin receptors expressed in an oocyte. SK, Substance K; SP, substance P; NK, neuromedin K.

For the ligand-binding study the receptor cDNA was inserted into a eukaryotic expression vector, which was then introduced into COS cells (Yokota *et al.*, 1989; Shigemoto *et al.*, 1990). We then determined displacement of radiolabeled tachykinin binding to either receptor cDNA-transfected cells or membranes prepared from these cells by the three tachykinins. Figure 8 shows an example of the ligand-binding experiments by indicating competition analysis of radiolabeled eledoisin binding to the neuromedin K receptor expressed in COS cells by the three tachykinins (Shigemoto *et al.*, 1990). The result indicated that binding of eledoisin to this receptor was most effectively inhibited by neuromedin K and less effectively displaced by substance K and substance P. The ligand-binding and electrophysiological characterization of the three receptors explicitly demonstrated that the three receptors differ in rank orders of affinities to the three tachykinins. For substance P receptor the rank order of affinities is substance P, substance K, and neuromedin K; for substance K receptor, substance K, neuromedin K, and substance P; for neuromedin K receptor, neuromedin K, substance K, and substance P.

Figure 9 shows electrophysiological responses of the neuromedin K receptor expressed in an oocyte after repeated applications of neuromedin K (Shigemoto *et al.*, 1990). A potent response was observed by the first application of neuromedin K. This response was reduced by a following application of the same peptide after a short washing and was recovered by a longer washing. Similar characterization of the other two tachykinin receptors shows that the

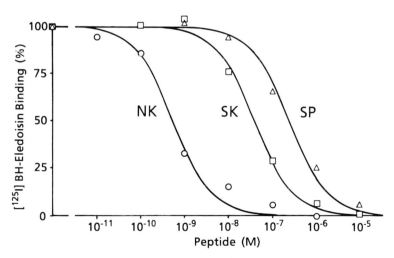

FIG. 8.   Displacement of ^{125}I-labeled Bolton–Hunter (BH) eledoisin binding to membranes of neuromedin K (NK) receptor cDNA-transfected cells by three tachykinins. SK, Substance K; SP, substance P. (Data from Shigemoto *et al.*, 1990.)

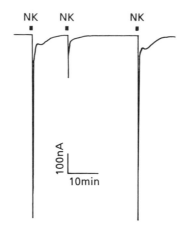

FIG. 9.   Desensitization effect of an agonist on the neuromedin K (NK) receptor expressed in an oocyte. Responses to repeated application of NK (10^{-7} M) were recorded under voltage clamp at -60 mV in an oocyte injected with the *in vitro* synthesized mRNA for NK receptor. (Data from Shigemoto *et al.*, 1990.)

desensitization behavior differs among the three receptors: The desensitization effect is manifested in the order of substance P, neuromedin K, and substance K receptors. The mechanisms of different densensitization behaviors of the three tachykinin receptors remain to be clarified. However, because the ionic mechanisms underlying the activation of the three receptors are associated primarily with an activation of a common secondary message, it is likely that the desensitization occurs at the receptor level, rather than via subsequent intracellular effectors.

F.   PRIMARY STRUCTURES OF TACHYKININ RECEPTORS

Figures 10 and 11 show the alignment of the amino acid sequences of the three rat tachykinin receptors and a schematic representation of the amino acids conserved in these three receptors (Yokota *et al.*, 1989; Shigemoto *et al.*, 1990; Sasai and Nakanishi, 1989). The three receptors have seven hydrophobic, presumably membrane-spanning, domains. The amino acid sequences are strikingly similar among the three tachykinin receptors, and the similarity is particularly remarkable in the putative transmembrane domains and their extending cytoplasmic portions close to the transmembrane helices. This similarity is in contrast to the sequence divergence in the amino- and carboxy-terminal regions. However, similar to other G protein-coupled receptors (O'Dowd *et al.*, 1989a), all three receptors possess potential N-glycosylation sites at their amino termini and many serine and threonine residues as possible phosphorylation sites at their

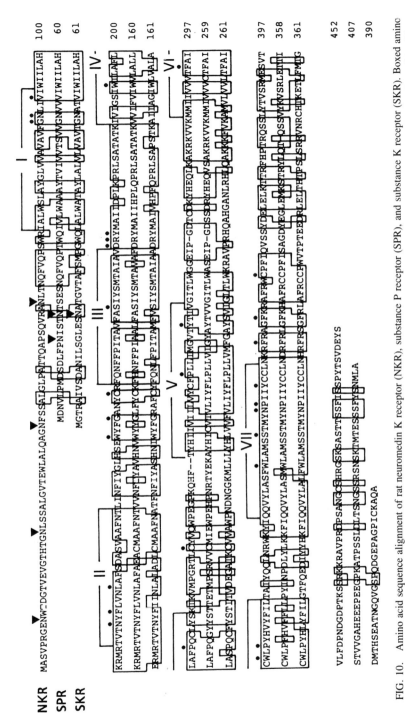

FIG. 10. Amino acid sequence alignment of rat neuromedin K receptor (NKR), substance P receptor (SPR), and substance K receptor (SKR). Boxed amino acids represent identical residues in two or all of the three sequences; dashes represent deletions of amino acid residues; solid circles indicate amino acid residues conserved in the sequences of the tachykinin, adrenergic, and muscarinic receptors; solid triangles indicate potential N-glycosylation sites. (Data from Shigemoto et al., 1990.)

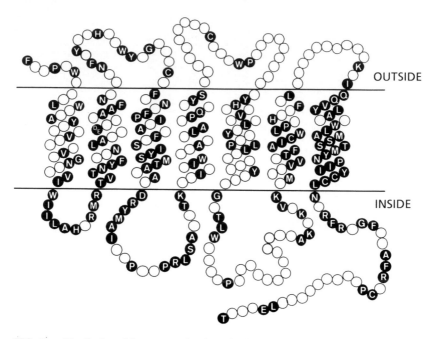

FIG. 11.   Distribution of the conserved amino acids in the core segments covering seven putative transmembrane regions of the three tachykinin receptors. Black circles indicate identical amino acids in the three tachykinin receptors. (Data taken from Shigemoto *et al.*, 1990.)

carboxy termini. Thus, all three tachykinin receptors belong to the family of G protein-coupled receptors.

The core sequences covering the seven putative transmembrane regions (Fig. 11) are identical at 157 positions of the three tachykinin receptors, and the percentages of homology in these core segments are 66.3% between substance P and neuromedin K receptors, 54.9% between substance K and neuromedin K receptors, and 53.7% between substance P and substance K receptors. Among these identical amino acids, certain amino acids, such as cysteine, proline, and glycine, are conserved in the sequences of all of the members of the adrenergic and muscarinic receptors (O'Dowd *et al.*, 1989a; Bonner *et al.*, 1987). Among the three cysteine residues, which are conserved throughout all three families of receptors, it has been suggested by β_2-adrenergic receptor analysis (Dixon *et al.*, 1987) that a disulfide bond is formed by two of the conserved cysteine residues, which are situated in the first and second extracellular loops. The third cysteine residue, which immediately follows transmembrane segment VII, is evidenced to be palmitoylated, and this results in the anchoring of the receptor to the plasma membrane (O'Dowd *et al.*, 1989b).

It has also been suggested that the proline and glycine residues in the membrane-spanning domains induce bends in the transmembrane helix, thus facilitating the interlock of adjacent helices (O'Dowd *et al.*, 1989a). The three amino acids with aromatic side chains are conserved in the three families of receptors, and these amino acids can be characterized as possessing the property to interact with their adjacent aromatic or charged amino acids. Thus, these conserved amino acids should play a crucial role in the formation of a fundamental structure of the G protein-coupled receptors.

In addition to these structural characteristics, several interesting sequence conservations and divergences are also notable in the three tachykinin receptors (Yokota *et al.*, 1989; Shigemoto *et al.*, 1990). (1) Within the seven putative transmembrane domains transmembrane segments II of both substance K and neuromedin K receptors contain an aspartic acid, as observed for other G protein-coupled receptors (O'Dowd *et al.*, 1989a). In contrast, this aspartic acid is replaced with a glutamic acid in the substance P receptor (Yokota *et al.*, 1989). (2) All three receptors contain one histidine residue each in transmembrane segments V and VI, and the presence of these two histidine residues is characteristic of the tachykinin receptors and thus could be important in the interaction with the tachykinin peptides. (3) The substance P and neuromedin K receptors are highly conserved not only throughout the third cytoplasmic loops, but also in portions of the carboxy-terminal regions. In contrast, most of these regions diverge between the substance K receptor and each of the other two receptors. As discussed above, all three tachykinin receptors are thought to be coupled to a phosphatidylinositol–calcium secondary message system. Therefore, as reported for β-adrenergic and muscarinic receptors (Strader *et al.*, 1987; Kubo *et al.*, 1988), the short homologous sequences near transmembrane segments V and VI could be important in the coupling of the receptors to a G protein. (4) The number of serine and threonine residues in the third cytoplasmic loops and the carboxy-terminal cytoplasmic regions differs among the three tachykinin receptors. Substance P, neuromedin K, and substance K receptors possess five, two, and one residue of these amino acids in their third cytoplasmic loops, respectively, and 26, 28, and 14 residues in their carboxy-terminal regions, respectively. The three tachykinin receptors show differing desensitization behaviors in response to the repeated application of agonists. Thus, it is possible that the sequence divergence and/or the different distribution of threonine and serine residues in the third cytoplasmic loops and the carboxy-terminal regions could participate in evoking differing desensitization behaviors of the three tachykinin receptors, probably as a result of different phosphorylations.

In summary, the three tachykinin receptors possess seven putative transmembrane domains with extracellular amino termini and cytoplasmic carboxy-termini and belong to the family of G protein-coupled receptors. The results described here thus demonstrate that the structures and functions of these peptide receptors are fundamentally similar to those of the receptors for classical small-molecule neurotransmitters such as catecholamines and acetylcholine. The three receptors differ in affinities to the tachykinin peptides and in desensitization behaviors, but are coupled to the same secondary message system. These similar but distinct properties of the three receptors should result from the sequence similarities and divergences which are distinctly segmented from one another. Our results thus provide the first comprehensive analysis of the molecular nature of the multiple peptide receptors, which exhibit similar but clearly distinguishable biological activities. Therefore, the tachykinin receptors provide an intriguing system to characterize the structure–function relationships of the diversified multiple peptide receptors.

Furthermore, autoradiographic localization of radiolabeled tachykinins showed different patterns of distribution of the three tachykinin-binding sites, suggesting different tissue and regional distribution of these receptors (Mantyh *et al.*, 1989). In addition, the expressions of the genes for the three tachykinin receptors could be regulated differently in response to external stimuli or during development. Further investigations by using the cDNA clones of the three receptors are likely to prove fruitful in understanding the mechanisms of the functional diversity of the same group of peptides at the level of peptide receptors.

III. Possible Epithelial Potassium Channel

A. DIVERSITY OF ION CHANNELS

Ion channels are essential not only for evoking electrical polarization of excitable cells, but also for optimal operation of many cellular functions in both excitable and nonexcitable cells (Hille, 1984; Jan and Jan, 1989). Figure 12 shows the schematic structures of Na^+, K^+, and Ca^{2+} channels which have been characterized at the molecular level (Noda *et al.*, 1984; Tanabe *et al.*, 1987; Tempel *et al.*, 1987). These proteins show significant similarities in their amino acid sequences and contain one or four structurally common motifs, each of which has the same pattern of six putative membrane-spanning domains. Among these membrane-spanning domains, one domain, called S4, bears positively charged amino acids every three residues, and this domain is thought to contribute the channel voltage sensor. These ion channels with different ion selectivities thus fall into a genetically related family and seem to have evolved from a common ancestor gene into their present forms (Stevens, 1987). However, ion channels are also known to exhibit a high degree of diversity, varying in electrophysiological and pharmacological properties (Hille, 1984; Kaczmarek and Levitan, 1987).

Furthermore, the above ion channels are involved in the excitability of nerve

● K^+ Channel

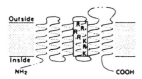

● Na^+ and Ca^{2+} Channels

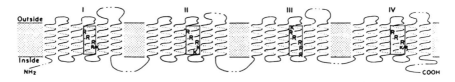

FIG. 12. Structural characteristics common to K^+, Na^+, and Ca^{2+} channels. The fourth putative transmembrane segments (S4) are enclosed, and the arginine and/or lysine residues in these segments are shown in one-letter code (i.e., R and K, respectively). (Data modified from Tanabe *et al.*, 1987, and Tempel *et al.*, 1987.)

and muscle cells, and whether or not the same family of ion channels is responsible for ion permeations in nonexcitable cells seems open to question. It is therefore important to investigate the molecular nature of ion channels with distinct properties and their associated modulatory proteins.

B. CLONING AND CHARACTERIZATION OF A NOVEL MEMBRANE PROTEIN (I_{SK} PROTEIN) EXHIBITING A POTASSIUM CHANNEL ACTIVITY

The kidney is an intriguing tissue to characterize ion channel proteins, because it is involved in controlling various types of ion permeations to maintain the electrolyte balance (Schultz, 1986). We therefore began investigations by characterizing ionic currents expressed in oocytes after injection of rat kidney mRNAs (Takumi *et al.*, 1988). Figure 13 shows voltage-clamp records obtained from an oocyte after injection of rat kidney mRNAs (Takumi *et al.*, 1988). In this oocyte depolarization induced a slowly activating outward current, and this current was always much greater than that of control oocytes injected with distilled water. The kidney mRNA was size-fractionated by sucrose density gradient centrifugation, and the activity of the mRNA was found in a fraction with an average mRNA size of ~800 nucleotides (Takumi *et al.*, 1988), which was considerably

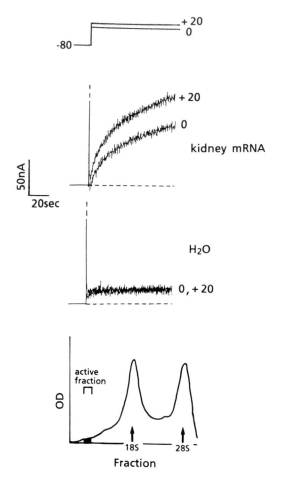

FIG. 13. Voltage-clamp records of oocytes injected with kidney mRNAs (top) and distilled water (middle), and the location of the mRNA inducing a K$^+$ channel activity by centrifugation on sucrose density gradient (bottom). In a bath solution containing 2 mM K$^+$, oocytes were held at -80 mV and depolarized stepwise to test potentials. OD, Optical density. (Data from Takumi *et al.*, 1988.)

smaller than those of other ion channel mRNAs so far reported (Noda *et al.*, 1984; Tanabe *et al.*, 1987; Tempel *et al.*, 1987). We therefore attempted isolation of a functional cDNA clone responsible for induction of the outward current, essentially according to the procedures described above, and then obtained such a functional cDNA clone (Takumi *et al.*, 1988).

The currents induced by the mRNA synthesized *in vitro* from the cloned cDNA were characterized in the oocyte expression system (Takumi *et al.*, 1988). As shown in Fig. 14, depolarization from a holding potential of -80 mV elicited large voltage- and time-dependent outward currents. On repolarization to -80 mV, slow outward tail currents were observed. When a clamp voltage to positive potentials was held longer, the outward current lasted for at least 20 minutes, suggesting that the channel responsible for the outward current does not undergo inactivation.

A series of electrophysiological and pharmacological experiments was performed to examine ionic mechanisms underlying the outward currents (Takumi *et al.*, 1988), and the properties of the outward currents are as follows: (1) In the medium containing 2 mM K^+, reversal of the tail currents occurred at ~ -100 mV, similar to the K^+ equilibrium potential in *Xenopus* oocytes (Lotan *et al.*, 1982). (2) In the external medium containing 20 mM K^+, the tail currents were reversed at -42 mV, in good agreement with the shift predicted by the Nernst equation for K^+. (3) The outward current was reduced by K^+ channel blockers, tetraethylammonium, and Ba^{2+}. (4) Reversal potential was insensitive to changes in external Cl^-, Na^+, or Ca^{2+} concentration. We thus conclude that the slowly activating outward current is carried selectively by K^+.

C. PRIMARY STRUCTURE OF I_{SK} PROTEIN

Figure 15 shows the amino acid sequence deduced for the rat protein from the cloned cDNA (Takumi *et al.*, 1988). We named this the I_{SK} protein. The rat I_{SK} protein is a polypeptide consisting of 130 amino acids with a clear hydrophobic

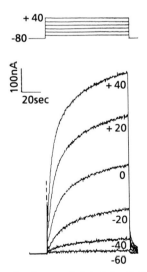

FIG. 14.   Voltage-clamp records of an oocyte injected with the mRNA synthesized *in vitro* from the cloned cDNA. The oocyte was held at -80 mV, depolarized stepwise to test potentials for 90 seconds, and repolarized to -80 mV. (Data from Takumi *et al.*, 1988.)

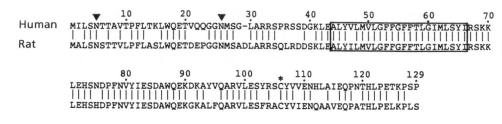

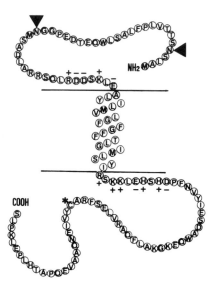

FIG. 15.   Amino acid sequences of rat and human I_{SK} proteins and a transmembrane model of rat I_{SK} protein. Bars represent amino acids identical between the two sequences; the dash represents a deletion of the amino acid in the human sequence; solid triangles indicate potential N-glycosylation sites. (Data from Takumi *et al.*, 1988, and Murai *et al.*, 1989.)

segment of 23 continuous uncharged amino acids, as illustrated in Fig. 15. Consistent with this finding, the translation product of the mRNA was located in the membrane fraction of oocytes (Takumi *et al.*, 1988). Our preliminary study indicated that the I_{SK} protein is probably glycosylated at two potential sites of the amino terminus. It is therefore likely that the amino terminus of the I_{SK} protein is located on the extracellular side, while its carboxy terminus is on the cytoplasmic side.

This protein, however, did not show any sequence similarities to known protein sequences, including the ion channel proteins. Thus, despite the fact that the I_{SK} protein is capable of inducing selective permeation of K^+ by membrane polarization, it represents a novel membrane protein that differs from the conventional ion channel proteins.

Figure 15 also shows the amino acid sequence of the human I_{SK} protein which was deduced from the nucleotide sequence of the cloned genomic DNA (Murai *et al.*, 1989). The human I_{SK} protein, like the rat counterpart, contains a distinct hydrophobic segment in its middle portion. Interestingly, not only this putative transmembrane domain but also its following sequence is extremely homologous between the two sequences: 48 of the 50 amino acids in these regions are identical between the two sequences. Because the human I_{SK} protein also induces a K^+ channel activity indistinguishable from that of the rat I_{SK} protein in the oocyte system (Murai *et al.*, 1989), the region conserved between the two sequences should play a crucial role in eliciting a K^+ channel activity of the I_{SK} protein.

D. STRUCTURAL IMPLICATION OF I_{SK} PROTEIN

The structural feature of the I_{SK} protein differs from those of the conventional ion channels and suggests some similarities to simple channel-forming peptide ionophores. Figure 16 shows representative examples of the peptide ionophores alamethicin (Pressman, 1976; Fox and Richards, 1982) and a synthetic amphiphilic peptide exhibiting a channel activity (Lear *et al.*, 1988). Although these peptides are small, they are inserted into the membrane in the form of an

A   B

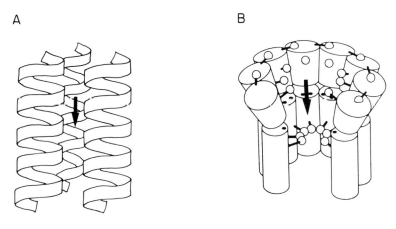

H_2N-(Leu-Ser-Ser-Leu-Leu-Ser-Leu)$_3$-CONH$_2$

1   10
Ac-Aib-Pro-Aib-Ala-Aib-Ala-Gln-Aib-Val-Aib-
11   20
Gly-Leu-Aib-Pro-Val-Aib-Aib-Glu-Gln-Phl

(Aib; α-aminoisobutyric acid)

FIG. 16. Schematic structures of channel-forming ionophores of (A) a synthetic peptide and (B) alamethicin. (Alamethicin structure from Fox and Richards, 1982.)

oligomeric structure and are able to make a pore which allows selectively monovalent cations to flow down along their electrochemical gradient. Furthermore, the channel formed by alamethicin is voltage dependent (Pressman, 1976). Therefore, analogous to these peptide ionophores, the simplest and most likely explanation for the function of the I_{SK} protein is that the I_{SK} protein per se functions as a discrete K^+-conducting ion channel, although it remains possible that this protein subserves as a modulatory protein.

If the I_{SK} protein indeed represents a new K^+ channel protein, the small simple structure of this protein provides an attractive system for investigating the molecular mechanism underlying the voltage-dependent K^+ channel activity. To address this question, we are currently investigating structure–function relationships of the I_{SK} protein by examining the effects of mutational changes of the I_{SK} protein on its channel activity. Individual amino acids surrounding the transmembrane domain were replaced with their structurally related amino acids by site-directed mutagenesis. The voltage-dependent channel activity of each of the resultant mutant proteins was then examined electrophysiologically in the oocyte expression system.

Consistent with the amino acid conservation in the transmembrane-following sequence, the result indicated that there is a marked difference in the effects of amino acid substitutions on the channel activity between the membrane-preceding and membrane-following regions (Takumi et al., in preparation). The substitutions of a single amino acid in many positions of the membrane-following region produced profound effects on the channel activity, whereas the same manipulation in the membrane-preceding region showed essentially no effect on the channel activity. Because K^+ permeate the membrane from the cytoplasmic side to the extracellular side, the finding of the crucial role of some amino acids in the membrane-following, presumably cytoplasmic, domain further supports the view that the I_{SK} protein functions as a K^+ channel protein.

E. CELLULAR LOCALIZATION OF I_{SK} PROTEIN

Blot hybridization analysis with the I_{SK} protein cDNA probe indicated that poly(A)$^+$ RNAs from the kidney, duodenum, stomach, pancreas, and submandibular gland gave rise to a common band with an estimated mRNA size of ~800 nucleotides (Takumi et al., 1988; Sugimoto et al., 1990). No appreciable amount of the mRNA was detected in the brain or the liver. The mRNA appears to be distributed in tissues where epithelial cells are actively involved in conducting K^+ permeations.

To determine the more precise localization of the I_{SK} protein, we prepared three types of antibody which specifically react with distinct parts of the rat I_{SK} protein. By using these three antibodies, we investigated the immunohistochemical localization of the I_{SK} protein in various tissues. Figure 17 represents immu-

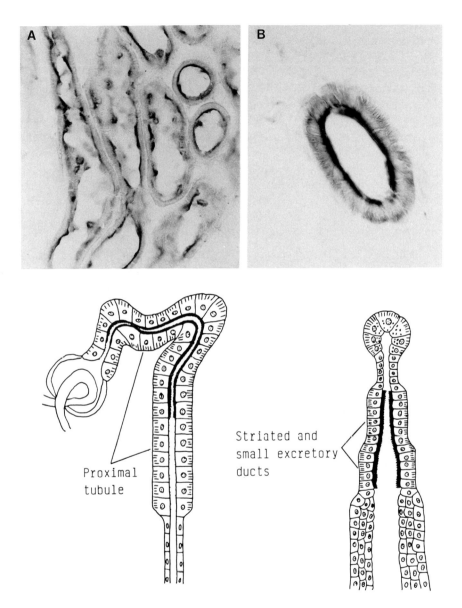

FIG. 17.   Immunostaining of sections of the (A) rat kidney and (B) submandibular gland. The darkened regions in the lower drawings represent positively immunostained apical membrane portions of the epithelial cells in the kidney proximal tubule and in the striated and small excretory ducts of the submandibular gland.

nostained sections of the kidney and the submandibular gland. The detailed immunohistochemical analyses indicated that the I_{SK} protein is localized in epithelial cells of the proximal convoluted and early proximal straight tubules of the kidney and in those of the striated and small excretory ducts of the submandibular gland (Sugimoto et al., 1990). Furthermore, the immunostained material is confined to the apical membrane portion of the epithelial cells (Sugimoto et al., 1990).

The epithelial cells in the renal proximal tubule and in the submandibular duct are known to show a similar morphology and to share many functional properties (Junqueira et al., 1986). Both of these epithelial cells actively resorb Na^+ and amino acids from tubular fluid following ultrafiltration of these compositions from glomerular cells or acinar cells (Giebisch and Aronson, 1986; Young and van Lennep, 1979). Both also actively secrete urea into the lumen. In the submandibular duct K^+ permeate from epithelial cells to the lumen, and K^+ concentrations increase along the duct (Young and van Lennep, 1979). Similarly, K^+ secretion into the lumen was found in proximal tubules (Giebisch and Aronson, 1986).

F.   MODEL OF I_{SK} PROTEIN FUNCTION

All of the above transports in the epithelial cells are thought to result from the asymmetrical distribution of the transport systems and to depend energetically on the electrochemical Na^+ gradient which is driven by the Na^+,K^+-ATPase pump located in the basolateral membrane of epithelial cells (Schultz, 1986). Therefore, taking into account the distinct cellular localization of the I_{SK} protein, together with the direction of the Na^+ transport across the epithelium, a model of the I_{SK} protein function is illustrated in Fig. 18 (Sugimoto et al., 1990). The

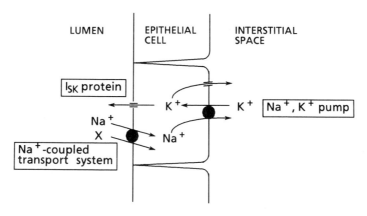

FIG. 18.   Model of the function of the I_{SK} protein. (Data from Sugimoto et al., 1990.)

Na^+,K^+-ATPase pump generates a lower intracellular Na^+ concentration. The resultant Na^+ gradient across the apical membrane causes the entry of Na^+ into the cell from the lumen through the Na^+/sugar or amino acid cotransport system (Schultz, 1986). This flow of Na^+ induces depolarization of 10–15 mV over the stable apical membrane potential on the order of -70 mV (Frömter, 1984). Under the magnitude of this depolarization, the I_{SK} protein is capable of inducing a slowly activating K^+ current (Takumi *et al.*, 1988).

Therefore, the depolarizing effect on the apical membrane can stimulate the K^+ channel activity of the I_{SK} protein and thus results in permeations of K^+ from the epithelial cells to the lumen. This model of the function of the I_{SK} protein can now be tested by comparing the properties of the possible K^+ channel in the epithelial apical membrane with those of the I_{SK} protein, which have been well characterized in the oocyte expression system.

The function of K^+ permeation in nonexcitable epithelial cells could be different from that of excitable cells such as nerve and skeletal muscle cells. In the excitable cells a rapid activation/deactivation of the K^+ channel activity must occur in response to membrane potential changes to control cell excitability and synaptic transmission. In contrast, in epithelial cells the rapid response of the K^+ channel activity is not necessarily needed to control the intracellular K^+ concentrations. Thus, it is tempting to hypothesize that the I_{SK} protein, though small and simple, is able to fulfill the function of permeating K^+ in nonexcitable epithelial cells and thus could differ from the ion channel proteins in excitable cells not only in the structural and electrophysiological properties, but also in the evolutionary relationship.

Finally, the oocyte expression system has been shown to be capable of producing a large number of foreign channels and receptors, depending on the sources of mRNA injected (Dascal, 1987). Because the conventional approach through protein purification is not readily available for most of these membrane proteins, the method we developed will be widely applicable as a direct approach to characterize these proteins. Furthermore, the oocyte expression system combined with electrophysiological measurements is extremely sensitive for identifying the mRNA which is capable of inducing electrophysiological responses by either ligand application or membrane polarization. Thus, the extension of the method discussed here might also be useful for revealing further novel receptors and ion channels.

IV. Concluding Remarks

This article summarizes our studies concerning the molecular and genetic aspects of the mammalian tachykinin receptors. The studies indicate that the neuropeptide system is diversified not only at the peptide level, but also at the receptor level, through various cellular mechanisms characteristic of higher eukaryotic cells. This article also includes our studies concerning the molecular characterization of a probable epithelial K$^+$ channel. In addition, a new strategy to characterize receptors and ion channels at the molecular level is discussed. It is hoped that these molecular and genetic studies on the receptors and the ion channel will contribute to the understanding of the detailed mechanisms underlying the regulation of transmembrane signaling.

ACKNOWLEDGMENTS

We thank Dr. Tetsuo Sugimoto for collaboration in the immunohistochemical investigations. Works described here was supported in part by research grants from the Ministry of Education, Science and Culture of Japan; the Institute of Physical and Chemical Research; and the Science and Technology Agency of Japan.

REFERENCES

Barnard, E. A., Miledi, R., and Sumikawa, K. (1982). *Proc. R. Soc. London, B* **215,** 241–246.
Bonner, T. I., Buckley, N. J., Young, A. C., and Brann, M. R. (1987). *Science* **237,** 527–532.
Buck, S. H., and Burcher, E. (1986). *Trends Pharmacol. Sci.* **7,** 65–68.
Dascal, N. (1987). *CRC Crit. Rev. Biochem.* **22,** 317–387.
Dixon, R. A. F., Sigal, I. S., Candelore, M. R., Register, R. B., Scattergood, W., Rands, E., and Strader, C. D. (1987). *EMBO J.* **6,** 3269–3275.
Fox, R. O., Jr., and Richards, F. M. (1982). *Nature (London)* **300,** 325–330.
Frömter, E. (1984). *Am. J. Physiol.* **247,** F695–F705.
Giebisch, G., and Aronson, P. S. (1986). *In* "Membrane Transport Processes in Organized Systems" (T. E. Andreoli, J. F. Hoffman, D. D. Fanestil, and S. G. Schultz, eds.), pp. 285–316. Plenum, New York.
Harada, Y., Takahashi, T., Kuno, M., Nakayama, K., Masu, Y., and Nakanishi, S. (1987). *J. Neurosci.* **7,** 3265–3273.
Hille, B. (1984). "Ionic Channels of Excitable Membranes," pp. 99–116. Sinauer, Sunderland, Massachusetts.
Jan, L. Y., and Jan, Y. N. (1989). *Cell (Cambridge, Mass.)* **56,** 13–25.
Junqueira, L. C., Carneiro, J., and Long, J. A. (1986). "Basic Histology," pp. 359–360. Lange, Los Altos, California.
Kaczmarek, L. K., and Levitan, I. B. (1987). "Neuromodulation: The Biochemical Control of Neuronal Excitability." Oxford Univ. Press, New York.
Kangawa, K., Minamino, N., Fukuda, A., and Matsuo, H. (1983). *Biochem. Biophys. Res. Commun.* **114,** 533–540.
Kawaguchi, Y., Hoshimaru, M., Nawa, H., and Nakanishi, S. (1986). *Biochem. Biophys. Res. Commun.* **139,** 1040–1046.
Kimura, S., Okada, M., Sugita, Y., Kanazawa, I., and Munekata, E. (1983). *Proc. Jpn. Acad.* **59,** 101–104.
Kotani, H., Hoshimaru, M., Nawa, H., and Nakanishi, S. (1986). *Proc. Natl. Acad. Sci. U.S.A.* **83,** 7074–7078.
Kubo, T., Bujo, H., Akiba, I., Nakai, J., Mishina, M., and Numa, S. (1988). *FEBS Lett.* **241,** 119–125.
Kusano, K., Miledi, R., and Stinnakre, J. (1982). *J. Physiol. (London)* **328,** 143–170.
Lear, J. D., Wasserman, Z. R., and DeGrado, W. F. (1988). *Science* **240,** 1177–1181.

Lotan, I., Dascal, N., Cohen, S., and Lass, Y. (1982). *Nature (London)* **298**, 572–574.

Mantyh, P. W., Gates, T., Mantyh, C. R., and Maggio, J. E. (1989). *J. Neurosci.* **9**, 258–279.

Masu, Y., Nakayama, K., Tamaki, H., Harada, Y., Kuno, M., and Nakanishi, S. (1987). *Nature (London)* **329**, 836–838.

Matsuto, T., Yanagisawa, M., Otsuka, M., Kanazawa, I., and Munekata, E. (1984). *Neurosci. Res.* **2**, 105–110.

Murai, T., Kakizuka, A., Takumi, T., Ohkubo, H., and Nakanishi, S. (1989). *Biochem. Biophys. Res. Commun.* **161**, 176–181.

Nakanishi, S. (1986). *Trends NeuroSci. (Pers. Ed.)* **9**, 41–44.

Nakanishi, S. (1987). *Physiol. Rev.* **67**, 1117–1142.

Nawa, H., Hirose, T., Takashima, H., Inayama, S., and Nakanishi, S. (1983). *Nature (London)* **306**, 32–36.

Nawa, H., Kotani, H., and Nakanishi, S. (1984a). *Nature (London)* **312**, 729–734.

Nawa, H., Doteuchi, M., Igano, K., Inouye, K., and Nakanishi, S. (1984b). *Life Sci.* **34**, 1153–1160.

Noda, M., Shimizu, S., Tanabe, T., Takai, T., Kayano, T., Ikeda, T., Takahashi, H., Nakayama, H., Kanaoka, Y., Minamino, N., Kangawa, K., Matsuo, H., Raftery, M. A., Hirose, T., Inayama, S., Hayashida, H., Miyata, T., and Numa, S. (1984). *Nature (London)* **312**, 121–127.

O'Dowd, B. F., Lefkowitz, R. J., and Caron, M. G. (1989a). *Annu. Rev. Neurosci.* **12**, 67–83.

O'Dowd, B. F., Hnatowich, M., Caron, M. G., Lefkowitz, R. J., and Bouvier, M. (1989b). *J. Biol. Chem.* **264**, 7564–7569.

Ohtsuka, M., and Konishi, S. (1975). *Cold Spring Harbor Symp. Quant. Biol.* **40**, 135–143.

Pressman, B. C. (1976). *Annu. Rev. Biochem.* **55**, 501–530.

Quirion, R. (1985). *Trends NeuroSci. (Pers. Ed.)* **8**, 183–185.

Regoli, D., Drapeau, G., Dion, S., and Couture, R. (1988). *Trends Pharmacol. Sci.* **9**, 290–295.

Sasai, Y., and Nakanishi, S. (1989). *Biochem. Biophys. Res. Commun.* **165**, 695–702.

Schultz, S. G. (1986). *In* "Membrane Transport Processes in Organized Systems" (T. E. Andreoli, J. F. Hoffman, D. D. Fanestil, and S. G. Shultz, eds.), pp. 135–150. Plenum, New York.

Shigemoto, R., Yokota, Y., Tsuchida, K., and Nakanishi, S. (1990). *J. Biol. Chem.* **265**, 623–628.

Stevens, C. F. (1987). *Nature (London)* **328**, 198–199.

Strader, C. D., Dixon, R. A. F., Cheung, A. H., Candelore, M. R., Blake, A. D., and Sigal, I. S. (1987). *J. Biol. Chem.* **262**, 16439–16443.

Sugimoto, T., Tanabe, Y., Shigemoto, R., Iwai, M., Takumi, T., Ohkubo, H., and Nakanishi, S. (1990). *J. Membr. Biol.* **113**, 39–47.

Takumi, T., Ohkubo, H., and Nakanishi, S. (1988). *Science* **242**, 1042–1045.

Takumi, T., Ohkubo, H., and Nakanishi, S. (1990). Manuscript in preparation.

Tanabe, T., Takeshima, H., Mikami, A., Flockerzi, V., Takahashi, H., Kangawa, K., Kojima, M., Matsuo, H., Hirose, T., and Numa, S. (1987). *Nature (London)* **328**, 313–318.

Tempel, B. L., Papazian, D. M., Schwarz, T. L., Jan, Y. N., and Jan, L. Y. (1987). *Science* **237**, 770–775.

Yokota, Y., Sasai, Y., Tanaka, K., Fujiwara, T., Tsuchida, K., Shigemoto, R., Kakizuka, A., Ohkubo, H., and Nakanishi, S. (1989). *J. Biol. Chem.* **264**, 17649–17652.

Young, J. A., and van Lennep, E. W. (1979). *Membr. Transp. Biol.* **4B**, 563–692.

DISCUSSION

S. I. Taylor. I noticed that there was a lot of mRNA for the protein in the pancreas. Is the cell type in the pancreas it is found in known?

S. Nakanishi. We have not yet extensively examined immunohistochemical localization of the

I_{SK} protein in the pancreas, but one of the antibodies showed the immunostained material at the epithelial cells of the secretory ducts of the pancreas.

A. R. Means.   The finding of a small potassium channel that only spans the membrane once is similar to what has recently been shown by Larry Jones from the University of Indiana for calcium. A protein of a similar size, called phospholamban, has been demonstrated to serve as a single membrane-spanning calcium transport protein. Maybe this type of topology will be more common than we might have previously anticipated.

S. Nakanishi.   The calcium channel activity of the phospholamban has been shown by reconstituting an oligopeptide corresponding to a single membrane-spanning domain of phospholamban in liposomes.

A. R. Means.   Larry Jones has now been able to utilize bacterially expressed phospholamban to reconstitute into liposomes. The vesicles will transport calcium, and phosphorylation by cAMP-dependent protein kinase affects transport rate.

W. Vale.   What is the mechanism of desensitization to the tachykinins?

S. Nakanishi.   We have not done experiments on the mechanism of desensitization yet, but we expect that, like adrenergic and muscarinic receptors, phosphorylation may be involved in the desensitization. The three tachykinin receptors differ in their effects on desensitization to agonists. Thus, we are interested in what mechanisms and what types of phosphorylation are involved in causing these differences.

J. Kirkland.   How does one determine that it is the single protein itself which is forming the channel, rather than perhaps a collection of the proteins in the oligomeric form?

S. Nakanishi.   We also assume that the I_{SK} protein forms an oligomeric structure, but we do not have the answer yet. We need a more detailed analysis of the biophysical properties of the I_{SK} protein.

A. R. Means.   In the case of Larry Jones' experiments with phospholamban, it is very clearly a pentamer. It is the association of the five subunits that results in ion movement.

Guanylate Cyclase Receptor Family

DAVID L. GARBERS

Departments of Pharmacology and Molecular Physiology and Biophysics, Howard Hughes Medical Institute, Vanderbilt University Medical Center, Nashville, Tennessee 37232

I. Introduction

Many different hormones, neurotransmitters, and drugs were tested for their effects on guanylate cyclase activity following the discovery of the enzyme in 1969 (Hardman and Sutherland, 1969; Schultz *et al.*, 1969; White and Aurbach, 1969). Initially, it was felt that the mechanisms by which the enzyme was regulated might follow a path similar to that of adenylate cyclase, but failures to directly activate guanylate cyclase in broken-cell preparations with agents known to elevate intracellular cGMP concentrations suggested that the enzyme was activated by indirect mechanisms (Goldberg and Haddox, 1977).

Research in 1974 and 1975 demonstrated that guanylate cyclase activity found in the soluble fractions of cell lysates was represented by a different protein than that found in the particulate fractions (Kimura and Murad, 1974; Garbers *et al.*, 1974; Chrisman *et al.*, 1975), and soon after these studies it became clear that nitric oxide, nitrosamines, and similar agents could activate the soluble form of guanylate cyclase (Mittal and Murad, 1977). Later work by Gerzer *et al.* (1981), showing that the soluble form of the enzyme contained heme, led to models in which the enzyme-bound heme was suggested to be a receptor for endothelial cell-derived relaxing factor (Ignarro, 1989). The plasma membrane form of guanylate cyclase found on sea urchin spermatozoa was not activated by these agents, however, suggesting that regulatory mechanisms would be different for this form of the enzyme (Garbers and Kopf, 1980).

In the late 1970s *Escherichia coli* heat-stable enterotoxin was shown to activate a particulate form of guanylate cyclase (Field *et al.*, 1978); these were the first studies to definitively demonstrate activation of a particulate enzyme in broken-cell preparations. However, the form activated appeared to be a detergent-insoluble, not a plasma membrane, form of the enzyme.

Research from two different areas resulted in the eventual identification of natural regulators of a plasma membrane form of guanylate cyclase. The first involved research undertaken to study mechanisms by which eggs communicate with spermatozoa. In 1979 Kopf *et al.* reported that a low-molecular-weight factor in the egg conditioned media of sea urchins could markedly elevate cGMP concentrations of sea urchin spermatozoa. Subsequently, the low-molecular-weight factor was purified and shown to be a decapeptide, named speract (Gly–Phe–Asp–Leu–Asn–Gly–Gly–Gly–Val–Gly) (Hansbrough and Garbers, 1981a; Suzuki *et al.*, 1981; Garbers *et al.*, 1982). Soon it became clear that speract could act in a species-specific manner, and the peptides from a number of other species were then isolated (Garbers, 1989a), all of which appeared to cause elevations of cGMP. The egg peptide, resact (Cys–Val–Thr–Gly–Ala–Pro–Gly–Cys–Val–Gly–Gly–Gly–Arg–Leu–NH$_2$), obtained from *Arbacia punctulata*, which shows no cross-reactivity with species reacting with speract, was then studied in considerable detail along with speract.

Both peptides increase the respiration rates and motility of sea urchin spermatozoa, particularly under slightly acidic seawater conditions. In addition, resact has been shown to act as a potent chemoattractant (Ward *et al.*, 1985a). Speract and resact are now known to cause a net proton afflux (Hansbrough and Garbers, 1981b; Repaske and Garbers, 1983), transient elevations of intracellular Ca^{2+} (Schackmann and Chock, 1986), and membrane potential changes (Lee and Garbers, 1986). In addition, the peptides cause marked elevations in both cAMP and cGMP concentrations (Hansbrough and Garbers, 1981a). Both peptides were subsequently shown to activate a plasma membrane form of guanylate cyclase (Suzuki *et al.*, 1984; Bentley *et al.*, 1986, 1988; Bentley and Garbers, 1986).

At about the same time the egg peptides were identified, an atrial natriuretic factor was discovered by deBold *et al.* (1981). Atrial natriuretic factor causes natriuresis, diuresis, and vasodilation, as well as other effects (Inagami, 1989). This factor (identified as a peptide), like the egg peptides, was shown to elevate intracellular cGMP and to activate a plasma membrane form of guanylate cyclase (Hamet *et al.*, 1984; Winquist *et al.*, 1984; Waldman *et al.*, 1984). Subsequently, other peptides were isolated which also displayed natriuretic properties (Sudoh *et al.*, 1988; Inagami, 1989; Garbers, 1989a).

Studies of sea urchin spermatozoa and of various mammalian somatic cells, to understand the mechanism by which the above peptides elevated intracellular cGMP, produced a similar conclusion: Guanylate cyclase appeared to interact directly with the peptides, thereby serving as a cell surface receptor.

II.   Sea Urchin Sperm Guanylate Cyclase

A.   CLONING

The plasma membrane form of guanylate cyclase was first purified from sea urchin spermatozoa (Garbers, 1976; Radany *et al.*, 1983), where it exists in extraordinarily high amounts. Early research had shown that the sea urchin enzyme behaved like the mammalian plasma membrane form with respect to metal ion specificity and kinetics (Garbers *et al.*, 1974), and antibody to the sea urchin enzyme could also immunoprecipitate the detergent-solubilized plasma membrane form from various rat tissues (Garbers, 1978). Therefore, the enzyme from spermatozoa has served as a model for that of mammalian somatic cells.

That guanylate cyclase might serve as a cell surface receptor in sea urchin spermatozoa was first recognized when an analog of resact was demonstrated to cross-link to the enzyme (Shimomura *et al.*, 1986). Three lines of evidence were used to establish that the ^{125}I-resact analog could be covalently coupled to guanylate cyclase in the presence of disuccinimidyl suberate: (1) The ^{125}I-cross-linked protein comigrated with the purified guanylate cyclase. (2) Antibody to guanylate cyclase immunoprecipitated the ^{125}I-cross-linked protein. (3) An apparent molecular weight shift of guanylate cyclase on sodium dodecyl sulfate gels, due to a loss of phosphate, could be reproduced with the ^{125}I-resact-labeled protein (Shimomura *et al.*, 1986).

The mRNA-encoding guanylate cyclase was first cloned by Singh *et al.* (1988). The predicted protein contained a single transmembrane domain which divided the protein approximately in half (Fig. 1). The proposed intracellular region contained a domain homologous with protein kinases (Yarden *et al.*, 1986; Hanks *et al.*, 1988) and a carboxy domain of unknown function.

The cDNA isolated from *A. punctulata* was then used to identify positive-hybridizing clones from a *Strongylocentrotus purpuratus* cDNA library (Thorpe and Garbers, 1989). *Strongylocentrotus purpuratus* spermatozoa do not respond to resact (Suzuki *et al.*, 1984). The guanylate cyclase from this sea urchin was similar to that of *Arbacia,* but was extended by about 136 amino acids at the carboxy terminus. The predicted protein from *S. purpuratus* was about 42% identical within the carboxy region (202 amino acids) with a cytoplasmic form of guanylate cyclase obtained from rat and bovine lung (Koesling *et al.*, 1988; Nakane *et al.*, 1988).

When the cDNA clones for the *A. punctulata* or *S. purpuratus* cyclases were expressed in COS-7 cells, however, neither peptide binding nor enzyme activity could be detected. The reasons for this are not known.

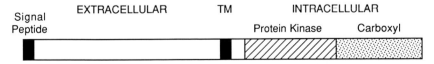

FIG. 1. *Strongylocentrotus purpuratus* guanylate cyclase. A single transmembrane (TM) domain divides the protein into an extracellular and an intracellular region. A predicted signal peptide would be cleaved to give the mature protein. Within the intracellular region at least two domains exist. One is homologous with the catalytic region of protein kinases, while the other, at the distal carboxy region, is homologous with the soluble form of guanylate cyclase and with two domains of the bovine brain adenylate cyclase.

B.   REGULATION OF ACTIVITY

Although the mechanism by which the sperm guanylate cyclase is activated by ligand has yet to be studied, desensitization mechanisms are understood to some extent. In the sea urchin spermatozoon phosphorylation dramatically affects guanylate cyclase activity. In 1983 Ward and Vacquier reported that egg jelly caused a rapid dephosphorylation of a protein with an apparent molecular weight of 160,000. Subsequently, this protein was identified as guanylate cyclase (Suzuki *et al.*, 1984; Ward *et al.*, 1985b), and the component of egg jelly that caused the rapid dephosphorylation was shown to be resact (Suzuki *et al.*, 1984). Vacquier and Moy (1986) subsequently found that the native guanylate cyclase contains 15–17 mol of phosphate per mole of enzyme and that jelly (resact) addition to cells causes a rapid and almost total loss of phosphate from the enzyme. The activity of the phosphorylated form of guanylate cyclase in detergent extracts, compared with that of the dephosphorylated form, is approximately 10-fold higher (Ramarao and Garbers, 1985).

The marked decrease in enzyme activity caused by resact was unexpected, since the peptide causes marked increases in sperm cGMP concentrations. The apparent paradox was resolved by subsequent experiments in which sperm plasma membranes were isolated under conditions in which guanylate cyclase remained in the phosphorylated form (Bentley *et al.*, 1986). The addition of resact to the membranes caused dephosphorylation of guanylate cyclase, as seen in interact cells, but large increases in guanylate cyclase activity occurred prior to the loss of phosphate. As the enzyme was dephosphorylated, its activity returned to basal levels, thereby desensitizing the system to the presence of the egg peptide. The loss of phosphate also explains the loss of positive cooperative kinetic behavior as a function of MeGTP concentration. The purified phosphorylated form of guanylate cyclase has a specific activity approximately 5-fold higher than that reported for the purified dephosphorylated form of the enzyme, and added protein phosphatases can cause a rapid decrease in enzyme activity (Ramarao and Garbers, 1988). The added protein phosphatases also cause a shift in kinetics from positively cooperative to linear as a function of added MeGTP (Ramarao and Garbers, 1988), which suggests that the phosphorylation state alters interactions between substrate-binding sites.

III.   Cloning and Expression of GC-A

While studies of spermatozoa were taking place, cross-linking studies of various mammalian cells and tissues suggested that atrial natriuretic peptide (ANP) coupled to at least two different receptors with apparent molecular weights of 66,000 and 120,000–180,000 (Inagami, 1989). The 66,000-molecular-weight protein appeared to exist as a homodimer, resulting in a third apparent receptor with an apparent molecular weight of 125,000–140,000 (Schenk *et al.*, 1987; Shimonaka *et al.*, 1987). It was also suggested by various groups that only the high-molecular-weight receptor was coupled to guanylate cyclase activation (Meloche *et al.*, 1988).

Four groups reported that the high-molecular-weight receptor copurified with guanylate cyclase activity (Kuno *et al.*, 1986; Paul *et al.*, 1987; Takayanagi *et al.*, 1987; Meloche *et al.*, 1988), but it remained unclear as to whether the two activities residued in the same or associated molecules. The specific activity of the purified guanylate cyclases appeared to be similar to that of the purified sea urchin enzyme, and ANP binding in some cases appeared close to the 1:1 stoichiometry predicted (Takayanagi *et al.*, 1987).

The low-molecular-weight ANP receptor was designated as the ANP clearance (ANP-C) receptor, and a cDNA encoding this receptor was subsequently cloned (Fuller *et al.*, 1988). The function of this binding protein has been suggested to be clearance of ANP from the circulation (Maack *et al.*, 1987), although others have claimed that it can couple to phospholipase C through a G protein (Hirata *et al.*, 1989) and therefore function in signaling. It appears to contain only 37 amino acids within the cytoplasm (Fuller *et al.*, 1988).

The above results suggested that if we could isolate the cDNA encoding a mammalian plasma membrane form of guanylate cyclase, that ANPs should be the first molecules studied for possible direct effects on the expressed enzyme. Both human and rat cDNA clones were subsequently isolated, initially using the sea urchin cDNA as a probe (Chinkers *et al.*, 1989; Lowe *et al.*, 1989). As expected, the intracellular domain contained regions closely related to those found in the sea urchin, whereas the extracellular domains were divergent.

The rat brain clone (labeled GC-A) was then transfected into COS-7 cells and demonstrated to express guanylate cyclase activity. The following experiments provided evidence that GC-A was a receptor for ANPs: (1) Membranes from COS-7 cells transfected with GC-A demonstrated large increases in specific ^{125}I-labeled ANP binding. (2) Atriopeptin I was approximately 1% as effective than ANP in competition assays, a specificity expected for the high-molecular-weight guanylate cyclase-coupled receptor. (3) ^{125}I-labeled ANP cross-linking studies showed the presence of a 130,000-molecular-weight cross-linked protein in the GC-A-transfected cells (Chinkers *et al.*, 1989). Lowe *et al.* (1989) performed similar experiments with the human clone at the same time and obtained essentially the same results.

IV. Cloning and Expression of GC-B

Since guanylate cyclase activity is found in many different tissues of the body (Hardman *et al.*, 1971), the question was raised as to whether multiple forms of the receptor existed, and if so, whether peptides other than ANP could serve as ligands for such members of this receptor family. The 3' region of the GC-A clone was used as a probe to search for other members of the family. Initially, the rat brain cDNA library was screened from which GC-A was isolated (Chinkers *et al.*, 1989). A number of positive-hybridizing clones were isolated which did not exhibit the same endonuclease restriction pattern as GC-A. One clone contained a small intron with an in-frame termination codon, while a second clone contained a small deletion in the 3' region; otherwise, the DNA sequences of both isolated clones were identical. The regions containing the intron and the deletion were removed to give a full-length clone named GC-B (Schulz *et al.*, 1989). The corresponding human clone was also obtained by others (Chang *et al.*, 1989).

A comparison of GC-A, GC-B, and the ANP-C receptor is given in Fig. 2. The ANP-C receptor, often the predominant ANP-binding protein of a given tissue, has been suggested to function as an ANP clearance receptor (Maack *et al.*, 1987), as mentioned in the previous section, while others have suggested that it functions in signaling (Hirata *et al.*, 1989). Whatever the case, it is a truncated member of the guanylate cyclase family, being approximately 33% identical to GC-A and 29% identical to GC-B within the extracellular domain (i.e., the amino acid level). GC-A and GC-B are similar within the distal carboxy regions, but the similarity then progressively decreases as one moves toward the amino terminus. However, the protein kinase-like domain is still approximately 72% identical and the extracellular domain is about 43% identical between GC-A and GC-B.

The divergence of GC-B and GC-A within the putative ligand-binding domain raised the obvious possibility that the ligand specificity would be different. Both ^{125}I-ANP (Chinkers *et al.*, 1989) and ^{125}I-labeled brain natriuretic peptide (BNP) (Sudoh *et al.*, 1988) bound to GC-B expressed in COS-7 cells; however, GC-A bound considerably greater amounts of ^{125}I-ANP and slightly greater amounts of ^{125}I-BNP than GC-B (Schulz *et al.*, 1989). Previously, we showed that basal cGMP concentrations remained low until ANP was added to COS-7 cells expressing GC-A. Therefore, we examined ANP, BNP, and atriopeptin I for their relative abilities to elevate cGMP concentrations in GC-A- and GC-B-transfected COS-7 cells (Fig. 3). Two important observations came from these studies: (1) BNP was relatively more potent than ANP in GC-B-transfected cells; the opposite was true in GC-A-transfected cells. (2) The relative concentrations of the three natriuretic peptides required to elevate cGMP were high and possibly not physiological in the GC-B-transfected cells. Although the data need to be interpreted with caution, since only COS-7 cells have been used in these expression studies, it is possible that the natural ligand for GC-B has not been discovered.

V. Identification of Catalytic Domain

The finding of a protein kinase-like domain in the sea urchin and mammalian guanylate cyclases prompted us to speculate that these domains might bind GTP

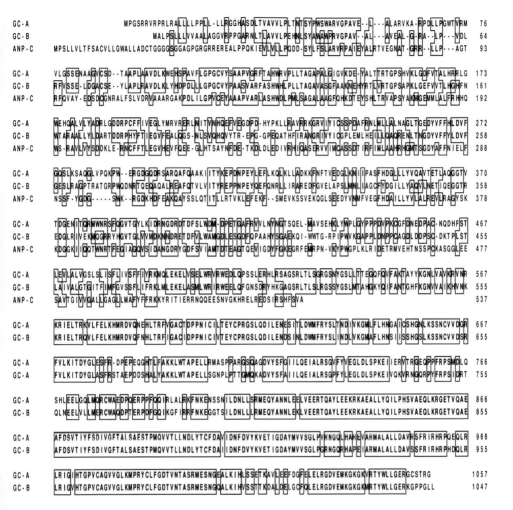

FIG. 2.   Comparison of GC-A (Chinkers *et al.*, 1989), GC-B (Schulz *et al.*, 1989), and ANP-C (Fuller *et al.*, 1988) receptors. Identities are boxed.

and catalyze the formation of cGMP (Singh *et al.*, 1988; Chinkers *et al.*, 1989). However, the subsequent data of Krupinski *et al.* (1989) on the bovine brain adenylate cyclase suggested otherwise. They found that adenylate cyclase contains two internally homologous domains which are also homologous with the distal carboxy domain of both the membrane and soluble forms of guanylate cyclase.

We then deleted the protein kinase-like domain from guanylate cyclase and found that the mutant GC-A expressed high guanylate cyclase activity (Chinkers and Garbers, 1989). Subsequently, we demonstrated that deletion of the carboxy

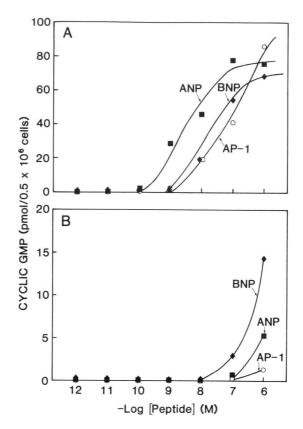

FIG. 3.   The effects of ANP, BNP, and atriopeptin I (AP-1) on cGMP concentrations. COS-7 cells were transfected with GC-A (A) or GC-B (B), and the various concentrations of natriuretic peptides, given on the abscissa, were then added. 3-Isobutyl-1-methylxanthine was included in the cell incubation mixtures. All reactions were for 5 minutes, after which they were terminated with 1 ml of 0.5N perchloric acid. cGMP concentrations were then quantitated by radioimmunoassay.

region homologous with adenylate cyclase resulted in a complete loss of guanylate cyclase activity. Therefore, the catalytic domain of guanylate cyclase is located within the distal carboxy region, a region homologous with the soluble form of the enzyme, as well as with adenylate cyclase (Krupinski *et al.*, 1989; Koesling *et al.*, 1988; Nakane *et al.*, 1988).

VI.   Function of the Protein Kinase-Like Domain

The same protein kinase deletion described above was studied in greater detail to determine whether it had a regulatory function. It should be emphasized that this domain might also possess its own catalytic function, thereby bestowing the receptor with multiple signaling properties. The expressed GC-A mutant contained high guanylate cyclase activity, but when membranes were treated with ANP, no stimulation of cyclase activity occurred (Chinkers and Garbers, 1989). Specific ANP binding, however, could easily be demonstrated. Subsequently, cGMP concentrations of intact COS-7 cells were determined. The cells transfected with the kinase deletion mutant contained high basal cGMP concentrations which were no longer affected by added ANP. Therefore, it appears that the protein kinase domain serves as a negative regulatory element and that the binding of ANP relieves inhibition of the catalytic domain.

VII. Summary

The plasma membrane forms of guanylate cyclase contain a highly conserved catalytic domain, which is also conserved in the soluble form of the enzyme and in mammalian adenylate cyclase (Fig. 4). A protein kinase-like domain lies to the amino-terminal side of the catalytic domain and appears to be required for signaling via cGMP; it might also signal, itself, through phosphotransferase activity. This domain is present in the growth factor receptors, but appears not to be a component of other guanylate cyclases or adenylate cyclases. A single

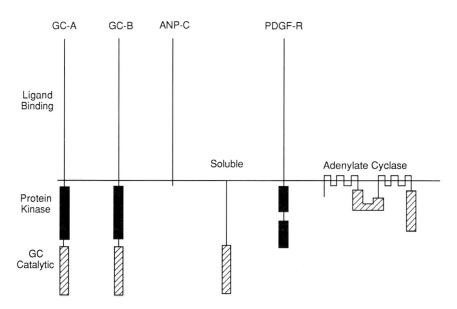

FIG. 4.   Comparison of GC-A and GC-B to other homologous proteins. ANP-C, The low-molecular-weight ANP-binding protein; soluble, the cytoplasmic form of guanylate cyclase; PDGF-R, the platelet-derived growth factor receptor; adenylate cyclase, the predicted structure based on the recently cloned mRNA from bovine brain (Krupinski et al., 1989).

transmembrane domain then separates the cyclase catalytic and protein kinase-like domains from the putative ligand-binding domain. At least two plasma membrane forms of gunaylate cyclase (i.e., GC-A and GC-B) have now been identified, and their ligand specificities appear to be distinctly different. The tissue/cellular distribution of this family of receptors is now of potential importance, since specific agonists might differentially regulate physiological processes via the secondary messenger, cGMP, dependent on cellular distribution of the receptors.

REFERENCES

Bentley, J. K., and Garbers, D. L. (1986). *Biol. Reprod.* **34,** 413–421.

Bentley, J. K., Shimomura, H., and Garbers, D. L. (1986). *Cell (Cambridge, Mass.)* **45,** 281–288.

Bentley, J. K., Khatra, A. S., and Garbers, D. L. (1988). *J. Biol. Chem.* **39,** 639–647.

Chang, M.-S., Lowe, D. G., Lewis, M., Hellmiss, R., Chen, E., and Goeddel, D. V. (1989). *Nature (London)* **341,** 68–72.

Chinkers, M., and Garbers, D. L. (1989). *Science* **245,** 1392–1394.

Chinkers, M., Garbers, D. L., Chang, M.-S., Lowe, D. G., Chin, H., Goeddel, D. V., and Schulz, S. (1989). *Nature (London)* **338,** 78–83.

Chrisman, T. D., Garbers, D. L., Parks, M. A., and Hardman, J. G. (1975). *J. Biol. Chem.* **250,** 374–381.

deBold, A. U., Bronstein, H. B., Veress, A. T., and Sonneberg, H. (1981). *Life Sci.* **28,** 89–94.

Field, M., Graf, L. H., Jr., Laird, W. J., and Smith, P. L. (1978). *Proc. Natl. Acad. Sci. U.S.A.* **75,** 2800–2804.

Fuller, F., Porter, J. G., Arfsten, A. E., Miller, J., Schilling, J. W., Scarborough, R. M., Lewicki, J. A., and Schenk, D. B. (1988). *J. Biol. Chem.* **263,** 9395–9401.

Garbers, D. L. (1976). *J. Biol. Chem.* **251,** 4071–4077.

Garbers, D. L. (1978). *J. Biol. Chem.* **253,** 1989–1901.

Garbers, D. L. (1989a). *Annu. Rev. Biochem.* **58,** 719–742.

Garbers, D. L. (1989b). *J. Biol. Chem.* **264,** 9103–9106.

Garbers, D. L., and Kopf, G. S. (1980). *Adv. Cyclic Nucleotide Res.* **13,** 251–306.

Garbers, D. L., Hardman, J. G., and Rudolph, F. B. (1974). *Biochemistry* **13,** 4166–4171.

Garbers, D. L., Watkins, H. D., Hansbrough, J. R., Smith, A., and Misono, K. (1982). *J. Biol. Chem.* **257,** 2734–2737.

Gerzer, R., Bohme, E., Hofmann, F., and Schultz, G. (1981). *FEBS Lett.* **132,** 71–74.

Goldberg, N. D., and Haddox, M. K. (1977). *Annu. Rev. Biochem.* **46,** 823–896.

Hamet, P., Tremblay, J., Pang, S. C., Garcia, R., Thibault, G., Gutkowska, J., Cantin, M., and Genest, J. (1984). *Biochem. Biophys. Res. Commun.* **123,** 515–527.

Hanks, S. K., Quinn, A. M., and Hunter, T. (1988). *Science* **241,** 42–53.

Hansbrough, J. R., and Garbers, D. L. (1981a). *J. Biol. Chem.* **256,** 1447–1452.

Hansbrough, J. R., and Garbers, D. L. (1981b). *J. Biol. Chem.* **256,** 2235–2241.

Hardman, J. G., and Sutherland, E. W. (1969). *J. Biol. Chem.* **244,** 6363–6370.

Hardman, J. G., Beavo, J. A., Gray, J. P., Chrisman, T. D., Patterson, W. D., and Sutherland, E. W. (1971). *Ann. N.Y. Acad. Sci.* **185,** 27–35.

Hirata, M., Chang, C. H., and Murad, F. (1989). *Biochim. Biophys. Acta* **1010,** 346–351.

Ignarro, L. J. (1989). *FASEB J.* **3,** 31–36.

Inagami, T. (1989). *J. Biol. Chem.* **264,** 3043–3046.

Kimura, H., and Murad, F. (1974). *J. Biol. Chem.* **249,** 6910–6916.

Koesling, D., Herz, J., Gausepohl, H., Niroomand, F., Hinsch, K.-D., Mulsch, A., Bohme, E., Schultz, G., and Frank, R. (1988). *FEBS Lett.* **239**, 29–34.

Kopf, G. S., Tubb, D. J., and Garbers, D. L. (1979). *J. Biol. Chem.* **254**, 8554–8560.

Krupinski, J., Coussen, F., Bakalyar, H. A., Tang, W.-J., Feinstein, P. G., Orth, K., Slaughter, C., Reed, R. R., and Gilman, A. G. (1989). *Science* **244**, 1558–1564.

Kuno, T., Andresen, J. W., Kamisaki, Y., Waldman, S. A., Chang, L. Y., Saheki, S., Leitman, D. C., Nakane, M., and Murad, F. (1986). *J. Biol. Chem.* **261**, 5817–5823.

Lee, H. C., and Garbers, D. L. (1986). *J. Biol. Chem.* **261**, 16026–16032.

Lowe, D. G., Chang, M.-S., Hellmiss, R., Chen, E., Singh, S., Garbers, D. L., and Goeddel, D. V. (1989). *EMBO J.* **8**, 1377–1384.

Maack, T., Suzuki, M., Almeida, F. A., Nussenzweig, D., Scarborough, M., McEnroe, G. A., and Lewicki, J. A. (1987). *Science* **238**, 675–678.

Meloche, S., McNicoll, N., Liu, B., Ong, H., and DeLean, A. (1988). *Biochemistry* **27**, 8151–8158.

Mittal, C. K., and Murad, F. (1977). *J. Cyclic Nucleotide Res.* **3**, 381–391.

Nakane, M., Saheki, S., Kuno, T., Ishii, K., and Murad, F. (1988). *Biochem. Biophys. Res. Commun.* **157**, 1139–1147.

Paul, A. K., Marala, R. B., Jaiswal, R. K., and Sharma, R. K. (1987). *Science* **235**, 1224–1226.

Radany, E. W., Gerzer, R., and Garbers, D. L. (1983). *J. Biol. Chem.* **258**, 8346–8351.

Ramarao, C. S., and Garbers, D. L. (1985). *J. Biol. Chem.* **260**, 8390–8396.

Ramarao, C. S., and Garbers, D. L. (1988). *J. Biol. Chem.* **263**, 1524–1529.

Repaske, D. R., and Garbers, D. L. (1983). *J. Biol. Chem.* **258**, 6025–6029.

Schackmann, R. W., and Chock, P. B. (1986). *J. Biol. Chem.* **261**, 8719–8728.

Schenk, D. G., Phelps, M. N., Porter, J. G., Fuller, F., Cordell, B., and Lewicki, J. A. (1987). *Proc. Natl. Acad. Sci. U.S.A.* **84**, 1521–1525.

Schultz, G., Bohme, E., and Muske, K. (1969). *Life Sci.* **8**, 1323–1332.

Schulz, S., Singh, S., Bellet, R. A., Singh, G., Tubb, D. J., Chin, H., and Garbers, D. L. (1989). *Cell (Cambridge, Mass.)* **58**, 1155–1162.

Shimomura, H., Dangott, L. J., and Garbers, D. L. (1986). *J. Biol. Chem.* **261**, 15778–15782.

Shimonaka, M., Saheki, T., Hagiwara, H., Ishido, M., Nogi, A., Fujita, T., Wakita, K., Inada, Y., Kondo, J., and Hirose, S. (1987). *J. Biol. Chem.* **262**, 5510–5514.

Singh, S., Lowe, D. G., Thorpe, D. S., Rodriguez, H., Kuang, W.-J., Dangott, L. J., Chinkers, M., Goeddel, D. V., and Garbers, D. L. (1988). *Nature (London)* **334**, 708–712.

Sudoh, T., Kangawa, K., Minamino, N., and Matsuo, H. (1988). *Nature (London)* **332**, 78–81.

Suzuki, N., Nomura, K., Ohtake, H., and Isaka, S. (1981). *Biochem. Biophys. Res. Commun.* **99**, 1238–1244.

Suzuki, N., Shimomura, H., Radany, E. W., Ramarao, C. S., Ward, G. E., Bentley, J. K., and Garbers, D. L. (1984). *J. Biol. Chem.* **259**, 14874–14879.

Takayanagi, R., Inagami, T., Snajdar, R. M., Imada, T., Tamura, M., and Misono, K. S. (1987). *J. Biol. Chem.* **262**, 12104–12113.

Thorpe, D. S., and Garbers, D. L. (1989). *J. Biol. Chem.* **264**, 6545–6549.

Vacquier, V. D., and Moy, G. W. (1986). *Biochem. Biophys. Res. Commun.* **137**, 1148–1152.

Waldman, S. A., Rapoport, R. M., and Murad, F. (1984). *J. Biol. Chem.* **259**, 14332–14334.

Ward, G. E., and Vacquier, V. D. (1983). *Proc. Natl. Acad. Sci. U.S.A.* **80**, 5578–5582.

Ward, G. E., Brokaw, C. J., Garbers, D. L., and Vacquier, V. D. (1985a). *J. Cell Biol.* **101**, 2324–2329.

Ward, G. E., Garbers, D. L., and Vacquier, V. D. (1985b). *Science* **227**, 768–770.

White, A. A., and Aurbach, G. D. (1969). *Biochim. Biophys. Acta* **191**, 686–697.

Winquist, R. J., Faison, E. P., Waldman, S. A., Schwartz, K., Murad, F., and Rapoport, R. M. (1984). *Proc. Natl. Acad. Sci. U.S.A.* **81**, 7661–7664.

Yarden, Y., Escobedo, J. A., Kuang, W.-J., Yang-Feng, T. L., Daniel, T. O., Tramble, P. M., Chen,
    E. Y., Ando, M. E., Harkins, R. N., Francke, U., Fried, V. A., Ullrich, A., and Williams, L.
    T. (1986). *Nature (London)* **323,** 226–232.

DISCUSSION

W. Vale.   Do ANP or BNP affect any metabolic parameters in sperm?

D. L. Garbers.   No, although I would not say that this has been extensively studied. ANP, as
you may know, does have dramatic effects in Leydig cells, but there are no effects that I know of on
spermatozoa.

W. Vale.   What are the tissue distributions of these receptors?

D. L. Garbers.   We are just starting to investigate this now. The B and the A cyclase receptors
are distributed differently, and many tissues seem to have some, but we obviously must use *in situ*
hybridization and other specific methods to determine whether different cell types are involved.

G. Ringold.   Have you made a point mutant in the lysine to assess whether ATP is required for
guanylate cyclase activity?

D. L. Garbers.   Yes, but we do not know if protein kinase activity is affected since we have yet
to determine whether the cyclase/receptor has protein kinase activity. However, the protein will still
signal with ANP in the face of a lysine mutation. These experiments have been done by Dr. Michael
Chinkers in our laboratory. This mutation may still bind ATP, even though it will not catalyze the
possible phosphotransferase activity. It could be argued that though ATP binding is required for
signaling to the catalytic domain, the catalytic in this case being cyclase activity, these results do not
rule out the possibility that there is also phosphoryl transferase activity which can function independent of the cyclase.

G. Ringold.   My impression was that in proteins that bind NAD or ATP lysine was essential for
the binding of ATP.

D. L. Garbers.   That was not my understanding. It is the catalytic activity that definitely is
destroyed, but the ATP-binding property in most cases has not been studied too well. We do not know
if ATP binds to the guanylate cyclase with or without the mutation.

A. R. Means.   Lysine is the residue that is covalently labeled by an azido-ATP. It has been
proposed that this lysine is one amino acid in the binding domain, but there is no evidence that it is
the only residue of the protein that is involved in binding ATP.

G. Ringold.   Is it conceivable that this protein catalyzes the reverse reaction and is, in fact, a
phosphatase?

D. L. Garbers.   If it were, it would be unusual. Granted, protein kinases can catalyze a reverse
reaction, but it would be unusual in that phosphatases, as we know them, certainly have their own
structures, which differ from those of protein kinases. When I say we have not been able to detect it, I
want to be very careful to state that we have not really tried to. We do not yet have all the reagents we
need, which are the stable cell lines and the antibodies in the mammalian system, to do these studies
effectively.

R. S. Swerdloff.   Do you have any more information on the mammalian sperm and its activating
factors?

D. L. Garbers.   If they exist, we may need to proceed with direct chemical purification, following such factors by the establishment of bioassay systems. I think the diversity in egg peptide
structure has eliminated the direct molecular approach. It still remains to be shown whether there are
active molecules other than those involved in the induction of the acrosome reaction in mammalian
germ cells.

S. Shenolikar.   As you examine the sequences for kinase homology, is the homology greater
with tyrosine kinases than with serine kinases?

D. L. Garbers.   Yes, it is.

S. Shenolikar.   Do you envisage this "kinase" autophosphorylating itself? Presumably, most of the endogenous phosphate is in serines and/or threonines, rather than tyrosine.

D. L. Garbers.   We have not yet done such studies.

S. Shenolikar.   I am fascinated by your finding of rapid dephosphorylation occurring on binding of ligand to the guanylate cyclase. Was this done in membranes?

D. L. Garbers.   This can be shown in intact cells or membranes. The first studies suggesting this were by Ward and Vacquier. We actually have also purified the phosphroylated form, and although you cannot add the peptide and induce dephosphorylation, you can add a phosphatase to dephosphorylate and see the same changes in enzyme activity predicted from the membrane studies.

S. Shenolikar.   Do you know what kind of phosphatase(s) is involved?

D. L. Garbers.   No.

S. Shenolikar.   Now that you know the sequence of the cyclase, having studied the consensus recognition sequences, do you have any inkling of what sort of kinases may be involved in putting on all those phosphates?

D. L. Garbers.   There are consensus sites for enzymes such as protein kinase C, and in fact there are a couple of reports in the literature that one can refer to on somatic cells in mammals. In somatic cells that have been studied, it seems that phosphorylation desensitizes similar to what has been found for other receptors.

C. Grunfeld.   Can you comment on one of your molecules from the sea urchin, which I believe was labeled AP sites, which appeared to have homology only in the proximal intracellular domain? Is that only in the tyrosine kinase domain? Does it lack a catalytic guanyl cyclase site?

D. L. Garbers.   You are very perceptive to pick that up. I did not discuss this, but for one of the sea urchin clones we do not have the entire apparent catalytic site.

M. Ascoli.   Is it correct that mammalian guanylate cyclase is not phosphorylated?

D. L. Garbers.   We do not know its state of phosphorylation either in the basal state or after addition of ADP. We will soon have the reagents (antibodies and stable lines) to do these studies.

M. Ascoli.   What is known about the cGMP protein kinases?

D. L. Garbers.   Do you want to know about the cGMP-dependent protein kinases?

M. Ascoli.   I was just interested in knowing if it would work in the same way cAMP does.

D. L. Garbers.   Possibly. Certainly there is a cGMP-dependent protein kinase in most tissues. Its substrate specificity often appears essentially the same as the A kinase. But based principally on retinal research, we might also suggest cGMP-dependent, and specific, ion channels. In addition, the cGMP-dependent phosphodiesterases may have a signaling function.

Insulinlike Growth Factor-Binding Proteins

Ron G. Rosenfeld,* George Lamson,* Hung Pham,* Youngman Oh,* Cheryl Conover,* Daisy D. De Leon,* Sharon M. Donovan,* Ian Ocrant,† and Linda Giudice‡

*Departments of Pediatrics and ‡Gynecology and Obstetrics, Stanford University Medical Center, Stanford, California 94305 and the †Department of Pediatrics, Rhode Island Hospital, Providence Rhode Island 02902

I. Insulinlike Growth Factors

A. HISTORICAL PERSPECTIVE

The insulinlike growth factors (IGFs), or somatomedins, constitute a family of growth hormone (GH)-dependent peptides with both anabolic and mitogenic activities for a wide variety of tissues and cell lines. Their initial identification represents a confluency of research on three seemingly distinct groups of peptides: (1) the observation by Salmon and Daughaday (1957) that GH, itself, could not directly stimulate [^{35}S]sulfate incorporation into rat chondrocyte proteoglycans (on the other hand, serum from hypophysectomized rats treated with GH could stimulate sulfation, leading to the terminology "sulfation factors" for these GH-dependent peptides); (2) studies by Froesch et al. (1963), showing that only a minor fraction of the insulinlike action of normal serum on muscle and adipose tissue could be neutralized by the addition of antiinsulin antibodies, leading to the identification of "nonsuppressible insulinlike activity" (NSILA); and (3) the discovery by Dulak and Temin (1973) that serum-free medium conditioned by BRL-3A rat hepatoma cells contained mitogenic activity, which they termed "multiplication-stimulating activity" (MSA).

In 1972 these seemingly diverse peptides were unified under the term "somatomedin," with the criteria that serum concentrations (1) must be GH dependent; (2) must possess insulinlike activity in extraskeletal tissues; (3) must promote the incorporation of sulfate into proteoglycans; and (4) must be capable of stimulating DNA synthesis and cell replication (Daughaday et al., 1972). By 1978 Rinderknecht and Humbel (1978a,b) had purified from human serum two

99

distinct somatomedin peptides, which they termed "insulinlike growth factors" I and II. IGF-I was found to have a molecular weight (M_r) of 7649, and consisted of 70 amino acids, while IGF-II had an M_r of 7471 and had 67 amino acids. Both growth factors are single-chain polypeptides, with three intrachain disulfide bridges. Forty-five amino acid positions are shared by the two peptides (with 70% identity). Furthermore, IGF-I and -II are characterized by a striking structural homology with human proinsulin. All three peptides are composed of A- and B-chain regions, with a connecting C peptide. Substantial sequence identity between proinsulin and the IGFs exists in the A- and B-chain regions; 20 of insulin's 51 amino acids are identical in IGF-I and -II, including the critical disulfide-bond-forming cysteines. The C peptide region of IGF-I and -II, which is 12 and eight amino acids long, respectively, is significantly smaller than the 35-amino-acid C peptide of proinsulin. Additionally, both IGFs possess unique carboxy-terminal D-peptide regions (eight residues for IGF-I and six residues for IGF-II).

B.   MOLECULAR BIOLOGY

The cloning of the human IGF-I cDNA by Jansen *et al.* (1983) was immediately followed by several reports of cloning of the human and rat IGF-II genes (Dull *et al.*, 1984; Bell *et al.*, 1984). It has become clear that IGF-I is encoded as a preprohormone, with an amino-terminal signal peptide and a carboxy-terminal E-peptide domain. The human IGF-I gene contains a minimum of five exons, which are separated by four introns, ranging in size from 1.9 to 50 kb. Alternative splicing of the primary IGF-I RNA transcript results in the formation of two distinct IGF-I mRNAs (Rotwein *et al.*, 1986). IGF-IB mRNA is composed of exons 1–3 and 5, encoding 153 amino acids; IGF-IA mRNA is composed of exons 1–4, encoding 195 residues. The human IGF-I gene is located on the long arm of chromosome 12, and spans over 100 kb of chromosomal DNA (Brissenden *et al.*, 1984; Tricoli *et al.*, 1984).

The human gene for IGF-II is located on the short arm of chromosome 11, in close proximity to the gene for insulin, and spans over 30 kb of DNA (Brissenden *et al.*, 1984; Tricoli *et al.*, 1984; Bell *et al.*, 1985). This gene is composed of at least eight exons (Jansen *et al.*, 1985; de Pagter-Holthuizen *et al.*, 1985; Daughaday and Rotwein, 1989). The preprohormone consists of a 24-amino-acid signal peptide, a 67-amino-acid mature peptide, and a carboxy-terminal peptide of 89 amino acids. Significant diversity exists in the 5'-untranslated regions, where different mRNA species arise as a result of distinct promoters and alternative RNA splicing (Frunzio *et al.*, 1986; de Pagter-Holthuizen *et al.*, 1987). Both IGF-I and -II are synthesized in a wide variety of tissues, and the regulation of their synthesis and secretion is currently a subject of great interest.

II. IGF Receptors

A. HISTORICAL PERSPECTIVE

Like insulin, with which they share structural homology, the IGFs bind with high affinity to specific membrane receptors (Rosenfeld and Hintz, 1986). Although both IGF-I and -II are capable of binding with lower affinity to the insulin receptor, distinct plasma membrane receptors for each peptide have been identified by competitive binding experiments, affinity cross-linking, purification of membrane receptors, and cloning receptor cDNAs.

Initial identification of specific receptors for IGf-I and -II was confirmed by structural characterization, using affinity cross-linking of receptors with [^{125}I]IGF, followed by polyacrylamide gel electrophoresis in sodium dodecyl sulfate (SDS–PAGE) (Kasuga et al., 1981; Chernausek et al., 1981; Bhaumick et al., 1981; Massague and Czech, 1982). These studies demonstrated that insulin and IGF-I bound preferentially to structurally similar receptors (type 1), comprising two $M_r = 135,000$ α subunits and two $M_r = 90,000$ β subunits. Both the α and β subunits are present on the cell membrane surface, are glycosylated, and are linked by interchain disulfide bonds. The α subunits contain the binding sites for either insulin or IGF-I; the β subunits contain a transmembrane domain, an ATP-binding site, and a tyrosine kinase domain. Interestingly, while IGF-II can bind to both the insulin and type 1 IGF receptor, it also binds with high affinity and specificity to a distinct type 2 receptor. This receptor is both structurally and immunologically distinct from the type 1 receptor. On SDS–PAGE, under nonreducing conditions, it migrates with an M_r of 220,000 and appears to be a single-chain polypeptide.

B. MOLECULAR BIOLOGY

In 1986 Ullrich et al. determined the complete primary structure of the human IGF-I receptor from cloned cDNA obtained from a human placental library. The resulting primary sequence contains a 30-residue signal peptide, followed by a 1337-amino-acid sequence, with a predicted M_r of 151,868. As is the case with the insulin receptor, the α and β subunits are contiguous and are generated following cleavage of an Arg–Lys–Arg–Arg sequence at positions 707–710. As anticipated, the β subunit contains a hydrophobic transmembrane domain, an ATP-binding site, and a tyrosine kinase domain. The insulin and type 1 IGF receptors show striking structural homology, especially in the region of the tyrosine kinase domain on the β subunit.

The close relationship between the insulin and IGF-I receptors was not surprising, given the binding affinities and structural similarities of the two receptors.

However, the cloning of the cDNA for the IGF-II receptor by Morgan *et al.* (1987) resulted in an unexpected observation. Unlike the insulin and IGF-I receptors, the type 2 IGF receptor is characterized by a long extracellular domain, containing 15 repeat sequences of approximately 150 residues, a 23-residue transmembrane domain, and a small 164-residue cytoplasmic domain. The mature peptide, without glycosylation, has a calculated M_r of 270,294.

No homology exists between the type 2 IGF receptor and the insulin or type 1 receptor. Furthermore, no ATP-binding site or kinase activity could be identified within the brief cytoplasmic domain. However, the type 2 IGF receptor is identical to the cation-independent mannose 6-phosphate receptor, which is involved in the cellular transport of lysosomal enzymes. The significance of a single receptor having discrete binding sites for IGF-II and mannose 6-phosphate remains unknown (Roth, 1988; Rosenfeld, 1989). Furthermore, it is not clear whether this receptor mediates any of the anabolic/mitogenic actions of IGF-II, or whether these actions are mediated via the binding of IGF-II to either the type 1 or insulin receptor.

III. IGF-Binding Proteins

A. HISTORICAL PERSPECTIVE

Despite the significant structural homology characteristic of insulin and the IGFs, and the structural–functional similarity of the insulin and type I IGF receptors, the IGFs differ from insulin in one important respect. Unlike insulin, both IGF-I and -II circulate in plasma complexed to a family of binding proteins (BPs). These carrier proteins not only serve to transport the IGFs to target cells, but might also modulate the interaction of the IGFs with their surface membrane receptors (Nissley and Rechler, 1984).

Although the existence of IGF-BPs was suspected over 20 years ago, the complexity of the interactions among multiple BPs, the IGF peptides, and their receptors has only recently been appreciated. Indeed, it has only been in the last two years that the first three human IGF-BPs have been cloned and sequenced, and it remains uncertain as to how many additional discrete IGF-BPs actually exist.

Early studies indicated that, when plasma was fractionated according to molecular size by gel chromatography under neutral conditions, both the NSILA and the sulfation activity comigrated in high-M_r fractions (Daughaday and Kipnis, 1966). This observation was difficult to reconcile with the fact that somatomedins purified from plasma were estimated to have M_rs of 5000–10,000. Burgi *et al.* (1966) estimated the M_r of human serum NSILA to be between 70,000 and 150,000. However, when serum was treated with 5 M acetic acid, the NSILA "dissociated into one uniform species of molecules," with an estimated

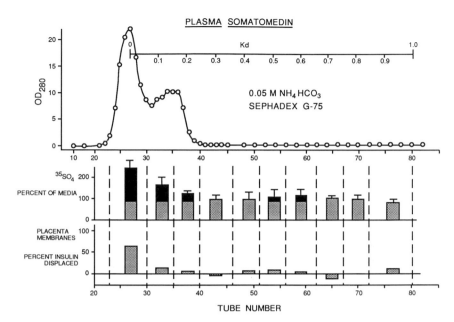

FIG. 1. Chromatography of whole plasma at neutral pH on Sephadex G-75. Somatomedin activity, measured by porcine bioassay and competition with [^{125}I]insulin, appeared at $K_d \geq 0.2$. OD, Optical density. (From Hintz and Liu, 1977.)

M_r between 6000 and 10,000, suggesting that the somatomedin peptides were originally complexed with larger plasma carrier proteins.

Similarly, Hintz and Liu (1977) demonstrated, by both porcine bioassay and competitive binding studies with [^{125}I]insulin, that, under neutral conditions, the somatomedin activity of whole human serum could be found at an M_r of over 60,000; acid treatment resulted in the migration of somatomedin bioactivity at an M_r of 5000–10,000 (Figs. 1 and 2). However, when plasma was incubated with [^{125}I]IGF and then chromatographed under neutral conditions, the major peak was found at an M_r of approximately 40,000, as first reported by Zapf *et al.* (1975). This binding was found to be of high affinity (with a K_d of less than 1 nM, saturable, and highly specific for the IGFs, with no demonstrable ability of insulin to compete for occupancy. These results demonstrated that the IGFs bind reversibly and with high affinity and specificity to at least two BPs: (1) an $M_r =$ 150,000 "large" BP, which is generally saturated by endogenous IGFs, and (2) a 40,000-molecular-weight "small" BP, which is generally unsaturated and capable of binding [^{125}I]IGF.

Moses *et al.* (1976) demonstrated the presence of similar-sized BPs in rat serum. As shown in Fig. 3, specific binding of [^{125}I]MSA was found in peaks II and III of normal rat serum. Peak I binding activity represented nonspecific

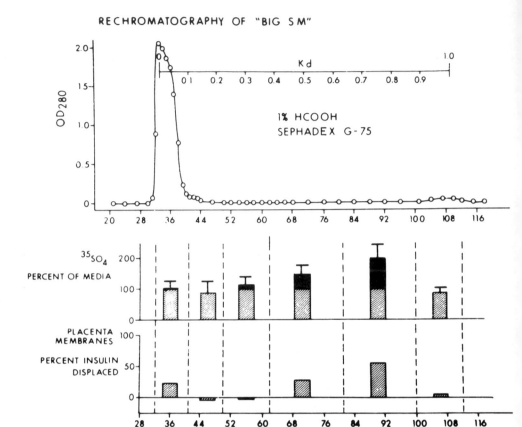

FIG. 2.   Chromatography of whole plasma at acid pH on Sephadex G-75. Somatomedin activity, measured by porcine bioassay and competition with [^{125}I]insulin, migrated in the molecular weight range 5000–10,000. OD, Optical density. (From Hintz and Liu, 1977.)

binding, since it was not displacable by excess unlabeled MSA. Peak IV represented free [^{125}I]MSA, while peak V was free [^{125}I]. The binding patterns of normal and hypophysectomized rat sera differed significantly. Peak II represented the major binding species in normal rat serum (Fig. 3a), while peak III was the only binding species present in hypophysectomized rat serum (Fig. 3b). Restoration of the binding pattern of normal serum was observed following treatment with GH (Fig. 3c and d). White *et al.* (1982) extended these studies by demonstrating that incubation of [^{125}I]MSA with adult rat serum primarily identified the large BP (peak II), while similar experiments with fetal rat serum resulted in primary labeling of the small BP (peak III) (Fig. 4). These experi-

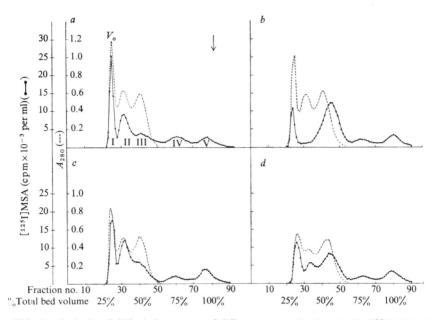

FIG. 3. Sephadex G-200 elution pattern of different rat sera incubated with [^{125}I]MSA. (*a*) Normal rat serum. (*b*) Hypophysectomized rat serum. (*c*) Serum from a hypophysectomized rat after 10 days of twice-daily intraperitoneal injections of bovine GH. (*d*) Serum from a hypophysectomized rat after intraperitoneal injections of bovine GH every 8 hours for 24 hours. Peaks II and III represent specific binding. Peak IV is unbound [^{125}I]MSA; peak V is free [^{125}I]; peak I is nonspecific binding. (From Moses *et al.*, 1976.)

ments were the first to demonstrate developmental regulation of both the IGF peptides and their BPs.

The presence of specific BPs for the IGFs was consistent with a series of investigations on the half-life of somatomedin activity in the serum. Daughaday *et al.* (1968) had originally reported that, following hypophysectomy in the rat, plasma somatomedin activity disappeared, with a half-life of 3–4 hours, a significantly greater half-life than that of insulin. Cohen and Nissley (1976), using a chick embryo fibroblast DNA synthesis bioassay, demonstrated rapid decay of somatomedin activity in hypophysectomized rats following acute GH treatment, but a prolonged half-life of 3–4 hours when hypohysectomized rats were treated with GH for 10 days. They proposed that prolongation of the half-life of somatomedin activity was the result of high-M_r carrier proteins. Subsequently, Kaufmann *et al.* (1977) demonstrated that the half-life of [^{125}I]NSILA following injection into normal rats was 3 hours. When excess unlabeled NSILA was injected simultaneously, the half-life of [^{125}I]NSILA was reduced to 10 minutes, consistent with its displacement from IGF carrier proteins.

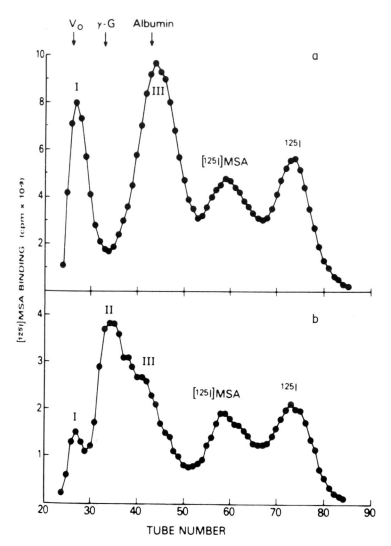

FIG. 4.   Chromatography of sera from (a) fetal (19-day) and (b) 40-day-old rats on Sephadex G-200 under neutral conditions. Peaks II and III represent specific binding of [^{125}I]MSA. (From White *et al.*, 1982.)

B.   METHODS OF DETECTION

1.   Gel Chromatography

As discussed above, initial characterization of IGF-BPs was by gel filtration chromatography. These studies demonstrated the presence of both a large and a small BP, with approximate M_rs of 150,000 and 40,000, respectively. The distribution of binding activity between these BPs was shown to be under both developmental and hormonal regulation. However, incubation of BPs or biological fluids with radioiodinated IGF, followed by gel chromatography for size fractionation, can only detect unsaturated binding sites and can, consequently, provide misleading information about the total BP activity. This is most evident in gel filtration studies of normal plasma, in which the large BP is typically saturated, while the small BP represents the majority of unsaturated binding activity (Hintz and Liu, 1977).

To circumvent this problem, samples must first be chromatographed under acid conditions, to remove bound endogenous IGF peptides. However, acid treatment can result in significant alterations in BP structure, with a decrease in size of the $M_r = 150,000$ large BP to approximately 40,000. The appearance of this $M_r = 40,000$ BP naturally led to the question of whether this acid-dissociated BP was the same as the unsaturated $M_r = 40,000$ BP found most prominently in hypophysectomized serum. To address this issue, Furlanetto (1980) used diethylaminoethyl (DEAE)–Sephadex chromatography to identify three protein peaks in human serum. Peak 2 bound [125I]somatomedin-C and was acid stable, while peak 3 was acid labile and did not bind radioiodinated somatomedin-C. An $M_r = 150,000$ complex could be formed by combining peaks 2 and 3 under neutral conditions. However, combination of peak 3 with the $M_r = 40,000$ BP found in normal, and especially hypopituitary, serum did not result in formation of the $M_r = 150,000$ complex. These experiments indicated that (1) the large $M_r = 150,000$ complex comprised an acid-labile component and a GH-dependent $M_r = 40,000$ acid-stable binding component and (2) the $M_r = 40,000$ GH-dependent subunit of the large BP was apparently different from the similar-sized non-GH-dependent BP found in hypopituitary serum.

2. Radioreceptor Assays for BPs

The ability of the BPs to specifically bind IGF with high affinity has been used as the basis for detecting and quantifying IGF-BP activity (Zapf et al., 1975; Moses et al., 1976; Hintz and Liu, 1977; Schalch et al., 1978). This methodology is dependent on the ability to separate free and carrier protein-bound [125I]IGF. Zapf et al. (1975) used activated charcoal to selectively precipitate free [125I]IGF, leaving the [125I]IGF–carrier protein complex in the supernatant. Alternatively, the [125I]IGF–carrier protein complex can be precipitated by polyethylene glycol (Hintz and Liu, 1980) or, if glycosylated, by concanavalin A plus polyethylene glycol (Martin and Baxter, 1986). As was the case with gel chromatography, however, this methodology only allows detection of *unoccupied* binding sites, and does not accurately measure total binding activity, unless endogenous IGF peptides are first removed by acid chromatography.

The ability of the carrier proteins to bind IGFs with high affinity and specificity has been the basis of a number of assays for IGF-I and -II (Schalch et al., 1978). Although all of the identified BPs have no affinity for insulin, it gradually became apparent that they comprise a heterogeneous population of proteins, with significant variability in their relative affinities for IGF-I and -II. With [^{125}I]IGF-I as the ligand, Binoux *et al.* (1984) demonstrated that BPs extracted from the culture media of livers from 4-week-old rats preferentially bound IGF-I over IGF-II. On the other hand, these same investigators identified a BP in human cerebrospinal fluid (CSF), with a selective affinity for IGF-II (Binoux *et al.*, 1982; Hossenlopp *et al.*, 1986a), and used the extracted CSF BP preparation in a relatively specific and highly sensitive IGF-II assay (Binoux *et al.*, 1986).

3. Affinity Labeling

Covalent cross-linking of [^{125}I]IGF by disuccinimidyl suberate, followed by SDS–PAGE, has been invaluable in our understanding of the structures of IGF and insulin receptors. D'Ercole and Wilkins (1984) adapted these methodologies to the study of IGF-BPs in rat sera and identified binding activity migrating with apparent M_rs of 95,000, 49,000, 36,000–33,000, and 26,000–23,000, with less intense complexes at M_rs of 175,000 and 115,000. Additionally, they were able to demonstrate an intense increase in the $M_r = 36,000–33,000$ complex following hypophysectomy, with accompanying reduction of the $M_r = 49,000$ complex (Fig. 5).

These methodologies could also be readily adapted for the identification and characterization of IGF-BPs in conditioned media of a wide variety of cells, as shown in Fig. 6.

Affinity cross-linking studies have sharper discriminatory capabilities than gel chromatography and represent a significant advancement in the characterization of BP structure. When combined with competitive binding studies, affinity labeling could, additionally, be used to investigate the affinity for IGF-I and -II of a variety of BPs coexisting in biological fluids (e.g., serum, CSF, and conditioned media). On the other hand, such methodologies are semiquantitative at best, since the intensity of the autoradiographic signal could be influenced by other factors besides the number of available binding sites. Additionally, binding of the radioligand to a specific BP will be affected by occupancy of the binding site by endogenous IGF. Finally, although representing a significant advance over gel filtration studies, sharper discrimination of BPs of similar size could be achieved by other methodologies, such as Western ligand blotting, discussed in the next section.

4. Western Ligand Blotting

This methodology, first developed by Hossenlopp *et al.* (1986b), has proved to be invaluable for the detection and characterization of IGF-BPs. As with affinity labeling, the biological sample of interest is subjected to SDS–PAGE, but subsequently is electroblotted to either nitrocellulose or nylon membrane. After drying, the membrane is soaked at 4°C in saline (0.15 M NaCl, 0.01 M Tris–HCl,

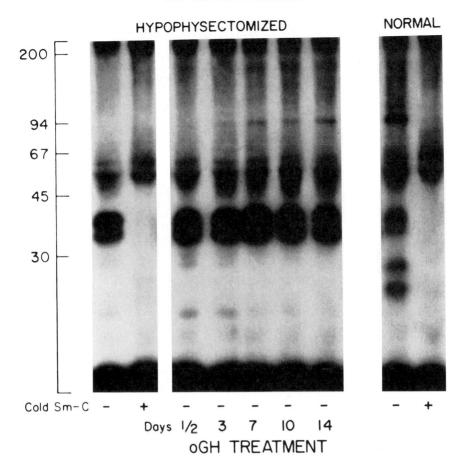

FIG. 5. Affinity-labeled [^{125}I]somatomedin-C complexes in rat serum. (From D-Ercole and Wilkins, 1984.)

pH 7.4, 0.5 mg/ml of sodium azide, supplemented with 3% Nonidet-P40). This is followed by a second soak in saline, 1% bovine serum albumin (BSA), followed by a third soak in saline, 0.1% Tween 20. The membrane is then incubated overnight with [^{125}I]IGF in a sealed plastic bag with saline, 1% BSA, 0.1% Tween 20. The membrane can then be washed and autoradiographed. Although apparently less sensitive than affinity labeling, this methodology permits sharp discrimination among IGF-BPs which might migrate with an apparent M_r within 1000 of each other. Additionally, the band seen on autoradiography is that of the BP, itself, without the addition of cross-linked [^{125}I]IGF (Fig. 7).

These techniques can be adapted to determine the affinity of each BP by cutting the band corresponding to a specific BP and incubating each band separately with [^{125}I]IGF and various concentrations of unlabeled ligand. An

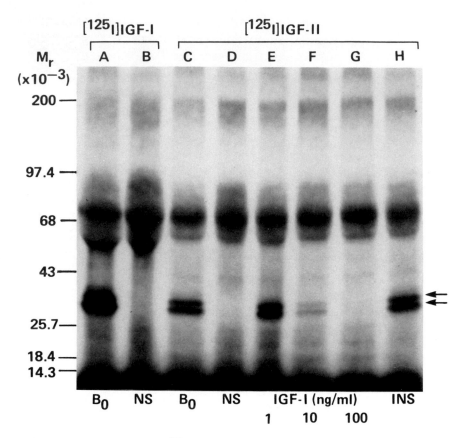

FIG. 6. SDS–PAGE of both [^{125}I]IGF-I (lanes A and B) and [^{125}I]IGF-II (lanes C–H) cross-linked to serum-free con\..tioned media from B104 cells and run under reducing conditions on a 6–12.5% gradient gel. Incubations of [^{125}I]IGF-I and [^{125}I]IGF-II with medium were performed as follows: lanes A and C (B_0), without competing peptides; lanes B and D [nonspecific (NS)], excess unlabeled IGF; lanes E–G (IGF-I), 1, 10, and 100 ng/ml unlabeled IGF-I, respectively; lane H [insulin (INS)], 10 μg/ml of unlabeled insulin. The arrows indicate the presence of cross-linked BPs, with apparent molecular weights of 33,000 and 35,000. (From Sturm et al., 1989.)

additional major advantage of this methodlogy, compared to affinity labeling, is that it appears to be unaffected by endogenous IGFs, which generally are dissociated from the BP complex during electrophoresis in SDS. This remains, however, to be rigorously demonstrated. One problem which should be noted with the Western ligand blot methodology is that not all IGF-BPs transfer with the same efficiency during electroblotting, and caution should therefore be used when making quantitative conclusions with this technique (Rosenfeld et al., 1989b).

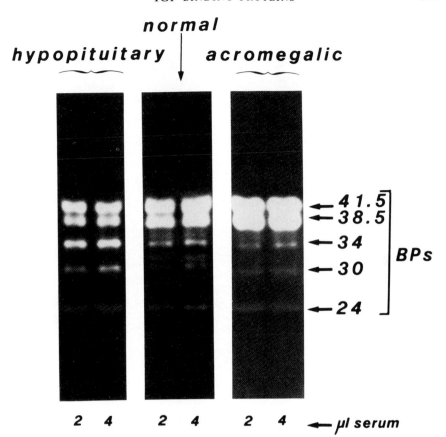

FIG. 7. Western ligand blot analysis of normal, hypopituitary, and acromegalic serum IGF-BPs. (From Hardouin *et al.*, 1987.)

5. *Immunoprecipitation*

The purification of the IGF-BPs has permitted the production of a variety of polyclonal and monoclonal antibodies, which have, in turn, allowed for more precise structural determination and measurement. Immunoprecipitation can be combined with affinity labeling of BPs with [^{125}I]IGF (Fig. 8), or the immunoprecipitated BP can be solubilized, subjected to SDS–PAGE, and then Western ligand blotted, as described in the previous section (Fig. 9). The latter technique combines immunological specificity with the discriminatory capability of ligand blotting and has been of particular value. Alternatively, metabolically labeled newly synthesized BPs can be immunoprecipitated and run on SDS–

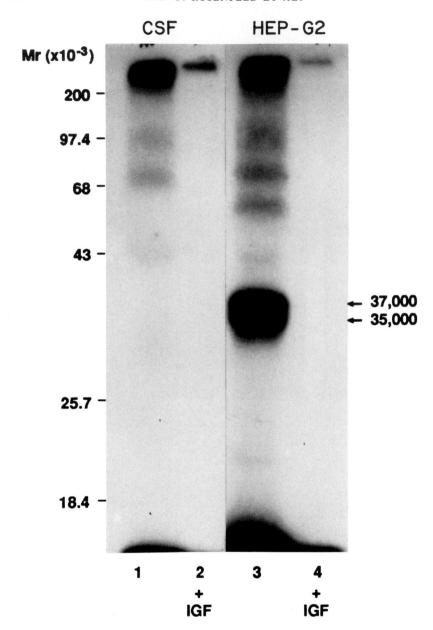

FIG. 8. SDS–PAGE of 12% gel of immunoprecipitates of CSF (lanes 1 and 2) and HEP-G2-conditioned medium (lanes 3 and 4) run under reducing conditions. [^{125}I]IGF-II was cross-linked to CSF and HEP-G2-conditioned medium in the absence (lanes 1 and 3) or presence (lanes 2 and 4) of excess IGF, and then immunoprecipitated with an antibody directed against IGF-BP-1. The arrows indicate the apparent 37,000- and 35,000-molecular-weight HEP-G2 doublet. (From Rosenfeld *et al.*, 1989a.)

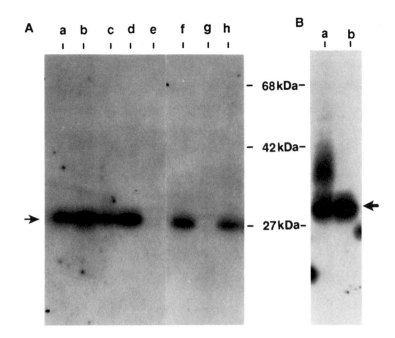

FIG. 9. Autoradiograph of a Western ligand blot of fluid or conditioned media immunoprecipi-tated with α-HEC-1 antiserum. Immunoprecipitates were electrophoresed on a 10% gel, and the blotted proteins were incubated with [^{125}I]IGF-II. (A) Rat CSF (lane a), conditioned media from BRL-3A cells (lane b), newborn astrocytes (lane c), fetal neuronal cells (lane d), adult anterior pituitary cells (lane e), adult pituitary neurointermediate lobe cells (lane f), B104 cells (lane g), and rat amniotic fluid (lane h). (B) HEC-1A-conditioned medium (lane a) and human CSF (lane b). Arrows indicate rat (A) and human (B) IGF-BP-2. (From Lamson *et al.*, 1989a.)

PAGE (Fig. 10). These methods are all potentially limited by the specificity of the antibodies used.

6. Western Blotting

Antibodics directed against the IGF-BPs can also be used in conventional Western immunoblotting, following size separation by SDS–PAGE (Fig. 11). Theoretical limitations of this methodology includc (1) poor transfer of BPs during the electroblotting procedure, (2) concealment of the epitope of interest during electroblotting, and (3) limitations in the specificity of the antibody(ies) used.

7. Radioimmunoassay

In addition to their use in immunoprecipitation and Western blot procedures, specific anti-BP antibodies have permitted the development of radioim-munoassays (RIAs) for several purified IGF-BPs. At this time specific RIAs have

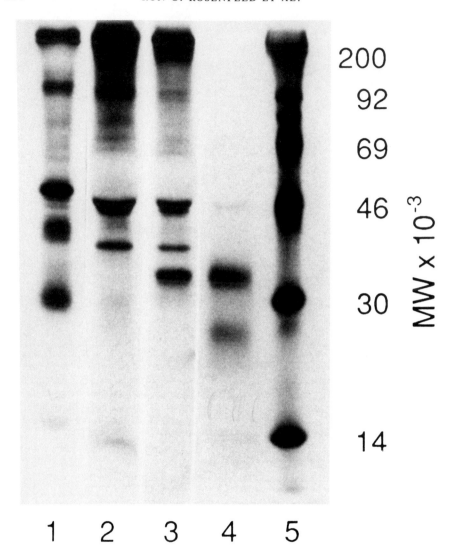

FIG. 10. Fluorography of total [35S]-labeled proteins and immunoprecipitated [35S]IGF-BP-1 from human granulosa cell culture medium. (Lane 1) total [35S]-labeled proteins; (lane 2) total [35S]-labeled proteins plus normal rabbit serum (nonspecific binding); (lane 3) immunoprecipitated [35S]IGF-BP-1; (lane 4) purified [125I]IGF-BP-1; (lane 5) 14C-methylated marker proteins. (From Suikkari *et al.*, 1989.)

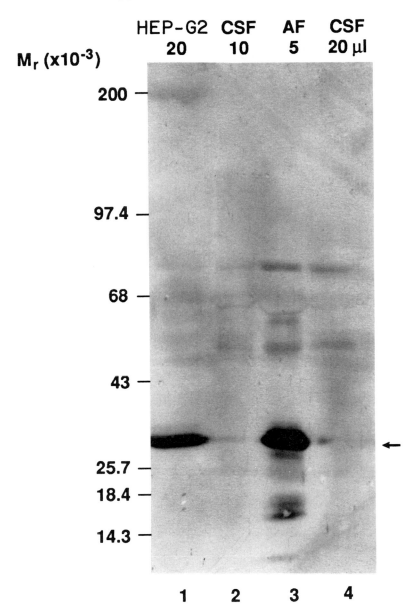

FIG. 11. Western immunoblot of HEP-G2-conditioned medium (lane 1), CSF (lanes 2 and 4), and amniotic fluid (AF) (lane 3) exposed to a polyclonal antibody to IGF-BP-1. The arrow indicates the apparent M_r = 30,000 band seen in HEP-G2-conditioned medium and the amniotic fluid, but not the CSF. (From Rosenfeld *et al.*, 1989a.)

TABLE I
Sources of IGF-BP-1

Source	Name	Established M_r	Reference
Amniotic fluid (AF)	AFBP	35,000–40,000	Chochinov et al. (1977)
	AFBP	35,000–40,000	Drop et al. (1979, 1984)
	AFBP	35,000	Povoa et al. (1984a)
	BP-28	28,000	Baxter et al. (1987)
Hepatoma	HEP-G2-BP	30,000–50,000	Moses et al. (1983)
Placenta/decidua	PP12	51,000	Bohn and Kraus (1980)
	PP12	34,000	Koistinen et al. (1986)
Endometrium	α_1-PEG	32,000	Bell et al. (1988)

been reported for human IGF-BP-1 (amniotic fluid BP) (Drop *et al.*, 1984; Povoa *et al.*, 1984b; Baxter *et al.*, 1987; Busby *et al.*, 1988b), human IGF-BP-3 (GH-dependent large BP) (Baxter and Martin, 1986), and rat IGF-BP-2 (BRL-3A BP) (Romanus *et al.*, 1986). These RIAs have already provided important new information on the physiological and hormonal regulation of the IGF-BPs.

C. BINDING PROTEIN STRUCTURE

As discussed above, early identification and characterization of IGF-BPs was by gel chromatogrpahy, with the resulting demonstration of two apparently discrete BPs: a large GH-dependent plasma BP and a small GH-independent BP. Further structural characterization awaited the development of affinity labeling and ligand blotting techniques, as well as the production of specific antibodies.

1. *IGF-BP-1 (BP-28)*

The identification of IGF-BP-1 resulted from studies of at least four seemingly distinct proteins (Table I): (1) an IGF-BP found in amniotic fluid (Chochinov *et al.*, 1977; Drop *et al.*, 1979); (2) an IGF-BP identified in the conditioned media of a human hepatoma cell line, HEP-G2 (Moses *et al.*, 1983); (3) PP12, a placental protein originally isolated from soluble extracts of term human placenta and adjacent membranes (Bohn and Kraus, 1980; Koistinen *et al.*, 1986); and (4) pregnancy-associated endometrial α_1-globulin (α_1-PEG), originally termed "endometrial protein 14" (Bell and Bohn, 1986; Bell *et al.*, 1988), a major secretory protein of the stromal cells of the decidua.

An acid-stable IGF-BP with an estimated M_r of 35,000–40,000 was first identified by Chochinov *et al.* (1977). This IGF-BP was subsequently further characterized by Drop *et al.* (1984), Povoa *et al.* (1984a,b), and Baxter *et al.* (1987), with the generation of polyclonal antibodies against partially purified BP preparations. These antibodies were found to cross-react with BP activity in fetal and cord sera (Povoa *et al.*, 1984b; D'Ercole *et al.*, 1985), suggesting that the amniotic fluid BP and the small BP found in fetal and newborn sera were the same. Baxter *et al.* (1987) subsequently purified this IGF-BP by a combination of IGF-I affinity chromatography and reversed-phase high-performance liquid chromatography, and termed it "BP-28," because of its apparent M_r on SDS–PAGE under nonreducing conditions (28,000 nonreduced, 34,000 reduced).

Concurrently, Moses *et al.* (1983) identified an IGF carrier protein in media conditioned by the human hepatoma cell line HEP-G2. This protein was found to be acid stable and nonglycosylated, with an M_r of 30,000–50,000. Povoa *et al.* (1985) purified the HEP-G2 IGF-BP to homogeneity through immunoaffinity chromatography, using a polyclonal antibody against purified amniotic fluid BP. Purified HEP-G2 and amniotic fluid IGF-BPs both migrated at apparent M_rs of 32,000 on SDS–PAGE under denaturing conditions. Additionally, the amino acid compositions of the two proteins were equivalent, and the amino-terminal sequences were identical (i.e., Ala–Pro–Trp–Gln). Powell *et al.* (1987) subsequently demonstrated identity between the first 10 amino acids of the amniotic fluid BP and the HEP-G2 IGF-BP.

Concurrently, Bohn and Kraus (1980) had isolated PP12 from soluble extracts of human placenta. M_r estimates ranged from 25,200 by ultracentrifugation to 51,000 by SDS–PAGE. Rutanen *et al.* (1985, 1986b) subsequently demonstrated that PP12 was a decidual, rather than a placental, protein, since decidual explants released significantly more PP12 than did explants from chorion and amnion; placental explants released no detectable PP12. Maternal and fetal serum PP12 levels ranged from 40 to 460 ng/ml, with levels 100- to 1000-fold higher in amniotic fluid (Rutanen *et al.*, 1982). In 1986 Koistinen *et al.* (1986, 1987) determined the amino-terminal amino acid sequence of PP12 and demonstrated that the first 15 amino acids were identical to the IGF-BP isolated from amniotic fluid. Additionally, PP12 was shown to specifically bind [^{125}I]IGF-I, confirming that this placental protein was, in fact, the major amniotic fluid IGF-BP.

α_1-PEG is a monomeric protein with an estimated M_r of 29,000–32,000. Originally termed "endometrial protein 14" (Bell and Bohn, 1986), it has been shown to be a minor secretory product during the menstrual cycle, but, perhaps, the major secretory protein of the endometrium during pregnancy. α_1-PEG has been shown to be immunochemically similar to PP12 (Bell and Bohn, 1986) and, like PP12, binds IGF-I with high affinity (Bell *et al.*, 1988). However, Bell and Keyte (1988) have suggested that these two proteins might be closely related, but not identical, peptides. Immunohistochemical studies of PP12 localization during the menstrual cycle have identified PP12 primarily in the glandular epithelium of the secretory endometrium (Waites *et al.*, 1988); α_1-PEG is principally associated with stromal cell populations. Although PP12 and α_1-PEG were first reported as differing in amino acid positions 11 and 12 (Koistinen *et al.*, 1986; Bell and Keyte, 1988), the amino-terminal sequence of α_1-PEG reported by Bell and Keyte (1988) corresponds to the primary structure predicted by the cDNA for PP12 (Julkunen *et al.*, 1988).

2. IGF-BP-3 (BP-53)

As described above, investigations using gel chromatography under neutral conditions demonstrated that endogenous IGF activity in both human and rat plasma was predominantly associated with an $M_r = 150,000$ complex. However, when plasma was incubated with [^{125}I]IGF, binding was primarily observed to an $M_r = 40,000$ protein. Hintz and Liu (1977, 1980) demonstrated that when plasma was chromatographed on Sephadex G-200 and individual fractions then either incubated with [^{125}I]IGF or chromatographed in acid prior to incubation with radioligand, both $M_r = 150,000$ and $M_r = 40,000$ IGF-BPs could be identified. They concluded that the larger BP is typically saturated with endogenous IGF, while the smaller BP is largely unsaturated. Treatment of the larger BP with acid results in the irreversible breakdown of the complex and the release of bound IGF. Furlanetto (1980) confirmed that the $M_r = 150,000$ BP complex has a three-subunit structure, which includes IGF, a binding subunit, and an acid-labile subunit.

Only limited additional insight into the nature of plasma IGF-BPs was provided by affinity labeling methodologies, which are only capable of identifying unsaturated BPs. Wilkins and D'Ercole (1985) used disuccinimidyl suberate to cross-link [^{125}I]IGF-I to human plasma and identified complexes with M_rs 160,000, 135,000, 110,000, 80,000, 50,000, 43,000–35,000, and 28,000–24,000. The $M_r = 43,000–35,000$ complex was most prominent in hypopituitary plasma and was the only IGF-BP not adsorbed by concanavalin A–Sepharose. These investigators hypothesized that all of the other IGF-BPs in plasma represented oligomers of the GH-dependent $M_r = 28,000–24,000$ complex.

The development of Western ligand blotting techniques by Hossenlopp *et al.* (1986b) permitted a more definitive elucidation of the IGF-BPs. Hardouin *et al.* (1987) demonstrated five molecular forms of BPs, with M_rs 41,500, 38,500, 34,000, 30,000, and 24,000. They size-fractionated human serum by neutral gel filtration on Sephadex G-200 and again identified large and small complexes (Fig. 12). Each complex was then subjected to SDS–PAGE, transfer onto nitrocellulose, and incubation with [^{125}I]IGF-I. As shown in Fig. 13, the large complex contained only the $M_r = 41,500$ and $M_r = 38,500$ IGF-BPs, while the small complex contained all five IGF-BPs. They suggested that the $M_r = 41,500$ and $M_r = 38,500$ BPs are involved in the formation of the large $M_r = 150,000$ complex.

Martin and Baxter (1986) purified a GH-dependent IGF-BP from Cohn fraction IV of human plasma by affinity chromatography on agarose–IGF-II. On SDS–PAGE under nonreducing conditions, two bands were visualized, a major

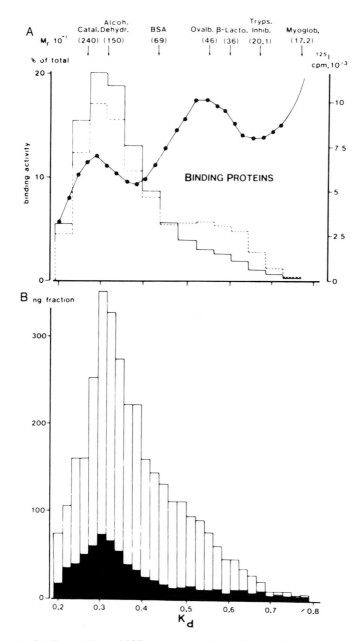

FIG. 12. Binding activity and IGF measurements in the eluates of neutral-pH Sephadex G-200 filtration of normal serum. The BPs and IGFs in each fraction were separated by acidic gel filtration prior to assay. (A) Binding activity measured using [^{125}I]IGF-I (——) or [^{125}I]IGF-II (– – – –). •——•, The elution profile of [^{125}I]IGF-I incubated with serum prior to chromatography $K_d = 0.43$ was taken as the borderline between the large and small complexes. (B) IGF-I (■) and IGF-II (□) levels, measured by radioimmunoassay and protein binding assay, respectively. (From Hardouin *et al.*, 1987.)

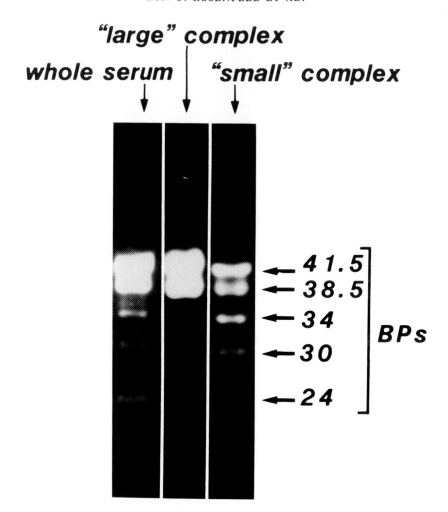

FIG. 13.   Western ligand blot analysis of IGF-BPs. Comparison of whole serum and the large and small complexes identified in Fig. 12. (From Hardouin *et al.*, 1987.)

band at $M_r = 53,000$ and a minor band at $M_r = 47,000$. Under reducing conditions these bands migrated at $M_r = 43,000$ and 40,000, respectively. Both BPs were glycosylated, were capable of binding both IGFs, and shared a common amino-terminal sequence, which was significantly different from that of the amniotic fluid BP. It seems reasonable to assume that these BPs are the same as the $M_r = 41,500$ and $M_r = 38,500$ IGF-BPs detected by Western ligand blotting (Hardouin *et al.*, 1987). It is further conceivable that some of the small serum

BPs, with apparent M_rs ranging from 18,000 to 30,000, represent proteolyzed forms of this IGF-BP, since several laboratories have reported the generation of BP fragments following prolonged storage or acid treatment (Ooi and Herington, 1986).

Baxter *et al.* (1986) and Baxter and Martin (1987) subsequently purified similar proteins from adult rat serum, with M_rs of 56,000 and 50,000 nonreduced and 48,000 and 44,000 reduced. Ten of the first 13 amino-terminal amino acids were identical in the rat and human GH-dependent IGF-BPs. Zapf *et al.* (1988) isolated three N-glycosylated IGF-BPs from adult rat serum, with estimated M_rs of 45,000, 42,000, and 32,000–30,000. These three peptides share the same amino terminus through position 31 and match the first 15 amino-terminal amino acids reported by Baxter and Martin (1987).

How these low-M_r BPs can be reconstituted to form the large $M_r = 150,000$ plasma IGF-BP has been difficult to elucidate. Martin and Baxter (1985) had demonstrated that an antibody against the $M_r = 60,000$ acid-treated plasma BP recognized the GH-dependent $M_r = 150,000$ IGF-BP. As stated above, Wilkins and D'Ercole (1985) had suggested that the $M_r = 150,000$ complex is actually a hexamer of the $M_r = 24,000–28,000$ IGF-BP found in serum on affinity cross-linking. Alternatively, it had been suggested by several groups that the $M_r = 150,000$ complex consists of IGF plus the acid-stable IGF-BP plus an acid-labile non-IGF-binding component (Furlanetto, 1980; Hintz and Liu, 1980). The latter hypothesis has been recently proved by Baxter (1988), who used an assay based on the ability of fractions to convert cross-linked BP-53–[^{125}I]IGF-I from an apparent M_r of 60,000 to approximately 150,000. This component was acid labile, losing activity irreversibly at pH <4.5. According to the model proposed by Baxter (1988), the $M_r = 150,000$ IGF-BP complex consists of (1) an acid-labile α subunit with an M_r of 80,000–85,000, (2) an acid-stable β subunit with binding activity, and (3) the IGF peptide, itself, which constitutes the γ subunit (Fig. 14). The β–γ complex can form in the absence of the α subunit. However, formation of the α–β complex only occurs in the presence of IGF-I or -II (γ subunit).

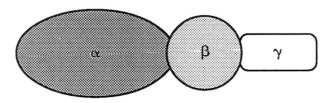

FIG. 14.   Proposed structure of circulating form of IGF-BP-3. The ternary complex consists of an acid-labile α subunit, a β subunit (which can be either IGF-BP-3 or related BPs), and a γ subunit, which represents the IGF peptide itself. (From Baxter and Martin, 1989.)

3. IGF-BP-2

In 1979 Moses *et al.* reported that BRL-3A cells synthesize and secrete both IGF-II and an IGF carrier protein. Two years later Knauer *et al.* (1981) purified the BRL-3A IGF-BP from serum-free conditioned media, by use of an MSA–Sepharose 4B affinity column. A single protein band was observed, with an M_r of 31,500. Mottola *et al.* (1986) reported that the IGF-II affinity-purified BRL-3A IGF-BP migrated with an apparent M_r of 36,300 under reducing conditions and was capable of binding both IGF-I and -II. Interestingly, a polyclonal antibody raised against the BRL-3A IGF-BP did not recognize a similarly sized IGF-BP from conditioned media of the rat hepatoma cell H-35. Thirty-one amino acids from the amino terminus were sequenced and found to have limited identity with the sequence from the human amniotic fluid/HEP-G2 IGF-BP. Concurrently, Romanus *et al.* (1986) purified the BRL-3A IGF-BP and estimated the M_r to be 33,000 on SDS–PAGE. A polyclonal antiserum generated against the purified IGF-BP recognized the $M_r = 40,000$ BP in neonatal rat serum, but failed to recognize the $M_r = 150,000$ complex in adult rat serum. When combined, the results of these studies suggested that the BRL-3A rat BP was potentially distinct from both IGF-BP-1 and IGF-BP-3.

Recently, Szabo *et al.* (1988) have purified an IGF-BP from conditioned media of Madin–Darby bovine kidney (MDBK) cells. Like the BRL-3A IGF-BP, the isolated BP had significantly higher affinity for IGF-II than for IGF-I. The purified BP migrated as a single band of $M_r = 40,000$ on SDS–PAGE. Amino-terminal amino acid sequencing demonstrated identity with rat IGF-BP-2 in the first 21 amino acids, with the exceptions of a cysteine-for-arginine substitution at position 13, and a lysine-for-glycine substitution at position 18. The MDBK BP amino-terminal sequence contains a nine-amino-acid insertion, but the following eight amino acids are identical to rat IGF-BP-2. An internal peptide fragment of the MDBK BP corresponds to residues 262–284 of the rat IGF-BP-2 and is identical at 22 of the 23 loci.

The human equivalent of the rat IGF-BP-2 has been difficult to identify. Rosenfeld *et al.* (1989a) showed that the major IGF-BP present in human CSF, originally identified by Hossenlopp *et al.* (1986a), was slightly larger than the BP found in amniotic fluid and HEP-G2-conditioned media and did not react with antibodies generated against IGF-BP-1. Recently, Lamson *et al.* (1989b) have identified an IGF-BP of similar size in the conditioned media of the human endometrial carcinoma cell line, HEC-1A. This BP did not react with antibodies to IGF-BP-1, and HEC-1A cells appeared to contain no mRNA for IGF-BP-1. An antibody generated against partially purified BPs from HEC-1A-conditioned media, as well as an antibody generated against purified rat IGF-BP-2, immunoprecipitated a similar-sized BP from both human CSF- and HEC-1A-conditioned media (Fig. 15). HEC-1A cells were subsequently shown to contain

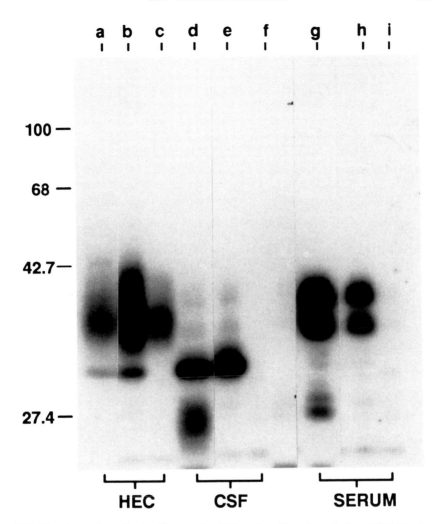

FIG. 15. Autoradiograph of a Western ligand blot of conditioned media from HEC-1A cells, CSF, or serum. Each sample has been run alone on a Western ligand blot (lanes a, d, and g), immunoprecipitated with rabbit polyclonal antibody to HEC-1A BPs (IGF-BP-2 and -3; lanes b, e, and h), or immunoprecipitated with normal rabbit serum (lanes c, f, and h). (From Lamson *et al.*, 1989b.)

mRNA for IGF-BP-2, strongly suggesting that the $M_r = 31,000–34,000$ complex is IGF-BP-2 (see below).

4. BP-24

A low-M_r IGF-BP has been identified in both rat and human sera (Figs. 7 and 13) (Hardouin et al., 1987; Zapf et al., 1988; Donovan et al., 1989). A similar-sized BP has also been found in conditioned media from human fibroblasts (Conover et al., 1989), human breast cancer cells (De Leon et al., 1989a), and seminal plasma (Rosenfeld et al., 1990) (see below). While it has been suggested that this BP might be a subunit or degradation product of a larger BP (e.g., IGF-BP-3), it does not appear to be recognized by antibodies generated against IGF-BP-1, -2, or -3 (De Leon et al., 1989a; Rosenfeld et al., 1990).

5. BP-16

Smaller proteins, capable of binding [^{125}I]IGF, have been reported. Ooi and Herington (1986) have identified a serum inhibitor of IGF activity which was acid stable, heat labile, and glycosylated, with an apparent M_r of 16,000–18,000. The precise relationship of these BPs/inhibitors to the low-M_r BPs identified by affinity cross-linking and Western ligand blotting remains to be established. However, Ooi and Herington (1986) have shown that $M_r = 16,000$ inhibitory activity could be generated by acid treatment of larger serum BPs. It has been demonstrated that a polyclonal antiserum generated against purified IGF-BP-3 recognizes this inhibitory binding subunit, by both RIA and Western blotting techniques (Baxter and Martin, 1986).

6. IGF-II Receptor as a Serum-Binding Protein

In studies of IGF carrier proteins in fetal rat serum, White et al. (1982) identified a high-M_r protein capable of specifically binding [^{125}I]IGF-II. This protein appeared to be significantly larger than both the $M_r = 40,000$ and the $M_r = 150,000$ classical IGF-BPs. Butler and Gluckman (1986) identified a similar $M_r > 200,000$ BP in fetal lamb serum. In both the rat and the sheep, serum levels of this BP decreased rapidly with age.

Recently, Kiess et al. (1987) have demonstrated that this fetal rat BP has all of the binding characteristics of a classical type 2 IGF receptor (i.e., a significantly greater affinity for IGF-II than for IGF-I and no affinity for insulin). Gelato et al. described a similar phenomenon in fetal sheep (Gelato et al., 1989) and monkey (Gelato et al., 1988) sera. By affinity cross-linking techniques the rat BP was found to migrate at $M_r = 210,000$ without reduction and at $M_r = 240,000$ following reduction, slightly smaller than the membrane IGF-II receptor. However, the BP was recognized by a polyclonal serum generated against rat chondrosarcoma IGF-II receptors (Kiess et al., 1987).

MacDonald et al. (1989) have elegantly demonstrated that this serum BP is, in

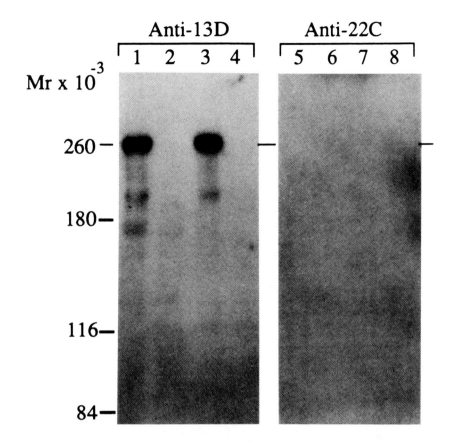

FIG. 16. Neonatal rat serum (lanes 1, 2, 5, and 6) and dilute neonatal plasma (lanes 3, 4, 7, and 8) were immunoadsorbed with antireceptor (odd numbers) or nonimmune (even numbers) immunoglobulin Affi-Gel resins. The washed resins were reduced and alkylated, electrophoresed on SDS–PAGE, and immunoblotted with anti-13D (extracellular receptor domain, lanes 1–4) or anti-22C (cytoplasmic domain, lanes 5–8). (From MacDonald et al., 1989.)

fact, the IGF-II receptor, which has been truncated in the carboxy-terminal domain. They generated antibodies against a 13-amino-acid sequence (13D) located amino terminal to the transmembrane domain and to a 22-residue peptide located in the cytoplasmic domain (22C). Both the circulating IGF-II receptor and the membrane-associated receptor could be recognized by the antibody against 13D; anti-22C recognized the membrane receptor, but not the serum receptor (Fig. 16). These results suggest that the serum form of the IGF-II receptor lacks both the carboxy-terminal intracellular and transmembrane domains, which involves removal of 189 amino acids.

The type II IGF receptor thus joins a group of soluble peptide hormone receptors that can be found in the circulation. This group includes the GH receptor (Baumann *et al.*, 1986; Herington *et al.*, 1986) and the transferrin receptor (Beguin *et al.*, 1988). The precise source and function of the circulating type II receptor, as well as what controls its ontogenic expression, remain unknown.

D. MOLECULAR BIOLOGY OF THE IGF-BPs

1. cDNA Clones

Studies of the molecular biology of the IGF-BPs have revealed extensive information about the structure of these proteins, indicating that they are members of a large gene family. Over the last 2 years several groups have reported cloning and sequencing human IGF-BP-1 (Lee *et al.*, 1988; Brinkman *et al.*, 1988b; Brewer *et al.*, 1988; Julkunen *et al.*, 1988), human IGF-BP-3 (Wood *et al.*, 1988), and both human (Schwander *et al.*, 1989) and rat (Brown *et al.*, 1989; Margot *et al.*, 1989) IGF-BP-2. It is from the amino acid sequences predicted by the cloned cDNAs for these BPs that most of our current knowledge of the structure of these proteins has been derived.

The first IGF-BP to be cloned and sequenced was human IGF-BP-1. The sequence was reported simultaneously by Lee *et al.* (1988) and by Brewer *et al.* (1988) from cDNAs isolated from two major sources of this protein: HEP-G2 cells and human decidua, respectively. Minor differences exist in the amino-terminal regions of the two sequences, but the sequence reported by Lee *et al.* (1988) has now been confirmed by several other groups. Brinkman *et al.* (1988b) isolated the cDNA for human IGF-BP-1 from a human placental library; Julkunen *et al.* (1988), from a decidual library. The complete human IGF-BP-1 (Lee *et al.*, 1988) is a 1553-bp DNA, with a 164-bp 5'-untranslated region, a 777-bp coding region, and a 612-bp 3'-untranslated region. The coding region thus encodes a total propeptide of 259 amino acids, 25 of which constitute a signal peptide (Table II). The mature protein consists of 234 amino acids, with a predicted M_r of 25,274.

The cDNA for the GH-dependent large serum BP, human IGF-BP-3, was cloned and sequenced by Wood *et al.* (1988). The complete cDNA is approximately 2500 bp in length. It contains an approximately 120-bp 5'-untranslated region, a 873-bp coding region, and approximately 1500 bp of 3'-untranslated sequence. A total propeptide of 291 amino acids, with a 27-amino-acid signal peptide, is predicted by the coding region sequence. The mature peptide of 264 amino acids has a predicted M_r of 28,500.

The cDNAs for a third class of BP, IGF-BP-2, have recently been isolated and sequenced, first in rats (Brown *et al.*, 1989; Margot *et al.*, 1989) and then

TABLE II
IGF-BP Sizes Predicted from cDNA Sequences

IGF-BP	Predicted sizes (amino acids)			M_r
	Total	Signal peptide	Mature peptide	
Human IGF-BP-1	259	25	234	25,274
Human IGF-BP-2	328	39	289	31,300
Rat IGF-BP-2	304	34	270	29,564
Human IGF-BP-3	291	27	264	28,500

in humans (Binkert *et al.*, 1989). In fact, Binkert *et al.* (1989) used the rat cDNA, isolated from a rat liver cDNA library (Margot *et al.*, 1989), to subsequently isolate the human cDNA. The rat and human cDNAs are 83% homologous (Binkert *et al.*, 1989). The rat cDNA is approximately 1500 bp in length, containing about 250 bp of 5'-untranslated region, 912 bp of coding region, and approximately 250 bp of 3'-untranslated region. A total propeptide of 304 amino acid residues is predicted, with a 34-residue signal peptide. The mature protein of 270 amino acids has a predicted M_r of 29,564. The human IGF-BP-2 cDNA is approximately the same size as the rat cDNA, but the coding region is 984 bp. The complete propeptide is 328 amino acids, with a 39-residue signal peptide. The mature protein consists of 289 amino acids, with a predicted M_r of 31,300.

2. Protein Structure

The determination of the primary amino acid sequences from the cloned cDNAs of the IGF-BPs reveals several interesting relationships. The most striking similarity in the BP structures is the conservation of cysteine residues. As shown in Fig. 17, each of the IGF-BPs has a cysteine-rich region at both the amino and carboxy termini of the proteins. In each of the IGF-BPs, there are 18 conserved cysteines, which are arranged in approximately the same spatial relationship in each BP. Only human IGF-BP-2 differs in the number of cysteines, having 20, but, nevertheless, it has the same conserved spacing of the common 18 cysteine residues. Conservation of the spatial relationships of the cysteines indicates that the secondary structure of the IGF-BPs, as dictated by disulfide bonds, must also be well conserved. Formation of a peptide-binding site in the molecule is dependent on disulfide bonds, as evidenced by the failure of the IGF-BPs to bind IGF-I or -II when the BPs are reduced. Other conformation-dependent functions of the IGF-BPs might also be the result of conserved disulfide bonds.

An analysis of the amino acid sequence of the IGF-BPs also revealed the presence of a conserved Arg–Gly–Asp sequence near the carboxy termini of all

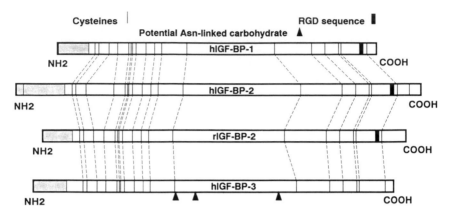

FIG. 17. Structural comparison of sequenced human (h) and rat (r) IGF-BPs. Shaded regions correspond to signal peptides.

of the IGF-BPs, with the exception of human IGF-BP-3. The Arg–Gly–Asp sequence has been shown to be the minimum required sequence in many extra-cellular matrix proteins that are bound by membrane receptors of the integrin protein family (Ruoslahti and Pierschbacher, 1987). It has been proposed that the IGF-BPs could bind to cell membranes through their Arg–Gly–Asp sequences. This hypothesis is supported by a report that a synthetic Arg–Gly–Asp sequence could block the binding of human IGF-BP-1 to cell membranes (Brewer *et al.*, 1988).

Despite these shared features, there are several significant differences among the primary amino acid sequences of the IGF-BPs. The sequences of the "spacer" regions between the conserved cysteines are not well conserved. Significant variability also exists in the signal peptide sequences. Perhaps the most significant difference among the IGF-BPs is in their glycosylation. Only human and rat IGF-BP-3s have been shown to be glycosylated through N-linked carbohydrates (Wood *et al.*, 1988; Zapf *et al.*, 1988; Lamson *et al.*, 1989b). Amino acid sequence analysis confirms that only the human IGF-BP-3 sequence possesses potential N-linked asparagine residues (Wood *et al.*, 1988). The significance of this glycosylation is unknown, but it might be related to the fact that only IGF-BP-3 is bound to an acid-labile subunit, thus constituting the large $M_r = 150,000$ serum complex.

Recombinant DNA techniques should facilitate more detailed structure–function characterization of each of the IGF-BPs. Current investigations using site-specific mutagenesis of the cloned cDNAs should be capable of pinpointing the regions of the BP molecules involved in the specific binding of IGF peptides, as well as other potential functions (e.g., membrane binding and secretion).

TABLE III
IGF-BP mRNA Expression

IGF-BP	mRNA size (kb)	Tissues expressed in
Human IGF-BP-1	1.5–1.6	Decidua, placenta, liver, HEP-G2 cells, breast cancer cells
Human IGF-BP-2	Unpublished	HEC-1A cells, breast cancer cells, secretory-phase endometrium
Rat IGF-BP-2	1.4–2.0	BRL-3A cells; fetal: liver, kidney, lung, brain, placenta, intestine; adult: brain, pituitary, liver, kidney, testes
Human IGF-BP-3	2.5	Liver, placenta, proliferative-phase endometrium, breast cancer cells, HEC-1A cells

3. mRNA Expression

The use of IGF-BP cDNAs as probes for mRNA by Northern analysis and *in situ* hybridization has made it possible to characterize the tissue expression of the IGF-BPs. Table III lists the reported sizes and currently identified sources of the IGF-BP mRNAs.

The expression of human IGF-BP-1 has been characterized most extensively. This BP is most prominently expressed in decidualized endometrium and, to a lesser extent, in endometrium during the secretory phase of the menstrual cycle (Brewer *et al.*, 1988; Giudice *et al.*, 1990a). While mRNA for human IGF-BP-1 has reportedly been detected in human endometrium by *in situ* hybridization, Fazleabas *et al.* (1989) have reported that in the baboon, mRNA for human IGF-BP-1 was detected in the glandular cells. IGF-BP-1 mRNA has also been detected by Northern blot analysis of RNA from human placenta (Brewer *et al.*, 1988; Lamson *et al.*, 1989b). It is conceivable, however, that the identified mRNA were actually in decidualized endometrial tissue contaminating the placental samples. IGF-BP-1 has also been reported in some human breast cancer cell lines (De Leon *et al.*, 1989a; Yee *et al.*, 1989), but it is not clear whether normal human breast tissue expresses mRNA for this BP.

Human IGF-BP-3 mRNA has been reported in RNA isolated from human liver (Wood *et al.*, 1988), placenta, and a human endometrial adenocarcinoma cell line, HEC-1A (Lamson *et al.*, 1989b). Additionally, mRNA for human IGF-BP-3 has been identified in normal human endometrium (Giudice *et al.*, 1990) and in several human breast cancer cell lines (De Leon *et al.*, 1989b). The expression of human IGF-BP-3 in endometrium and placenta could indicate that human IGF-BP-3, like human IGF-BP-1, is produced locally and might serve a paracrine role in regulating IGF access to specific receptors during pregnancy and fetal development.

The expression of IGF-BP-2 mRNA has been characterized in rats, but not yet in humans. It is the major IGF-BP mRNA expressed by the BRL-3A cell line (Brown *et al.*, 1989) and has been reported to be expressed in a wide range of fetal and adult tissues. Brown *et al.* (1989) have reported a marked decrease in rat IGF-BP-2 mRNA in adult (as compared to fetal) liver, kidneys, intestine, and lungs. A similar age-dependent decline in mRNA has been reported by Margot *et al.* (1989). However, both groups have reported that rat IGF-BP-2 levels remain high in the brain. It has been suggested that IGF-BP-2 plays a specific role in the central nervous system, because of its persistent mRNA expression and because preliminary studies indicate that it might be present in CSF (Lamson *et al.*, 1989a,b). This hypothesis is further supported by the report that rat IGF-BP-2 mRNA is detected in brain and in cultured neurons and glial cells (Lamson *et al.*, 1989a). Orlowski *et al.* (1989) have identified rat IGF-BP-2 mRNA expression in the choroid plexus by *in situ* hybridization. Because of the close similarities in rat and human IGF-BP-2s, it seems reasonable to expect that the expression of mRNA for this protein will be similar in humans.

4. Genomic Organization

Currently, genomic organization has been determined only for human IGF-BP-1 (Brinkman *et al.*, 1988a; Cubbage *et al.*, 1989). The organization of this gene is depicted in Fig. 18. The gene spans 5.2 kb and contains four exons. The promoter region has the consensus TATA and CAAT box sequence elements. Sequence analyses to date do not show any known tissue-specific regulatory elements, although studies in progress with promoter–chloramphenicol acetyl-transferase (CAT) constructs should reveal possible regulatory regions of the promoter.

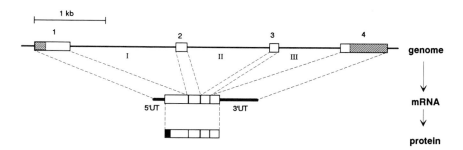

FIG. 18.   Genomic organization of the human IGF-BP-1 gene. ▨, Coding sequence; □, untranslated (UT) sequence; ■, signal peptide. [Adapted from Brinkman *et al.* (1988a) and from Cubbage *et al.* (1989).]

Analysis of the genomic DNA by restriction enzyme digestion with multiple enzymes has indicated that there is a single gene for human IGF-BP-1 (Brewer *et al.*, 1988; Brinkman *et al.*, 1988b; Julkunen *et al.*, 1988). S1 nuclease protection analysis of the promoter region showed the presence of a single transcription start site, arguing against the possibility of multiple promoters. Southern blot analysis of human–rodent somatic cell hybrids has indicated that the IGF-BP-1 gene is located on human chromosome 7 (Brinkman *et al.*, 1988a).

As the genomic organizations of the other IGF-BPs are determined, a number of questions concerning structural and functional relationships among the IGF-BPs should be answered. Promoter region analyses could reveal possible regulatory elements or factors. Comparison of genomic structure should determine whether the IGF-BP genes are derived from a common ancestral gene. Determination of chromosomal location of each of the IGF-BP genes should indicate whether the IGF-BP genes constitute a contiguous gene family on chromosome 7 or have translocated to other chromosomal locations. Comparisons of structure among species should also provide a measure of IGF-BP gene conservation through evolution.

E.   IGF-BPs IN BIOLOGICAL FLUIDS

1.   Human Serum

Characterization of the various IGF-BPs in human serum has been most convincingly performed by Hardouin *et al.* (1987), who combined gel chromatography and Western ligand blotting to identify five molecular forms of IGF-BPs in adult serum. As shown in Figs. 12 and 13, the large complex from gel chromatography contains only the $M_r = 41,500$ and $M_r = 38,500$ BPs, while the small complex contains all five BPs. The $M_r = 41,500$ and $M_r = 38,500$ BPs were found to be GH dependent, consistent with the binding subunits of the $M_r = 150,000$ IGF-BP-3. In hypopituitary serum the $M_r = 41,500$ and $M_r = 38,500$ BPs are diminished, while the $M_r = 34,000$ and $M_r = 30,000$ BPs are increased (Fig. 7). It seems probable that the $M_r = 30,000$ BP represents IGF-BP-1, while the $M_r = 34,000$ (which also appears prominently in CSF) potentially represents IGF-BP-2. The identity of the $M_r = 24,000$ BP remains uncertain at this time, although it is noteworthy that it appears prominently in human seminal fluid (Rosenfeld *et al.*, 1990) and in conditioned media from human fibroblasts (Conover *et al.*, 1989) and several human breast cancer cell lines (De Leon *et al.*, 1989a) (see below). This BP is not recognized by antibodies against IGF-BP-1, -2, and -3 (De Leon *et al.*, 1989, 1990; Rosenfeld *et al.*, 1990) and represents either a fourth IGF-BP or a proteolytic fragment of one of the other IGF-BPs.

2. Rat Serum

The existence of $M_r = 150,000$ and $M_r = 40,000$ BPs in rat serum was first demonstrated by Moses *et al.* (1976) (Fig. 3) and by Kaufmann *et al.* (1977). White *et al.* (1982) (Fig. 4) subsequently showed that the large BP predominated in adult serum, while the small BP appeared prominently in fetal serum. Romanus *et al.* (1986), using a polyclonal antibody generated against purified BP from BRL-3A-conditioned media, demonstrated that this antibody recognized the $M_r = 40,000$ BP from neonatal rat serum, suggesting that this small BP is related to IGF-BP-2.

The ontogeny of rat serum BPs has been further investigated by Donovan *et al.* (1989) (Figs. 19–21). Seven molecular forms of BP were identified by Western ligand blotting, with apparent M_rs of 42,000, 41,000, 40,000, 38,000, 28,000, 26,000, and 22,000. Following deglycosylation with endoglycosidase F, the four largest bands were reduced in size to two bands with apparent M_rs of 35,000 and 32,000; the $M_r = 28,000$, 26,000, and 22,000 BPs were unchanged. The $M_r =$

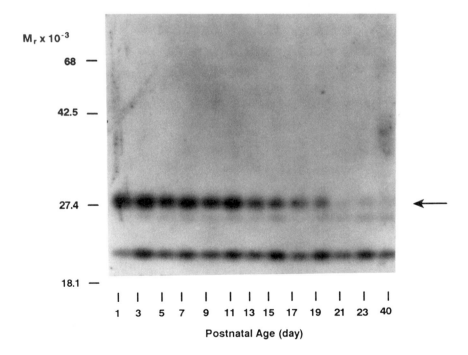

FIG. 19. Ontogenic pattern of rat serum BPs visualized with [^{125}I]IGF-I by Western ligand blot. The arrow indicates the predominant neonatal BP, with an apparent molecular weight of 28,000, presumably representing rat IGF-BP-2. (From Donovan *et al.*, 1989.)

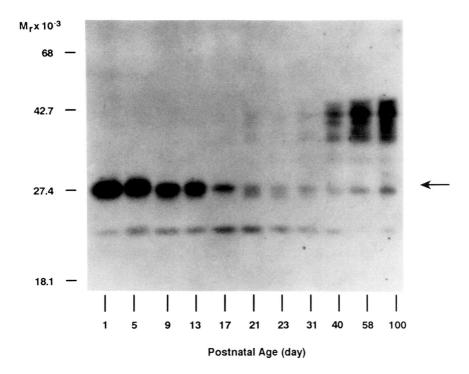

FIG. 20.   Ontogenic pattern of rat serum BPs visualized with [^{125}I]IGF-II by Western ligand blot. The arrow indicates the predominant neonatal BP, with an apparent molecular weight of 28,000, presumably representing rat IGF-BP-2. (From Donovan *et al.*, 1989.)

28,000, 26,000, and 22,000 BPs were found in neonatal rat serum, with the $M_r = 28,000$ BP predominating. With increasing age the $M_r = 28,000$ BP decreased in amount, and the four $M_r = 38,000–42,000$ BPs appeared at approximately 19 days of age.

Comparison of Western ligand blots of neonatal rat serum, BRL-3A-conditioned media, rat amniotic fluid, and rat CSF demonstrated that all contained a prominent $M_r = 28,000$ BP that was precipitated by antibody to purified rat IGF-BP-2 (data not shown) and by the polyclonal antibody α-HEC-1, generated against an $M_r = 31,000–34,000$ BP found in HEC-1A-conditioned media and believed to be human IGF-BP-2 (Lamson *et al.*, 1989a,b; Donovan *et al.*, 1989) (Fig. 21). These findings indicate that the predominant BP in neonatal rat serum is structurally and immunologically similar to the major BRL-3A, amniotic fluid, and CSF BPs. IGF-BP-3 in rat serum appears during the third week of life and gradually increases to adult levels.

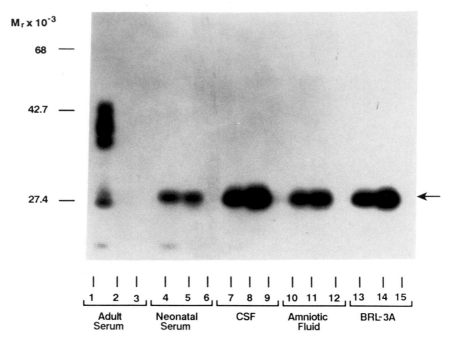

FIG. 21.   Immunoprecipitation of rat IGF-BPs with α-HEC-1. Autoradiograph of a Western ligand blot of adult rat serum (day 100 postnatal, lanes 1–3), neonatal rat serum (day 3 postnatal, lanes 4–6), rat CSF (lanes 7–9), rat amniotic fluid (lanes 10–12), and BRL-3A-conditioned media (lanes 13–15). Each sample is represented in three lanes, the first lane being a ligand blot of the original sample (lanes 1, 4, 7, 10, and 13), the second lane being an immunoprecipitation with α-HEC-1 (lanes 2, 5, 8, 11, and 14), and the third lane being an immunoprecipitation with normal rabbit serum (lanes 3, 6, 9, 12, and 15). The arrow indicates the presumptive rat IGF-BP-2. (From Donovan *et al.*, 1989.)

3.   Porcine Serum

McCusker *et al.* (1988, 1989) have studied the ontogeny and regulation of serum IGF-BPs in the pig. Fetal and postnatal sera were found to contain six molecular forms of IGF-BPs, with M_rs of 220,000, 43,000, 39,000, 34,000, 29,000, and 24,000. The serum concentrations of all six BPs appear to increase with gestational age. In the fetal pig the $M_r = 34,000$ and $M_r = 29,000$ forms predominate, while postnatally the major forms are $M_r = 43,000$ and $M_r = 39,000$, mirroring the findings in the rat.

Walton *et al.* (1989) have recently purified an acid-stable IGF-BP from adult porcine serum. This protein consisted of two major species, with $M_r = 45,000$ and $M_r = 41,000$. Amino-terminal sequence demonstrated that 11 of the first 12 residues from this porcine plasma BP were identical to those of rat IGF-BP-3; seven of 12 residues are identical to those of human IGF-BP-3.

4. Lymph

The presence of IGF peptides and IGF-BPs in lymph was originally reported by Cohen and Nissley (1976) and by Moses *et al.* (1979). Recently, Binoux and Hossenlopp (1988) demonstrated that concentrations of IGF-I and -II in human lymph were 10–30% of corresponding serum levels, with a similar proportion of each peptide. By Western ligand blotting they demonstrated the presence in lymph of the five molecular forms of IGF-BP which they identified in serum. However, less than 10% of the binding activity of lymph was found complexed to the large $M_r = 150,000$ IGF-BP. These data suggest that the $M_r = 150,000$ IGF-BP is not capable of crossing the capillary barrier and might act to retain IGF peptides within the vascular compartment. On the other hand, the $M_r = 34,000$, 30,000, and 24,000 molecular forms appear capable of crossing the capillary barrier and might be involved in transporting the IGFs to their target cells.

5. Cerebrospinal Fluid

In 1982 Binoux *et al.* identified IGF-binding activity in human CSF. By Western ligand blotting Hossenlopp *et al.* (1986a) demonstrated five molecular forms of IGF-BPs in human CSF. These BPs ranged from $M_r = 24,000$ to 41,000, as in serum, but with the major BP at $M_r = 34,000$. Rosenfeld *et al.* (1989a) confirmed the presence of these five molecular forms (Fig. 22) and showed that the major CSF IGF-BP migrated on SDS–PAGE at a slightly higher apparent molecular weight than did IGF-BP-1 from HEP-G2 cells (Fig. 23). They concluded that the major CSF IGF-BP was structurally and immunologically distinct from IGF-BP-1 on the basis of (1) the slightly higher apparent M_r of the CSF BP on SDS–PAGE; (2) the 10- to 20-fold higher affinity of the CSF BP for IGF-II over IGF-I; and (3) the failure of the major CSF BP to be recognized by several different antibodies directed against IGF-BP-1 (Figs. 8 and 11).

Whether the major CSF IGF-BP, which migrates at $M_r = 30,000–34,000$, represents IGF-BP-2 remains uncertain. Lamson *et al.* (1989a) demonstrated that the CSF BP resembles a BP found in conditioned media of the human endometrial adenocarcinoma cell line HEC-1A: (1) the HEC-1A BP and CSF-BP migrate identically on SDS–PAGE; (2) neither BP is glycosylated; and (3) antibodies generated against partially purified HEC-1A BPs immunoprecipitate the major CSF BP (Fig. 15), as well as a similar-sized BP in conditioned media from a number of neural primary cultures and cell lines (Fig. 9). Polyclonal antibodies against HEC-1A BPs and rat IGF-BP-2 apparently immunoprecipitate the same-sized BP in rat CSF and a slightly larger BP in human CSF (data not shown). Furthermore, *in situ* hybridization studies have demonstrated abundant mRNA

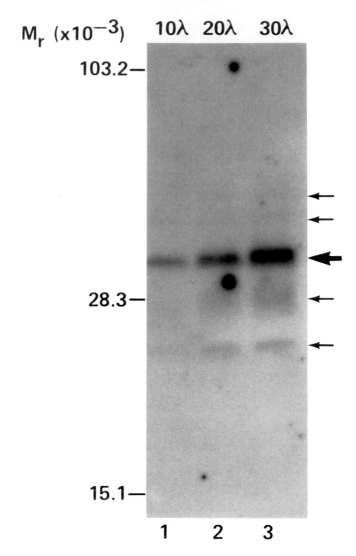

FIG. 22.   Western ligand blot of human CSF. Ten (lane 1), 20 (lane 2), or 30 (lane 3) microliters of CSF were electrophoresed through 12% SDS–PAGE, transferred onto nitrocellulose, incubated with [^{125}I]IGF-II, and visualized by autoradiography. Arrows indicate the five visualized bands, the large arrow indicating the major band, at an apparent molecular weight of 34,000. (From Rosenfeld *et al.*, 1989a.)

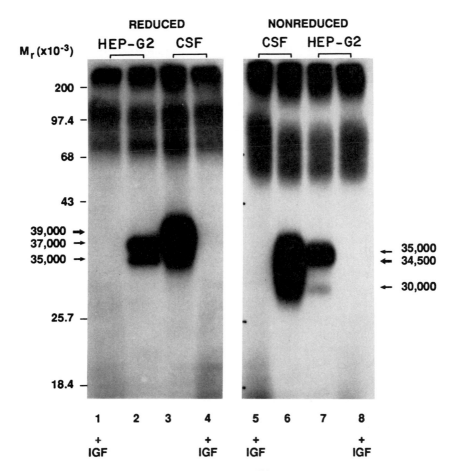

FIG. 23. Autoradiogram of 12% SDS–PAGE of [^{125}I]IGF-II cross-linked to HEP-G2-conditioned medium (lanes 1, 2, 7, and 8) and CSF (lanes 3–6) and run under reducing (lanes 1–4) and nonreducing (lanes 5–8) conditions. Lanes 1, 4, 5, and 8 indicate cross-linking in the presence of excess unlabeled IGF. (From Rosenfeld *et al.*, 1989a.)

for rat IGF-BP-2 in the choroid plexus, the site of CSF production (Orlowski *et al.*, 1989).

However, Roghani *et al.* (1989) recently reported purification of an apparently different IGF-BP from human CSF. Amino-terminal sequence data show nonidentity with the amino acid sequence deduced from the human IGF-BP-2 cDNA by Schwander *et al.* (1989). While it is possible that Roghani *et al.* (1989) have purified a minor BP component of the CSF, it is also conceivable that this BP shares epitopes with IGF-BP-2, resulting in its recognition by the two polyclonal antibodies described above.

6. Amniotic Fluid

Amniotic fluid has been shown to be, as described above, a rich source of IGF-BP-1, whether it be termed "amniotic fluid BP" (Drop *et al.*, 1984; Povoa *et al.*, 1984a), "PP12" (Koistinen *et al.*, 1986), or "α_1-PEG" (Bell *et al.*, 1988). Several groups have purified IGF-BP-1 from amniotic fluid and have demonstrated its identity with the BP found in conditioned media of HEP-G2 cells (D'Ercole *et al.*, 1985; Povoa *et al.*, 1985). Baxter *et al.* (1987) further demonstrated the presence of both BP-28 (IGF-BP-1) and BP-53 (IGF-BP-3) in amniotic fluid and showed that levels of both BPs decline with increasing fetal maturity.

The rat amniotic fluid BP has been less well characterized. Specifically, the rat equivalent of IGF-BP-1 has not yet been identified. Interestingly, Donovan *et al.* (1989) demonstrated that the major rat amniotic fluid BP is similar in size to the BRL-3A BP (rat IGF-BP-2) and to the major BP found in rat CSF. Furthermore, α-HEC-1 immunoprecipitates all three of these BPs, suggesting that the major BP in rat CSF and rat amniotic fluid is IGF-BP-2 (Fig. 21). Preliminary data indicate, however, that rat granulosa cells secrete an IGF-BP of the same approximate size as rat IGF-BP-2, but which does not immunoprecipitate with antibodies against rat IGF-BP-2 (Adashi *et al.*, 1990). Since human granulosa cells have been shown to secrete IGF-BP-1 (Suikkari *et al.*, 1989), it seems probable that rat granulosa cells are secreting a similar peptide.

7. Follicular Fluid

In 1984 Koistinen reported immunoreactive PP12 (IGF-BP-1) in preovulatory follicular fluid. Seppala *et al.* (1984) demonstrated by RIA that follicular fluid from women hyperstimulated for *in vitro* fertilization contained 6–230 μg/liter of PP12-like immunoreactive material. Follicular PP12 was indistinguishable from the PP12 found in amniotic fluid. These authors reported a positive correlation between PP12 and follicular fluid concentrations of estradiol or progesterone. Biopsies of hyperstimulated preovulatory follicles indicated that PP12 was identified only in lutenizied granulosa cells. More recently, Suikkari *et al.* (1989) demonstrated the synthesis of PP12 in [^{35}S]methionine-labeled granulosa cells obtained after ovarian hyperstimulation for *in vitro* fertilization and showed that media conditioned by such granulosa cells had increased PP12 concentrations over a 72-hour culture period.

It is probable that follicular fluid contains other IGF-BPs besides IGF-BP-1. Ui *et al.* (1989) have recently demonstrated that porcine follicular fluid contains an $M_r = 45,000$ inhibitor of follicle-stimulating hormone action on granulosa cells. Coincubation of stoichiometric amounts of either IGF-I or -II with the inhibitor neutralized its inhibitory effect. Amino-terminal sequence analysis showed identity with human IGF-BP-3 in 33 of the first 41 residues. Recent data from our laboratories indicate the presence of IGF-BP-1, -2, and -3 in follicular fluid, by both Western ligand blotting and immunoprecipitation (Giudice *et al.*, 1990b).

8. Seminal Plasma

The character and role of IGF-BPs in the male reproductive system have been less well studied than in the female reproductive system, although Baxter *et al.* (1984a) identified IGF-binding activity of $M_r = 40,000$ in human seminal plasma. Seppala *et al.* (1985) found PP12 (IGF-BP-1)-like immunoreactivity in human seminal plasma, and suggested that levels were similar to those found in normal male serum. We have recently characterized IGF-BPs in normal, oligospermic, and azospermic human seminal plasma by Western ligand blotting and immunoprecipitation (Rosenfeld *et al.*, 1990) (Fig. 24). No binding activity was observed at $M_r = 37,000-40,000$ unlike the glycosylated IGF-BP-3 found in serum. A prominent band was observed at $M_r = 31,000$ in all samples; immunoprecipitation with HEC-1 indicated that this band probably represents IGF-BP-2. An intense band was also observed at $M_r = 24,000$ in most, although not all, specimens. This band failed to react with antibodies against IGF-BP-1, -2, or -3 and possibly represents a fourth discrete IGF-BP (see above). A faint band observed at $M_r = 28,000$ was seen in some samples and might represent IGF-BP-1 or a degradation product of IGF-BP-2 or -3.

The source of seminal plasma IGF-BPs remains to be elucidated. Presumably, these proteins are synthesized within the male reproductive system, since their relative quantities do not resemble the IGF-BP pattern seen in normal adult male serum. Sertoli cells have been shown to produce IGF-I (Smith *et al.*, 1987), as well as other plasma proteins (e.g., transferrin and androgen BP), and are embryologically related to granulosa cells, which are known to produce IGF-BPs (see above). Preliminary data from our laboratory indicate that the prostate, too, might be a source of IGF-BPs.

9. Milk

The presence of growth factors in breast milk is of particular interest, since such factors could have important roles in the proliferation and maturation of the intestinal epithelium or, potentially, are absorbed intact from the gut and transferred to the infant. Alternatively, IGF peptides could represent excretory products of the lactating breast. Various growth factors, including epidermal growth factor, insulin, and IGF-I, have been reported in human milk (Baxter *et al.*, 1984b; Corps *et al.*, 1988). IGF-BPs in milk could play a role in the bioavailability of IGF peptides to the gut mucosa and/or the infant.

In 1984 Baxter *et al.* (1984b) reported the presence of immunoreactive IGF-I and carrier protein in human milk. Using an RIA for PP12/IGF-BP-1, Suikkari (1989) subsequently demonstrated the presence of IGF-BP-1 in human milk. Levels of milk IGF-BP-1 declined from 165 ± 80 μg/liter to 97 ± 70 μg/liter between postpartum hours 4 and 92, paralleling the decline in milk IGF-I levels. A positive correlation was identified between the milk levels or IGF-I and IGF-BP-1.

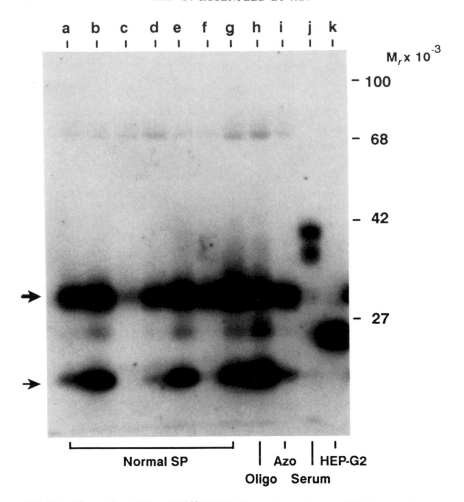

FIG. 24. Western ligand blot with [^{125}I]IGF-II of normal seminal plasma (SP, lanes a–g), and SP from an oligospermic subject (Oligo, lane h), and an azospermic subject (Azo, lane i). Lane j shows normal adult male serum, and lane k shows conditioned medium from HEP-G2 cells. The thick arrow indicates the 31,000-molecular-weight BP (presumably human IGF-BP-2); the thin arrow indicates the 24,000-molecular-weight BP. (From Rosenfeld *et al.*, 1990.)

It is noteworthy that previous studies of IGF-BPs in milk have been limited by assay methodologies. Charcoal assays or affinity cross-linking studies of non-acid-chromatographed milk only detect unsaturated BPs. RIAs for PP12 only detect those BPs with identical epitopes (i.e., IGF-BP-1). Our recent studies of rat milk have demonstrated the presence of IGF-BP-1, -2, and -3 on days 5–17 of lactation (Donovan *et al.*, 1990).

10. Endometrium

As described in Sections III,C,1 and III,E,6, there exists a considerable literature on IGF-BP-1 in decidualized endometrium (Rutanen *et al.*, 1985, 1986a,b; Koistinen *et al.*, 1986). Indeed, IGF-BP-1 was extensively studied in parallel investigations of amniotic fluid IGF-BP, PP12, and α_1-PEG. In a series of elegant studies, Rutanen *et al.* (1985, 1986a) demonstrated the synthesis and secretion of PP12 by early pregnancy decidua, showing that PP12 is primarily a protein of decidual, rather than trophoblastic, origin. Additionally, explants from secretory-phase endometrium produced immunoreactive PP12 and could be shown by metabolic labeling to synthesize *de novo* PP12 (Rutanen *et al.*, 1985). Proliferative-phase endometrium, on the other hand, contained no PP12, unless cultured and treated with progesterone (Rutanen *et al.*, 1986b).

Concurrently, Bell and colleagues demonstrated that α_1-PEG is a major secretory protein of stromal cells of the decidua in both humans and baboons (Bell *et al.*, 1988; Waites *et al.*, 1988). The proposed site of synthesis and/or storage is the perinuclear region of the hypertrophied stromal or decidual cell. In the nonpregnant baboon α_1-PEG is primarily localized to the deep glandular epithelium; in nonpregnant humans α_1-PEG is generally identified in stromal cells undergoing predecidual cell differentiation, characteristic of late secretory-phase endometrium.

The functional significance of this highly regulated production of IGF-BP-1 has not been established. It has been suggested that such BPs could be involved in the regulation of endometrial proliferation or, alternatively, in the regulation of trophoblastic proliferation following implantation (Rutanen *et al.*, 1988; Ritvos *et al.*, 1988).

Recent studies from our laboratories have demonstrated that the endometrial adenocarcinoma cell line HEC-1A synthesizes and secretes IGF-BP-2 and -3, but not IGF-BP-1 (Lamson *et al.*, 1989b) (Fig. 15). These observations suggested that endometrial tissue might be capable of producing other IGF-BPs besides IGF-BP-1. Giudice *et al.* (1990a) have recently shown concordant expression of mRNA for all three IGF-BPs in normal human secretory-phase endometrium, but with little detectable mRNA in the proliferative phase.

11. Breast Cancer

An extensive literature already exists on the production of IGF-I and -II by a variety of human breast cancer cell lines (Huff *et al.*, 1986, 1988; Dickson *et al.*, 1986; Minuto *et al.*, 1989). In some of these cell lines, a dramatic mitogenic effect of insulin and IGF-I and -II has been demonstrated, leading to a theory of autocrine stimulation of human breast cancer cell proliferation (Furlanetto and DiCarlo, 1984; Myal *et al.*, 1984; Lippman *et al.*, 1986; Dickson *et al.*, 1986). However, De Leon *et al.* (1988, 1989, 1990) have recently demonstrated the

TABLE IV
IGF-BPs in Human Breast Cancer Cell Lines

IGF-BP	Hs578T	MCF-7
IGF-BP-1		
Ligand blot	+	−
Immunoreactive	+	−
mRNA	+	−
IGF-BP-2		
Ligand blot	−	+
Immunoreactive	−	+
mRNA	−	+
IGF-BP-3		
Ligand blot	+	−
Immunoreactive	+	−
mRNA	+	−
BP-24[a]		
Ligand blot	+	+
Immunoreactive	ND	ND
mRNA	ND	ND

[a]Antibodies and cDNA for the $M_r = 24,000$ IGF-BP are not currently available. ND, Not done.

production of IGF-BPs by four human breast cancer cell lines: MCF-7, T-47D, MDA-231, and Hs578T (Table IV). Figure 25 demonstrates the presence of four molecular forms of IGF-BPs in conditioned media from two of these cell lines. mRNA for IGF-BP-1 has been identified in Hs578T and MDA-231 (De Leon *et al.*, 1989a; Yee *et al.*, 1989); mRNA for IGF-BP-3 has been demonstrated in Hs578T (De Leon *et al.*, 1990); mRNA for IGF-BP-2 has been identified in MCF-7 and T-47D (De Leon *et al.*, 1990). The M_r - 24,000 IGF-BP has also been identified in conditioned media from some of these cell lines.

The presence of IGF-binding activity in conditioned media from cultured human breast cancer cell lines has been confirmed by studies by Minuto *et al.* (1989) and by Yee *et al.* (1989). The latter study demonstrated immunoprecipitation of metabolically labeled IGF-BP-1 by MDA-231 cells. mRNA for IGF-BP-1 in Hs578T and MDA-231 cells was identified by RNase protection assay, confirming the observations of De Leon *et al.* (1989).

The presence of IGF-BPs in the conditioned media of these cell lines probably explains the wide discrepancies in the IGF-I and -II concentrations reported (Huff *et al.*, 1988; Karey and Sirbasku, 1988). IGF-BPs have been shown to result in the erroneous determination of IGF concentrations, unless the BPs are rigorously removed or saturated (De Leon *et al.*, 1990) (see Section III,G). Indeed, cell lines which have been previously reported to produce large quantities of IGFs have now been shown to lack mRNA for these peptides (Yee *et al.*, 1989; Peres

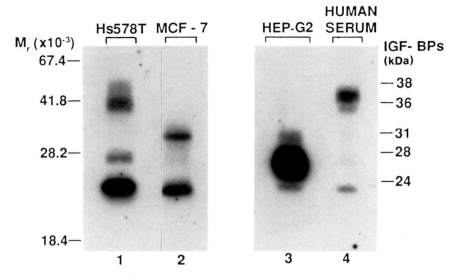

FIG. 25. Western ligand blot of conditioned medium from the human breast cell cancer lines Hs578T and MCF-7 (lanes 1 and 2, respectively), HEP-G2 cells (lane 3), and adult human serum (lane 4). [^{125}I]IGF-I was used as radioligand. (From De Leon *et al.*, 1990.)

et al., 1987). It is interesting to speculate that if the IGF system is involved in autocrine/paracrine/endocrine regulation of human breast cancer cell proliferation, it might be through the local production of IGF-BPs, which serve to modulate the effects of IGF-1 and/or -II on these cells.

12. Fibroblasts

Romanus *et al.* (1987) demonstrated that rat embryo fibroblasts produce an IGF carrier protein with a size similar to that of the rat IGF-BP-2 produced by BRL-3A cells. Antibodies against rat IGF-BP-2 immunoprecipitate a [^{35}S]cysteine-labeled $M_r = 33,000$ protein produced by these fibroblasts. This protein is synthesized as an $M_r = 35,000$ precursor in reticulocyte lysate translation systems directed by RNA from both BRL-3A cells and rat embryo fibroblasts.

Adams *et al.* (1983) first demonstrated the release of BP activity into the conditioned medium of cultured human fibroblasts. DeVroede *et al.* (1986) and Clemmons *et al.* (1986) showed that human fibroblasts secrete an $M_r = 35,000$ IGF-BP, which associates with the cell surface and can modulate binding of IGF-I to cell membrane receptors. Martin and Baxter (1988) subsequently demonstrated that neonatal human skin fibroblasts in monolayer culture produce no BP-28 (IGF-BP-1), but produce two IGF-BPs which resemble—in size, binding characteristics, and antibody reaction—plasma BP-53 (IGF-BP-3). Conover *et*

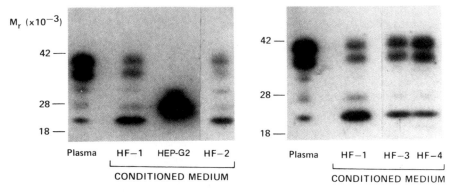

FIG. 26. Western ligand blots of conditioned medium from cultured human fibroblasts (HF), HEP-G2 cells, and normal human plasma, using [^{125}I]IGF-I as radioligand. (From Conover *et al.*, 1989.)

al. (1989), using Western ligand blotting, showed that human fibroblast-conditioned medium contains five molecular forms of IGF-BPs: $M_r = 41,500, 37,000, 32,000, 28,000$, and $23,000$ (Fig. 26), more or less resembling the BPs found in human serum by Hardouin *et al.* (1987). When compared with adult plasma, the lowest-M_r band, $M_r = 23,000$, was particularly prominent.

13. Central Nervous System

In 1981 Binoux *et al.* reported that explants of rat brain and pituitary produced IGF carrier proteins. However, except for characterization of BP activity in the CSF, there was little by way of further identification of BP activity in the central nervous system over the next 7 years. In 1988 Han *et al.* reported that conditioned media from cultured rat astroglial cells contained two species of IGF-BP of $M_r = 40,000$. The smaller of the two BPs was recognized by antibodies against the BRL-3A BP (IGF-BP-2). Concurrently, Sturm *et al.* (1989) reported that cross-linking studies of conditioned media from the B104 rat neuroblastoma cell line revealed two bands at $M_r = 36,500$ and $M_r = 39,000$, suggesting the production and secretion of low-M_r BPs.

Recent studies have extended our knowledge of IGF-BPs produced by various central nervous system tissues. Conditioned medium from primary cultures of rat anterior pituitary cells contained high-affinity IGF-BPs with apparent M_rs of 35,000, 27,000, and 24,000 (Rosenfeld *et al.*, 1989b). The $M_r = 27,000$ IGF-BP predominates in media from cultured neurointermediate pituitary cells. The $M_r = 35,000$ IGF-BP is glycosylated and probably represents IGF-BP-3. The $M_r = 27,000$ BP is nonglycosylated and resembles the BP of BRL-3A cells, suggesting that it is IGF-BP-2.

Western ligand blots of rat astrocytes, fetal rat neuronal cells, rat CSF, and

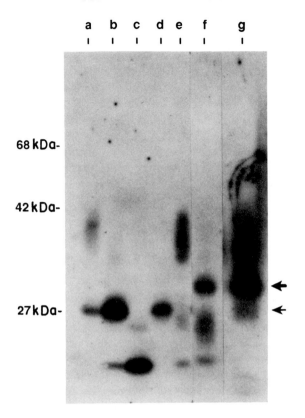

FIG. 27. Autoradiograph of a Western ligand blot (10% gel) of conditioned media from newborn rat astrocytes (lane a), fetal rat neuronal cells (lane b), B104 cells (lane c), BRL-3A cells (lane d), adult rat serum (lane e), human CSF (lane f), and HEC-1A cells (lane g). [^{125}I]IGF-I was used as radioligand. (From Lamson *et al.*, 1989a.)

BRL-3A cells identified an IGF-BP of identical size (Ocrant *et al.*, 1989; Lamson *et al.*, 1989a) (Fig. 27). Immunoprecipitation studies with α-HEC-1, a polyclonal antibody which recognizes the major BP in human CSF (presumably IGF-BP-2; see above), were positive for BRL-3A cells, neurons, astrocytes, neurointermediate pituitary, and rat CSF, suggesting that all produce IGF-BP-2 (Lamson *et al.*, 1989a) (Fig. 9). Both anterior pituitary and astrocyte cultures also produced the larger glycosylated BP, presumably IGF-BP-3. B104 neuroblastoma cells produced two smaller BPs, with $M_r = 26,000$ (minor band) and $M_r = 23,000$ (major band). This latter BP is also found in fetal neuronal cultures (Ocrant *et al.*, 1989; Lamson *et al.*, 1989a). The presence of IGF-BP-2 in the rat central nervous system is further documented by Northern blots, which show that total cellular RNA from BRL-3A cells, cultured fetal neurons, cultured newborn astroglial cells, adult rat brain, pituitary, and hypothalamus, and fetal rat brain and liver all demonstrate the same 1.4-kb single band when probed with a 36-base oligomer of the coding-region sequence of rat IGF-BP-2 (Lamson *et al.*, 1989a).

The role of IGF-BPs in the physiology of the pituitary and the central nervous system remains uncertain, due at least in part to the fact that the role of the IGFs in the central nervous system is still unknown. However, it is clear that these BPs can modulate the access of IGFs to the pituitary and the hypothalamus, thereby potentially influencing feedback control on GH production and secretion (Ceda *et al.*, 1987). Additionally, they might influence the access of brain IGF receptors to IGF peptides produced locally or delivered from the vascular compartment (Ocrant *et al.*, 1988).

F. REGULATION OF THE IGF-BPs

1. In Vitro

Hepatic production of IGF-BPs has been studied using liver explants, isolated liver perfusion systems, and primary hepatocyte cultures. Schwander *et al.* (1983) detected an M_r = 35,000 BP in rat liver perfusates, but attempts to evaluate GH dependency were equivocal. Secretion of this BP was 62% of normal in hypox rats, and 79% of normal in GH-treated hypox rats. Similarly, Scott *et al.* (1985a,b), studying adult rat hepatocytes in primary culture, demonstrated a 50% increase in BP activity following bovine GH treatment, but saw no effect when insulin was added to the cultures. On the other hand, Binoux *et al.* (1984) reported that the production of IGF and IGF-BP by rat liver explants was regulated differently. IGF levels were increased by GH or insulin treatment, but no significant effect on carrier production was observed.

Lewitt and Baxter (1989) have evaluated the regulation of BP-28 (IGF-BP-1) production by cultured human fetal liver explants. BP production was stimulated by theophylline, forskolin, and glucagon; BP levels were decreased following the addition of dexamethasone or insulin. Additionally, BP levels were inversely related to glucose concentrations in the medium, suggesting that intracellular glucose availability might be the critical factor in regulating hepatic IGF-BP-1 production. Recently, Hossenlopp *et al.* (1987) have demonstrated that human liver culture medium contains the same five molecular forms of BP seen in serum (M_rs of 41,500, 38,500, 34,000, 30,000, and 24,000). The exact nature and regulation of each of these forms remain to be elucidated.

Although HEP-G2 cells produce large quantities of IGF-BP-1 (Moses *et al.*, 1983; Powell *et al.*, 1987), they have not proved to be a particularly useful model for studying hormonal regulation *in vitro*. On the other hand, explants of secretory-phase endometrium have been shown to produce IGF-BP-1, and secretion can be significantly increased by the addition of progesterone (Rutanen *et al.*, 1986a). The same is true for uterine decidual cells and decidual explants (Rutanen *et al.*, 1985), but not for trophoblast cultures (Rutanen *et al.*, 1986b).

Schmid *et al.* (1989) evaluated the production of IGF-BPs by the rat osteoblast cell line PyMS. They determined that GH and IGF-I stimulate and cortisol inhibits an $M_r = 49,000–42,000$ species of BP, presumably representing rat IGF-BP-3. Interestingly, the addition of IGF-I also appeared to induce a nonglycosylated $M_r = 32,000$ BP, which is further stimulated by cortisol.

Martin and Baxter (1988) demonstrated that neonatal human skin fibroblasts produce BP-53 (IGF-BP-3), but no BP-28 (IGF-BP-1). Levels of immunoreactive IGF-BP-3 in conditioned media were stimulated in a dose-dependent manner by epidermal growth factor. Conover *et al.* (1989) recently reported that normal human dermal fibroblasts produce at least five molecular forms of IGF-BPs (M_rs of 41,500, 37,000, 32,000, 28,000, and 23,000). GH treatment resulted in an increase in BP activity, while glucocorticoids diminished binding activity. Insulin, epidermal growth factor, and platelet-derived growth factor had no effect. By comparison, HEP-G2 IGF-binding activity was enhanced by progesterone, decreased by insulin, and unaffected by GH.

2. *In Vivo*

a. Ontogeny.   The ontogeny of serum BPs in rats and pigs has been documented by Donovan *et al.* (1989) and by McCusker *et al.* (1988, 1989), respectively, and is described in Sections III,E,2 and III,E,3. The ontogeny of IGF-BPs in human sera has been less completely documented. Borsi *et al.* (1982) have reported that over 50% of the radioreceptor-assayable IGF peptide content in cord blood circulated as part of an $M_r = 50,000$ complex, in contrast to adult plasma, in which the majority of the IGF peptide content was found as part of an $M_r = 150,000$ complex. Unsaturated IGF-BP activity, with an $M_r = 40,000–50,000$, was strikingly elevated in newborns. These observations were extended by Drop *et al.* (1984), who, using an RIA for IGF-BP-1, showed that levels were elevated in fetal blood, fell significantly at birth, and declined further throughout childhood until adult life. It is not clear at this time, however, whether the major serum BP in the fetus/newborn is IGF-BP-2 [as suggested by Donovan *et al.* (1989) in the rat], IGF-BP-1, or both. Baxter and Martin (1986) developed an RIA for BP-53 (IGF-BP-3) and demonstrated that serum levels of this BP rise progressively during childhood, thus paralleling the increase in serum IGF-I levels. The estimated serum level of IGF-BP-3 in healthy adults is 6 μg/ml. This quantity of IGF-BP-3 is roughly equimolar with concentrations of total circulating IGF peptide, further suggesting that in serum this BP is saturated with endogenous IGFs.

b. Hormonal Regulation of IGF-BPs.   Multiple studies have demonstrated that IGF-BP-3 is GH dependent (Baxter and Martin, 1986; McCusker *et al.*,

1988). Levels are approximately doubled in acromegaly and significantly decreased in GH deficiency. It has been shown, however, that IGF-BP-3 and IGF-I responses to GH treatment are not necessarily coordinated. Unlike IGF-BP-1, IGF-BP-3 levels are not significantly affected by food intake and show little diurnal variability (Baxter and Cowell, 1987).

Early studies of the regulation of IGF-BP-1 involved clinical evaluation of PP12, before the eventual demonstration of identity between these two proteins. In 1982 Rutanen et al. developed an RIA for PP12 and demonstrated increasing serum levels during pregnancy and in patients with trophoblastic disease and ovarian cancer. Concomitantly, studies of the amniotic fluid BP also showed increasing serum levels during pregnancy, as well as dramatically high levels in amniotic fluid (Drop et al., 1984; Povoa et al., 1984a). Although some studies also suggest that IGF-BP-1 concentrations are inversely related to GH status (Hintz et al., 1981; Drop et al., 1984), it is possible that some of the unsaturated $M_r = 40,000$ BP activity might actually represent IGF-BP-2.

Busby et al. (1988b), however, using an RIA for IGF-BP-1, have shown that the mean plasma level of IGF-BP-1 in 15 normal fasting adults at 8:00 A.M. was 9.4 ng/ml, compared to a mean level of 19.5 ng/ml in GH-deficient subjects and 7.3 ng/ml in acromegalic patients. Baxter and Cowell (1987), on the other hand, showed that serum IGF-BP-1 levels have a marked diurnal rhythm and appear to be unaffected by GH status of the patient or by pulsatile GH secretory activity. Plasma levels of IGF-BP-1 can vary 10- to 20-fold over the course of a day, with levels achieving peak values of 50–500 ng/ml at 8:00 A.M.

Cotterill et al. (1988) have further demonstrated that this diurnal variation was unrelated to serum cortisol levels, but was inversely related to plasma insulin levels (Fig. 28). The typical diurnal variation of IGF-BP-1 could be altered by modifications of the eating pattern (Fig. 29). Fasting or induction of hypoglycemia with insulin treatment resulted in rapid increases in IGF-BP-1 levels. These studies indicate that serum levels of IGF-BP-1 vary according to the metabolic status of the subject and are potentially influenced by intracellular glucose concentrations. It is attractive to hypothesize that increasing serum levels of IGF-BP-1 during times of reduced serum glucose (e.g., fasting and insulin treatment) serve to protect the cells against the hypoglycemic actions of the IGFs. This hypothesis is further extended by the observation by Suikkari et al. (1988) that serum levels of IGF-BP-1 decrease by 40–70% during steady-state euglycemic hyperinsulinemia, when substrate availability is high.

G.   EFFECT OF IGF-BPs ON ASSAYS FOR IGF-I AND -II

The presence of high-affinity IGF-BPs in serum, other biological fluids, and conditioned media from a wide variety of normal and transformed cells compli-

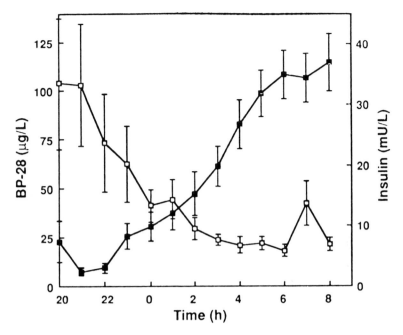

FIG. 28.   Mean (± SE) plasma BP-28 (human IGF-BP-1) (■) and insulin (□) concentrations in 21 short children during overnight sampling from 1:00–8:00 A.M. (From Cotterill *et al.,* 1988.)

cates assays of IGF peptides. Furlanetto *et al.* (1977) maintained that for RIA, preincubation of serum samples with antibody for 96 hours prior to addition of [^{125}I]IGF-I avoided the artifacts resulting from the continued presence of IGF-BPs in the samples assayed. Furlanetto and Marino (1987) also maintained that the addition of heparin allows IGF-I RIAs to be performed in plastic tubes without interference by BPs. Daughaday *et al.* (1980) subsequently developed an acid–ethanol extraction method which eliminated interference by BPs present in normal human serum, but was subject to difficulties in interpretation whenever BP levels were particularly high, as in rat serum or uremia.

Other investigators have maintained that the accurate assessment of IGF concentrations requires rigorous removal or saturation of all BP activity. Mesiano *et al.* (1988) demonstrated that significant amounts of IGF-binding activity in ovine plasma survive acid–ethanol extraction and can potentially interfere with both RIAs and radioreceptor assays. Similarly, Powell *et al.* (1986) showed that acid–ethanol extraction of uremic human plasma resulted in significant underestimation of radioimmunoassayable serum IGF-I concentrations and overestimation of serum radioreceptor-assayable IGF-II concentrations. Presumably, this is because

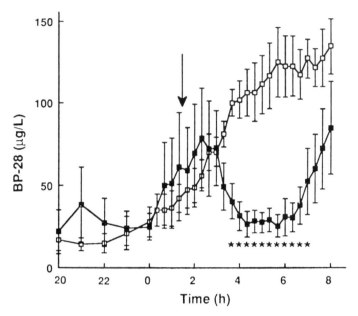

FIG. 29. Mean (± SE) plasma BP-28 (human IGF-BP-1) and insulin concentrations in 10 children during overnight sampling. Five children were given a small meal at 1:30 A.M. (■), and five were given water at the same time (□). *, Time points when the plasma human IGF-BP-1 levels in the two groups differed ($p < 0.01$). (From Cotterill *et al.*, 1988.)

BPs compete with membrane preparations for [^{125}I]IGF in the radioreceptor assays. On the other hand, [^{125}I]IGF-BP complexes can be precipitated by polyethylene glycol in RIAs, along with [^{125}I]IGF–antibody complexes and can result in artifactually low determinations of IGF peptide concentrations (Fig. 30).

Both Zapf *et al.* (1981) and Horner *et al.* (1978) suggested that accurate determination of IGF peptide concentrations necessitates acid chromatography (i.e., acidification of sample with either formic or acetic acid, followed by gel filtration). Chromatographic separation is typically over a Sephadex G-50 column, which separates both IGF-I and -II from their BPs. Blum *et al.* (1988) suggested that interference by BPs in RIAs for IGF-II can be prevented by saturating BP activity remaining after acid–ethanol extraction with excess unlabeled IGF-I. This method, however, can only be used when the antibody is highly specific for either IGF-I or -II.

Whatever methods are used, it is clearly necessary to document full removal of BP activity before assay. This is especially true in cell cultures, in which the amount of BP activity can be quite high, despite minimal measurable IGF peptide. In our own laboratories we are currently using acid chromatography prior to all IGF assays and documenting by Western ligand blots that all BP activity has

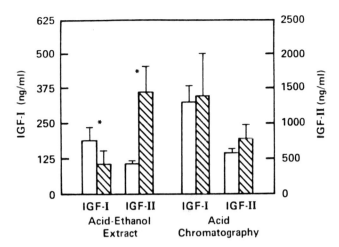

FIG. 30. Serum levels (mean ± SD) of IGF-I and -II in seven normal adults (□) and eight adults with chronic renal failure (▧). Somatomedins were separated from carrier proteins by acid–ethanol extraction of one aliquot of serum from each patient; this separation was also performed by acid chromatography of a second serum aliquot. The acid–ethanol extracts and the somatomedin fractions from acid-chromatographed serum were then assayed from IGF-I (by RIA) and IGF-II (rat placental membrane radioreceptor assay). *, Uremia different from normal ($p < 0.05$). (From Powell *et al.*, 1986.)

been removed from thc peptide fraction, in which intact $M_r = 7500$ IGF-I and -II elute (Rosenfeld *et al.*, 1990; De Leon *et al.*, 1990).

H. BIOLOGICAL ACTIONS OF THE IGF-BPs

Of all aspects of the IGF-BPs, their biological actions are probably the least well understood at this time. The ability of these proteins to specifically bind the IGF peptides with high affinity leads to the obvious hypothesis that the BPs act to modulate the actions of the IGFs by regulating their access to target membrane receptors. It is also conceivable, however, that the IGF-BPs might have some kind of regulatory or effector actions, independent of the IGFs. The presence of multiple IGF-BPs expressed differentially in various tissues suggests that each BP species could have a specific regulatory rolc(s). Thc experimental evidence to date supports at least three different roles for at least two forms of IGF-BP.

One role of IGF-BP-3 appears to be as a carrier for IGF peptides in the serum and, possibly, in other biological fluids. Under normal conditions the majority of IGF peptide content of serum is complexed with IGF-BP-3 and the acid-labile subunit in an $M_r = 150,000$ complex. As described above, binding of IGF peptides to this complex significantly increases the half-life of the peptide (Cohen and Nissley, 1976; Kaufmann *et al.*, 1977). It has therefore, been suggested that IGF-BP-3 acts to protect circulating IGF peptides from degradation, thereby increasing the amount of IGF potentially available to target tissues. It remains unclear, however, as to whether IGF peptides bound to IGF-BP-3 are capable of being delivered to target tissues, or whether they remain unavailably complexed in serum. Blum et al. (1989) recently reported that the mitogenic activity of IGF-I on baby hamster and human fibroblasts was enhanced when the IGF-I was first complexed to purified human IGF-BP-3. This finding supports the hypothesis that IGF-BP-3 acts as a reservoir for extended IGF peptide action.

The biological actions of human IGF-BP-1 have been best characterized at this time. Paradoxically, IGF-BP-1 has been shown to both inhibit and enhance the mitogenic actions of the IGFs in different cell systems.

Initial reports using impure preparations of this BP described an inhibitory effect on IGF-I and -II stimulation of DNA synthesis in human fibroblasts (Drop et al., 1979), and glucose transport in the adipocytes (Zapf et al., 1979). Subsequent studies, using purified preparations of human IGF-BP-1 have demonstrated that IGF-BP-1 competes with membrane receptors in endometrial tissue and placenta for the binding of IGF-I (Rutanen et al., 1988a; Pekonen et al., 1988). Furthermore, purified preparations of human IGF-BP-1 were shown to not only block the binding of IGF-I to its membrane receptors on the choriocarcinoma cell JEG-3, but also inhibit the IGF-I-stimulated uptake of amino acids by these cells (Ritvos et al., 1988). These studies have suggested that one action of IGF-BP-1 might be to inhibit IGF action by directly competing with membrane receptors.

On the other hand, an enhancing effect of IGF-BP-1 has been reported in the stimulation of DNA synthesis in a number of cell types, most notably in porcine aortic smooth muscle (Elgin et al., 1987; Busby et al., 1989), fibroblasts (Clemmons et al., 1987), and FRTL5 thyroid cells (Frauman et al., 1989). Stimulation of these cells by IGF-I in the presence of human IGF-BP-1 resulted in a 2- to 4-fold greater synthesis of DNA than that observed with IGF-I alone.

The potential availability of pure IGF-BPs produced by recombinant DNA technology should greatly facilitate investigations into the biological roles of these proteins. The surprising complexity of IGF-BPs, evidenced by the number of different forms, their ontogenic and hormonal regulation, and variable glycosylation suggests that they play important roles in the regulation of IGF action. Indeed, recent evidence suggests that these BPs are capable of acting as endocrine, paracrine, and autocrine factors, which modulate IGF stimulation of a variety of biological actions.

ACKNOWLEDGMENT

Supported in part by National Institutes of Health Grant DK28229 (to R.G.R.).

REFERENCES

Adams, S. O., Nissley, S. P., Greenstein, L. A., Yang, Y. W.-H., and Rechler, M. M. (1983). *Endocrinology (Baltimore)* **112**, 979–987.

Adashi, E. Y., Resnick, C. A., Hernandez, E. R., Hurwitz, A., and Rosenfeld, R. G. (1990). *Endocrinology (Baltimore)* **126**, 1305–1307.

Baumann, G., Shaw, M. A., and Amburn, K. (1986). *Metabolism* **38**, 683–689.

Baxter, R. C. (1988). *J. Clin. Endocrinol. Metab.* **67**, 265–272.

Baxter, R. C., and Cowell, C. T. (1987). *J. Clin. Endocrinol. Metab.* **65**, 432–440.

Baxter, R. C., and Martin, J. L. (1986). *J. Clin. Invest.* **78**, 1504–1512.

Baxter, R. C., and Martin, J. L. (1987). *Biochem. Biophys. Res. Commun.* **147**, 408–415.

Baxter, R. C., and Martin, J. L. (1989). *Prog. Growth Factor Res.* **1**, 49–68.

Baxter, R. C., Martin, J. L., and Handelsman, D. J. (1984a). *Acta Endocrinol. (Copenhagen)* **106**, 420–427.

Baxter, R. C., Zaltsman, Z., and Turtle, J. R. (1984b). *J. Clin. Endocrinol. Metab.* **58**, 955–959.

Baxter, R. C., Martin, J. L., Tyler, M. I., and Howden, E. H. (1986). *Biochem. Biophys. Res. Commun.* **139**, 1256–1261.

Baxter, R. C., Martin, J. L., and Wood, M. H. (1987). *J. Clin. Endocrinol. Metab.* **65**, 423–431.

Beguin, Y., Huebers, H. A., Josephson, N., and Finch, C. A. (1988). *Proc. Natl. Acad. Sci. U.S.A.* **85**, 637–640.

Bell, S. C., and Bohn, H. (1986). *Placenta* **7**, 283–294.

Bell, S. C., and Keyte, J. W. (1988). *Endocrinology (Baltimore)* **123**, 1202–1204.

Bell, G. I., Merryweather, J. P., Sanchez-Pescador, R., Stempien, M. M., Priestley, L., Scott, J., and Rall, L. B. (1984). *Nature (London)* **310**, 775–777.

Bell, G. I., Gerhard, D. S., Fong, N. M., Sanchez-Pescador, R., and Rall, L. B. (1985). *Proc. Natl. Acad. Sci. U.S.A.* **82**, 6450–6454.

Bell, S. C., Patel, S. R., Jackson, J. A., and Waites, G. T. (1988). *J. Endocrinol.* **118**, 317–328.

Bhaumick, B., Bala, R. M., and Hollenberg, M. D. (1981). *Proc. Natl. Acad. Sci. U.S.A.* **78**, 4279–4283.

Binkert, C., Landwehr, J., Mary, J.-L., Schwander, J., and Heinrich, G. (1989). *EMBO J.* **8**, 2497–2502.

Binoux, M., and Hossenlopp, P. (1988). *J. Clin. Endocrinol. Metab.* **67**, 509–514.

Binoux, M., Hossenlopp, P., Lassarre, C., and Hardouin, N. (1981). *FEBS Lett.* **124**, 178–184.

Binoux, M., Hardouin, S., Lassarre, C., and Hossenlopp, P. (1982). *J. Clin. Endocrinol. Metab.* **55**, 600–602.

Binoux, M., Seurin, D., Lassarre, C., and Gourmelen, M. (1984). *J. Clin. Endocrinol. Metab.* **59**, 453–462.

Binoux, M., Lassarre, C., and Gourmelen, M. (1986). *J. Clin. Endocrinol. Metab.* **63**, 1151–1155.

Blum, W. F., Ranke, M. B., and Bierich, J. R. (1988). *Acta Endocrinol. (Copenhegen)* **118**, 374–380.

Blum, W. F., Jenne, E. W., Reppin, F., Kietzmann, K., Ranke, M. B., and Bierich, J. R. (1989). *Endocrinology (Baltimore)* **125**, 766–772.

Bohn, H., and Kraus, W. (1980). *Arch. Gynecol.* **229**, 279–291.

Borsi, L., Rosenfeld, R. G., Liu, F., and Hintz, R. L. (1982). *J. Clin. Endocrinol. Metab.* **54**, 223–228.

Brewer, M. T., Stetler, G. L., Squires, C. H., Thompson, R. C., Busby, W. H., and Clemmons, D. R. (1988). *Biochem. Biophys. Res. Commun.* **152**, 1289–1297.

Brinkman, A., Groffen, C. A. H., Kortleve, D. J., and Drop, S. L. S. (1988a). *Biochem. Biophys. Res. Commun.* **157**, 898–907.

Brinkman, A., Groffen, C., Kortleve, D. J., Geurts, A., and Drop, S. L. S. (1988b). *EMBO J.* **7**, 2417–2423.

Brissenden, J. E., Ullrich, A., and Francke, U. (1984). *Nature (London)* **310**, 781–784.

Brown, A. L., Chiariotti, L., Orlowski, C. C., Mehlman, T., Burgess, W. H., Ackerman, E. J., Bruni, C. B., and Rechler, M. M. (1989). *J. Biol. Chem.* **264**, 5148–5154.

Burgi, H., Muller, W. A., Humbel, R. E., Labhart, A., and Froesch, E. R. (1966). *Biochim. Biophys. Acta* **121**, 349–359.

Busby, W. H., Snyder, D. K., and Clemmons, D. R. (1988). *J. Clin. Endocrinol. Metab.* **67**, 1225–1230.

Busby, W. H., Hossenlopp, P., Binoux, M., and Clemmons, D. R. (1989). *Endocrinology (Baltimore)* **125**, 773–777.

Butler, J. H., and Gluckman, P. D. (1986). *J. Endocrinol.* **109**, 333–338.

Ceda, G. P., Davis, R. D., Rosenfeld, R. G., and Hoffman, A. R. (1987). *Endocrinology (Baltimore)* **120**, 1658–1662.

Chernausek, S. D., Jacobs, S., and Van Wyk, J. J. (1981). *Biochemistry* **20**, 7345–7350.

Chochinov, R. H., Mariz, I. K., Hajek, A. S., and Daughaday, W. H. (1977). *J. Clin. Endocrinol. Metab.* **44**, 902–908.

Clemmons, D. R., Elgin, R. G., Han, V. K. M., Cassella, S. J., D'Ercole, A. J., and Van Wyk, J. J. (1986). *J. Clin. Invest.* **77**, 1548–1556.

Clemmons, D. R., Han, V. K. M., Elgin, R. G., and D'Ercole, A. J. (1987). *Mol. Endocrinol.* **1**, 339–347.

Cohen, K. L., and Nissley, S. P. (1976). *Acta Endocrinol. (Copenhagen)* **83**, 243–258.

Conover, C. A., Liu, F., Powell, D., Rosenfeld, R. G., and Hintz, R. L. (1989). *J. Clin. Invest.* **83**, 852–859.

Corps, A. N., Brown, K. D., Ress, L. H., Carr, J., and Prosser, C. G. (1988). *J. Clin. Endocrinol. Metab.* **67**, 25–29.

Cotterill, A. M., Cowell, C. T., Baxter, R. C., and Silink, M. (1988). *J. Clin. Endocrinol. Metab.* **67**, 882–887.

Cubbage, M. L., Suwanichkul, A., and Powell, D. R. (1989). *Mol. Endocrinol.* **3**, 846–851.

Daughaday, W. H., and Kipnis, D. M. (1966). *Recent Prog. Horm. Res.* **22**, 49–99.

Daughaday, W. H., and Rotwein, P. (1989). *Endocr. Rev.* **10**, 68–91.

Daughaday, W. H., Heins, J. N., Srivastava, L., and Hammer, C. (1968). *J. Lab. Clin. Med.* **72**, 803–812.

Daughaday, W. H., Hall, K., Raben, M. S., Salmon, W. D., Jr., Van den Brande, J. L., and Van Wyk, J. J. (1972). *Nature (London)* **235**, 107–109.

Daughaday, W. H., Mariz, I. K., and Blethen, S. L. (1980). *J. Clin. Endocrinol. Metab.* **51**, 781–788.

De Leon, D. D., Bakker, B., Wilson, D. M., Hintz, R. L., and Rosenfeld, R. G. (1988). *Biochem. Biophys. Res. Commun.* **152**, 398–405.

De Leon, D. D., Wilson, D. M., Bakker, B., Lamson, G., Hintz, R. L., and Rosenfeld, R. G. (1989). *Mol. Endocrinol.* **3**, 567–574.

De Leon, D. D., Bakker, B., Wilson, D. M., Lamson, G., and Rosenfeld, R. G. (1990). *Endocrinology (Baltimore)* (in press).

de Pagter-Holthuizen, P., Hoppener, J. W. M., Jansen, M., Guerts van Kessel, A. H. M., van Ommen, G. J. B., and Sussenbach, J. S. (1985). *Hum. Genet.* **69**, 170–173.

de Pagter-Holthuizen, P., van Schaik, F. M. A., Verduijn, G. M., van Ommen, G. J. B., Bouma, B. N., Jansen, M., and Sussenbach, J. S. (1987). *FEBS Lett.* **195**, 179–184.

D'Ercole, A. J., and Wilkins, J. R. (1984). *Endocrinology (Baltimore)* **114**, 1141–1144.

D'Ercole, A. J., Drop, S. L. S., and Kortleve, D. J. (1985). *J. Clin. Endocrinol. Metab.* **61**, 612–617.

DeVroede, M. A., Tseng, L. Y. H., Katsyannis, P. G., Nissley, S. P., and Rechler, M. M. (1986). *J. Clin. Invest.* **77**, 602–613.

Dickson, R. B., McManaway, E., and Lippman, M. E., (1986). *Science* **232**, 1540–1542.

Donovan, S. M., Oh, Y., Pham, H., and Rosenfeld, R. G. (1989). *Endocrinology (Baltimore)* **125**, 2621–2627.

Donovan, S. M., Wilson, D. M., Hintz, R. L., and Rosenfeld, R. G. (1990). Manuscript in preparation.

Drop, S. L. S., Valiquette, G., Guyda, H. J., Corvol, M. T., and Posner, B. I. (1979). *Acta Endocrinol. (Copenhagen)* **90**, 505–518.

Drop, S. L. S., Kortleve, D. J., and Guyda, H. J. (1984). *J. Clin. Endocrinol. Metab.* **59**, 899–907.

Dulak, N. C., and Temin, H. M. (1973). *J. Cell. Physiol.* **81**, 153–160.

Dull, T. J., Gray, A., Hayflick, J. S., and Ullrich, A. (1984). *Nature (London)* **310**, 777–781.

Elgin, R. G., Busby, W. H., Jr., and Clemmons, D. R. (1987). *Proc. Natl. Acad. Sci. U.S.A.* **84**, 3254–3258.

Fazleabas, A. T., Jaffe, R. C., Verhage, H. G., Waites, G., and Bell, S. C. (1989). *Endocrinology (Baltimore)* **124**, 2321–2329.

Frauman, A. G., Tsuzaki, S., and Moses, A. C. (1989). *Endocrinology (Baltimore)* **124**, 2289–2296.

Froesch, E. R., Burgi, H., Ramsier, E. B., Bally, P., and Labhart, A. (1963). *J. Clin. Invest.* **42**, 1816–1834.

Frunzio, R., Chiariotti, L., Brown, A. L., Graham, D. E., Rechler, M. M., and Bruni, C. B. (1986). *J. Biol. Chem.* **261**, 17138–17149.

Furlanetto, R. W. (1980). *J. Clin. Endocrinol. Metab.* **51**, 12–19.

Furlanetto, R. W., and DiCarlo, J. N. (1984). *Cancer Res.* **44**, 2122–2128.

Furlanetto, R. W., and Marino, J. M. (1987). *In* "Methods in Enzymology" (D. Barnes and D. A. Sirbasku, eds.), Vol. 146, p. 216. Academic Press, Orlando, Florida.

Furlanetto, R. W., Underwood, L. E., Van Wyk, J. J., and D'Ercole, A. J. (1977). *J. Clin. Invest.* **60**, 648–657.

Gelato, M. C., Kiess, W., Lee, L., Malozowski, S., Rechler, M. M., and Nissley, P. (1988). *J. Clin. Endocrinol. Metab.* **67**, 669–675.

Gelato, M. C., Rutherford, C., Stark, R. I., and Daniel, S. S. (1989). *Endocrinology (Baltimore)* **124**, 2935–2943.

Giudice, L. C., Mikowski, D. A., Lamson, G., Rosenfeld, R. G., and Irwin, J. C. (1990a). Submitted for publication.

Giudice, L. C., Farrell, E. M., Pham, H., and Rosenfeld, R. C. (1990b). Submitted for publication.

Han, V. K. M., Lauder, J. M., and D'Ercole, A. J. (1988). *J. Neurosci.* **8**, 3135–3143.

Hardouin, S., Hossenlopp, P., Segovia, B., Scurin, D., Portolan, G., Lassarre, C., and Binoux, M. (1987). *Eur. J. Biochem.* **170**, 121–132.

Herington, A. C., Ymer, S. I., and Stevenson, J. L. (1986). *Biochem. Biophys. Res. Commun.* **139**, 159–165.

Hintz, R. L., and Liu, F. (1977). *J. Clin. Endocrinol. Metab.* **45**, 988–995.

Hintz, R. L., and Liu, F. (1980). *In* "Growth Hormone and Other Biologically Active Peptides" (A. Pecile and E. E. Muller, eds.), pp. 133–143. Excerpta Medica, Amsterdam.

Hintz, R. L., Rosenfeld, R. G., and Kemp, S. F. (1981). *J. Clin. Endocrinol. Metab.* **53**, 100–104.

Horner, J. M., Liu, F., and Hintz, R. L. (1978). *J. Clin. Endocrinol. Metab.* **47**, 1287–1295.

Hossenlopp, P., Seurin, D., Segovia-Quinson, B., and Binoux, M. (1986a). *FEBS Lett.* **208**, 439–444.

Hossenlopp, P., Seurin, D., Segovia-Quinson, B., Hardouin, S., and Binoux, M. (1986b). *Anal. Biochem.* **154,** 138–143.

Hossenlopp, P., Seurin, D., Segovia, B., Portolan, G., and Binoux, M. (1987). *Eur. J. Biochem.* **170,** 133–142.

Huff, K. K., Kaufman, D., Gabbay, K. H., Spencer, E. M., Lippman, M. E., and Dickson, R. B. (1986). *Cancer Res.* **46,** 4613–4619.

Huff, K. K., Knabbe, C., Lindsey, R., Kaufman, D., Brozert, D., Lippman, M. E., and Dickson, R. B. (1988). *Mol. Endocrinol.* **2,** 200–208.

Jansen, M., van Schaik, F. M. A., Ricker, A. T., Bullock, B., Woods, D. E., Gabbay, K. H ., Nussbaum, A. L., Sussenbach, J. S., and Van den Brande, J. L. (1983). *Nature (London)* **306,** 609–611.

Jansen, M., van Schaik, F. M. A., van Tol, H., Van den Brande, J. L., and Sussenbach, J. S. (1985). *FEBS Lett.* **179,** 243–246.

Julkunen, M., Koistinen, R., Aalto-Setala, K., Seppala, M., Janne, O. A., and Kontula, K. (1988). *FEBS Lett.* **236,** 295–302.

Karey, K. P., and Sirbasku, D. A. (1988). *Cancer Res.* **48,** 4083–4092.

Kasuga, M., Van Obberghen, E., Nissley, S. P., and Rechler, M. M. (1981). *J. Biol. Chem.* **256,** 5305–5308.

Kaufmann, U., Zapf, J., Torretti, B., and Froesch, E. R. (1977). *J. Clin. Endocrinol. Metab.* **44,** 160–166.

Kiess, W., Greenstein, L. A., White, R. M., Lee, L., Rechler, M. M., and Nissley, S. P. (1987). *Proc. Natl. Acad. Sci. U.S.A.* **84,** 7720–7724.

Knauer, D. J., Wagner, F. W., and Smith, G. L. (1981). *J. Supramol. Struct. Cell. Biochem.* **15,** 177–191.

Koistinen, R. (1984). *Clin. Chim. Acta* **141,** 235–240.

Koistinen, R., Kalkkinen, N., Huhtala, M.-L., Seppala, M., Bohn, H., and Rutanen, E.-M. (1986). *Endocrinology (Baltimore)* **118,** 1375–1378.

Koistinen, R., Huhtala, M.-L., Stenman, U.-H., and Seppala, M. (1987). *Clin. Chim. Acta* **164,** 293–303.

Lamson, G., Pham, H., Oh, Y., Schwander, J., and Rosenfeld, R. G. (1989a). *Endocrinology (Baltimore)* **123,** 1100–1102.

Lamson, G., Oh, Y., Pham, H., Giudice, L. C., and Rosenfeld, R. G. (1989b). *J. Clin. Endocrinol. Metab.* **69,** 852–859.

Lee, Y.-L., Hintz, R. L., James, P. M., Lee, P. D. K., Shively, J. E., and Powell, D. R. (1988). *Mol. Endocrinol.* **2,** 404–411.

Lewitt, M. S., and Baxter, R. C. (1989). *J. Clin. Endocrinol. Metab.* **69,** 246–252.

Lippman, M. E., Dickson, R. B., Kasid, A., Gelmann, E., Davidson, N., McManaway, M., Huff, K., Bronzert, D., Bates, S., Swain, S., and Knabbe, C. (1986). *J. Steroid Biochem.* **24,** 147–154.

MacDonald, R. G., Tepper, M. A., Clairmont, K. B., Perregaux, S. B., and Czech, M. P. (1989). *J. Biol. Chem.* **264,** 3256–3261.

Margot, J. B., Binkert, C., Mary, J.-L., Landwehr, J., Heinrich, G., and Schwander, J. (1989). *Mol. Endocrinol.* **3,** 1053–1060.

Martin, J. L., and Baxter, R. C. (1985). *J. Clin. Endocrinol. Metab.* **61,** 799–801.

Martin, J. L., and Baxter, R. C. (1986). *J. Biol. Chem.* **261,** 8754–8760.

Martin, J. L., and Baxter, R. C. (1988). *Endocrinology (Baltimore)* **123,** 1907–1915.

Massague, J., and Czech, M. P. (1982). *J. Biol. Chem.* **257,** 5038–5045.

McCusker, R. H., Campion, D. R., and Clemmons, D. R. (1988). *Endocrinology (Baltimore)* **122,** 2071–2079.

McCusker, R. H., Campion, D. R., Jones, W. K., and Clemmons, D. R. (1989). *Endocrinology (Baltimore)* **125,** 501–509.

Mesiano, S., Young, I. R., Browne, C. A., and Thorburn, G. D. (1988). *J. Endocrinol.* **119,** 453–460.

Minuto, F., Barreca, A., Del Monte, P., Cariola, G., Torre, G. C., and Giordano, G. (1989). *J. Clin. Endocrinol. Metab.* **68,** 621–626.

Morgan, D. O., Edman, J. C., Standring, D. N., Fried, V. A., Smith, M. C., Roth, R. A., and Rutter, W. J. (1987). *Nature (London)* **329,** 301–307.

Moses, A. C., Nissley, S. P., Cohen, K. L., and Rechler, M. M. (1976). *Nature (London)* **263,** 137–140.

Moses, A. C., Nissley, S. P., Passamani, J., White, R. M., and Rechler, M. M. (1979). *Endocrinology (Baltimore)* **104,** 536–546.

Moses, A. C., Freinkel, A. J., Knowles, B. B., and Aden, D. P. (1983). *J. Clin. Endocrinol. Metab.* **56,** 1003–1008.

Mottola, C., MacDonald, R. G., Brackett, J. L., Mole, J. E., Anderson, J. K., and Czech, M. P. (1986). *J. Biol. Chem.* **261,** 11180–11188.

Myal, Y., Shiu, R. P. C., Bhaumick, N., and Bala, M. (1984). *Cancer Res.* **44,** 5486–5490.

Nissley, S. P., and Rechler, M. M. (1984). *In* "Hormonal Proteins and Peptides" (C. H. Li, ed.), pp. 127–203. Academic Press, Orlando, Florida.

Ocrant, I., Valentino, K. L., Eng, L. F., Hintz, R. L., Wilson, D. M., and Rosenfeld, R. G. (1988). *Endocrinology (Baltimore)* **123,** 1023–1034.

Ocrant, I., Pham, H., Oh, Y., and Rosenfeld, R. G. (1989). *Biochem. Biophys. Res. Commun.* **159,** 1316–1322.

Ooi, G. T., and Herington, A. C. (1986). *Biochem. Biophys. Res. Commun.* **137,** 411–417.

Orlowski, C. C., Tseng, L. Y.-H., Brown, A. L., Taylor, T., Yang, Y. W.-H., Romanus, J. A., and Rechler, M. M. (1989). *Proc. Annu. Meet. Endocr. Soc., 71st (Abst. 88A).*

Pekonen, F., Suikkari, A.-M., Makinen, T., and Rutanen, E.-M. (1988). *J. Clin. Endocrinol. Metab.* **67,** 1250–1257.

Peres, R., Betsholtz, C., Westermark, B., and Heldin, C.-H. (1987). *Cancer Res.* **47,** 3425–3429.

Povoa, G., Enberg, G., Jornvall, H., and Hall, K. (1984a). *Eur. J. Biochem.* **144,** 199–204.

Povoa, G., Roovete, A., and Hall, K. (1984b). *Acta Endocrinol. (Copenhagen)* **107,** 563–570.

Povoa, G., Isakkson, M., Jornvall, H., and Hall, K. (1985). *Biochem. Biophys. Res. Commun.* **128,** 1071–1078.

Powell, D. R., Rosenfeld, R. G., Baker, B. K., Liu, F., and Hintz, R. L. (1986). *J. Clin. Endocrinol. Metab.* **63,** 1186–1192.

Powell, D. R., Lee, P. D. K., Shively, J. E., Eckenhausen, M., and Hintz, R. L. (1987). *J. Chromatogr.* **420,** 163–170.

Rinderknecht, E., and Humbel, R. E. (1978a). *J. Biol. Chem.* **253,** 2769–2776.

Rinderknecht, E., and Humbel, R. E. (1978b). *FEBS Lett.* **89,** 283–286.

Ritvos, O., Ranta, T., Jalkanen, J., Suikkari, A.-M., Voutilainen, R., Bohn, H., and Rutanen, E.-M. (1988). *Endocrinology (Baltimore)* **122,** 2150–2157.

Roghani, M., Hossenlopp, P., Lepage, P., Balland, A., and Binoux, M. (1989). *FEBS Lett.* **255,** 253–258.

Romanus, J. A., Terrell, J. E., Yang, W.-H., Nissley, S. P., and Rechler, M. M. (1986). *Endocrinology (Baltimore)* **118,** 1743–1758.

Romanus, J. A., Yang, Y. W.-H., Nissley, S. P., and Rechler, M. M. (1987). *Endocrinology (Baltimore)* **121,** 1041–1050.

Rosenfeld, R. G. (1989). *In* "Hormonal Regulation of Growth" (H. Frisch and M. O. Thorner, eds.), pp. 113–126. Raven, New York.

Rosenfeld, R. G., and Hintz, R. L. (1986). *In* "The Receptors" (P. M. Conn, ed.), Vol. 3, pp. 281–329. Academic Press, Orlando, Florida.

Rosenfeld, R. G., Pham, H., Conover, C. A., Hintz, R. L., and Baxter, R. C. (1989a). *J. Clin. Endocrinol. Metab.* **68,** 638–646.

Rosenfeld, R. G., Pham, H., Oh, Y., and Ocrant, I. (1989b). *Endocrinology (Baltimore)* **124,** 2867–2874.

Rosenfeld, R. G., Pham, H., Oh, Y., Lamson, G., and Giudice, L. C. (1990). *J. Clin. Endocrinol. Metab.* **70,** 551–553.

Roth, R. A. (1988). *Science* **239,** 1269–1271.

Rotwein, P., Pollock, K. M., Didier, D. K., and Krivi, G. G. (1986). *J. Biol. Chem.* **261,** 4828–4832.

Ruoslahti, E., and Pierschbacher, M. D. (1987). *Science* **238,** 491–497.

Rutanen, E.-M., Bohn, H., and Seppala, M. (1982). *Am. J. Obstet. Gynecol.* **144,** 460–463.

Rutanen, E.-M., Koistinen, R., Wahlstrom, T., Bohn, H., Ranta, T., and Seppala, M. (1985). *Endocrinology (Baltimore)* **116,** 1304–1309.

Rutanen, E.-M., Koistinen, R., Sjoberg, J., Julkunen, M., Wahlstrom, T., Bohn, H., and Seppala, M. (1986a). *Endocrinology (Baltimore)* **118,** 1067–1071.

Rutanen, E.-M., Menabawey, M., Isaka, K., Bohn, H., Chard, T., and Grudzinskas, J. G. (1986b). *J. Clin. Endocrinol. Metab.* **63,** 675–679.

Rutanen, E.-M., Pekonen, F., and Makinen, T. (1988a). *J. Clin. Endocrinol. Metab.* **66,** 173–180.

Rutanen, E.-M., Karkkainen, T., Lundqvist, C., Pekonen, F., Ritvos, O., Tanner, P., Welin, M., and Weber, T. (1988b). *Biochem. Biophys. Res. Commun.* **152,** 208–215.

Salmon, W. D., Jr., and Daughaday, W. H. (1957). *J. Lab. Clin. Med.* **49,** 825–836.

Schalch, D. S., Heinrich, U. E., Koch, J. G., Johnson, C. J., and Schlueter, R. J. (1978). *J. Clin. Endocrinol. Metab.* **46,** 664–671.

Schmid, C., Zapf, J., and Froesch, E. R. (1989). *FEBS Lett.* (in press).

Schwander, J. C., Hauri, C., Zapf, J., and Froesch, E. R. (1983). *Endocrinology (Baltimore)* **113,** 297–302.

Scott, C. D., Martin, J. L., and Baxter, R. C. (1985a). *Endocrinology (Baltimore)* **116,** 1094–1101.

Scott, C. D., Martin, J. L., and Baxter, R. C. (1985b). *Endocrinology (Baltimore)* **116,** 1102–1107.

Seppala, M., Wahlstrom, T., Koskimies, A. I., Tenhunen, A., Rutanen, E.-M., Koistinen, R., Huhtaniemi, I., Bohn, H., and Stenman, U.-H. (1984). *J. Clin. Endocrinol. Metab.* **58,** 505–510.

Seppala, M., Koskimies, A. I., Tenhunen, A., Rutanen, E.-M., Sjoberg, J., Koistinen, R., Julkunen, M., and Wahlstrom, T. (1985). *Ann. N.Y. Acad. Sci.* **442,** 212–226.

Smith, E. P., Svoboda, M. E., Van Wyk, J. J., Kierszenbaum, A. L., and Tres, L. L. (1987). *Endocrinology (Baltimore)* **120,** 186–193.

Sturm, M. A., Conover, C. A., Pham, H., and Rosenfeld, R. G. (1989). *Endocrinology (Baltimore)* **124,** 388–396.

Suikkari, A.-M. (1989). *Eur. J. Obstet. Gynecol.* **30,** 19–25.

Suikkari, A.-M., Koivisto, V. A., Rutanen, E.-M., Yki-Jarvinen, H., Karonen, S.-L., and Seppala, M. (1988). *J. Clin. Endocrinol. Metab.* **66,** 266–272.

Suikkari, A.-M., Jalkanen, J., Koistinen, R., Butzow, R., Ritvos, O., Ranta, T., and Seppala, M. (1989). *Endocrinology (Baltimore)* **124,** 1088–1090.

Szabo, L., Mottershead, D. G., Ballard, F. J., and Wallace, J. C. (1988). *Biochem. Biophys. Res. Commun.* **151,** 207–214.

Tricoli, J. V., Rall, L. B., Scott, J., Bell, G. I., and Shows, T. B. (1984). *Nature (London)* **310,** 784–786.

Ui, M., Shimonaka, M., Shimasaki, S., and Ling, N. (1989). *Endocrinology (Baltimore)* **125,** 912–916.

Ullrich, A., Gray, A., Tam, A. W., Yang-Feng, T., Tsubokawa, M., Collins, C., Henzel, W., Le Bon, T., Kathuria, S., Chen, E., Jacobs, S., Francke, U., Ramachandran, J., and Fujita-Yamaguchi, Y. (1986). *EMBO J.* **5,** 2503–2512.

Waites, G. T., James, R. F. L., and Bell, S. C. (1988). *J. Clin. Endocrinol. Metab.* **67,** 1100–1104.

Walton, P. E., Baxter, R. C., Burleigh, B. D., and Etherton, T. D. (1989). *Comp. Biochem. Physiol. B* **92B,** 561–567.

White, R. M., Nissley, S. P., Short, P. A., Rechler, M. M., and Fennoy, I. (1982). *J. Clin. Invest.* **69,** 1239–1252.

Wilkins, J. R., and D'Ercole, A. J. (1985). *J. Clin. Invest.* **75,** 1350–1358.

Wood, W. I., Cachianes, G., Henzel, W. J., Winslow, G. A., Spencer, S. A., Hellmiss, R., Martin, J. L., and Baxter, R. C. (1988). *Mol. Endocrinol.* **2,** 1176–1185.

Yee, D., Favoni, R. E., Lupu, R., Cullen, K. J., Lebovic, G. S., Huff, K. K., Lee, P. D. K., Lee, Y. L., Powell, D. R., Dickson, R. B., Rosen, N., and Lippman, M. E. (1989). *Biochem. Biophys. Res. Commun.* **158,** 38–44.

Zapf, J., Waldvogel, M., and Froesch, E. R. (1975). *Arch. Biochem. Biophys.* **168,** 638–645.

Zapf, J., Schoenle, E., Jagars, G., Sand, I., Grunwald, J., and Froesch, E. R. (1979). *J. Clin. Invest.* **63,** 1077–1084.

Zapf, J., Walter, H., and Froesch, E. R. (1981). *J. Clin. Invest.* **68,** 1321–1330.

Zapf, J., Born, W., Chang, J.-Y., James, P., Froesch, E. R., and Fischer, J. A. (1988). *Biochem. Biophys. Res. Commun.* **156,** 1187–1194.

DISCUSSION

F. S. French. How do you suggest binding proteins might enhance the activity of IGF other than by prolonging half-life? Is there any evidence for possible enhancement at the cellular level?

R. G. Rosenfeld. The suggestions has been made, although it remains to be proved, that the binding proteins may be capable of not only delivering the peptide to the cell, but helping it bind to its receptor. Those binding proteins, for example, which have the RGD sequence may be capable of attaching to the cell membrane and thereby delivering the nondegraded peptide directly to the receptor. Alternatively, the binding proteins could be involved in the migration of the peptides from serum, where they are complexed to the large BP3, into biological fluids or into the intercellular region, where they could be delivered directly to the cell receptors.

F. S. French. Is there any evidence that the binding proteins might have receptors?

R. G. Rosenfeld. Data are very incomplete. We have attempted to find specific binding of BP-3 to cell membrane receptors, but our data are equivocal at this point. So far as I know, nobody has definitively established that there is a specific binding protein receptor.

S. P. Bottari. The IGF-II receptor seems to be mainly an intracellular receptor and may be a nuclear receptor.

R. G. Rosenfeld. It clearly is primarily an intracellular receptor. In most cells, about 90% of the receptor is found, not complexed with the nucleus, but in the Golgi apparatus in a perinuclear location. The hypothesis is that as lysosomal proteins are synthesized, a mannose 6-phosphate moiety is attached to the lysosomal proteins, which then allows them to be bound by the mannose 6-phosphate receptor and targeted for transport to the lysosomes. Why this receptor appears to be capable of specifically binding IGF-II with very high specificity and with quite surprisingly high affinity remains to be established. Some suggest that its role may be simply to bind IGF-II and clear it from biological fluids by having it degraded in the lysosomes. I would think that this is a rather prosaic and uninteresting role for the receptor. My guess is that it has some other biological role in terms of IGF-II action that remains to be established.

S. P. Bottari. Recent reports on IGF-I action at the nuclear level by Bob Irvine's group showed that it could stimulate incorporation of phosphate into the PI pool and also stimulate PIP_2 formation.

R. G. Rosenfeld. This has also been shown for IGF-II. Nishimoto and Koyima in Tokyo have in a series of studies demonstrated that IGF-II and the IGF-II receptor may be linked to a G protein and may be involved in the inositol phosphate pathway.

S. P. Bottari. I understand, but I wanted to stress that this was observed at the nuclear level, which is unaffected.

R. G. Rosenfeld. Correct.

S. P. Bottari. You have not found anything like this for the IGF-II receptor?

R. G. Rosenfeld. No. I would say that IGF-II is still a peptide in search of a role.

S. M. Rosenthal. I have a question on the breast cancer data and the possibility of an autocrine mechanism for IGF-1. I believe you said that on attempting to assay for IGF-I, what you actually measured turned out to be binding proteins. I wondered if Northern blots of that same tissue demonstrated the expression of IGF-I or if Western blots detected the presence of this peptide.

R. G. Rosenfeld. Some of the cell lines which have been putative producers of nanomolar concentrations of IGF-I have, in fact, been shown to not even contain message for IGF-I, not even by RNase protection methodologies. When we have rigorously removed all the detectable binding protein, we cannot assay any ICF activity either by radioimmunoassay or by immunoblotting techniques.

S. Shenolikar. Would you comment on your finding that several transformed cell lines produce IGF-binding protein(s) with RGD sequences. As I understood it, the cell adhesion receptors which recognize these sequences are actually down-regulated in cells transformed by tumor-promoting phorbol ester and in virtually transformed cells. These two effects appear to be somewhat contradictory. What, then, might be the role of the RGD sequences in the function of the binding proteins?

R. G. Rosenfeld. It remains to be put together in a logical way. The observation was made purely in the sense that when one cross-links iodinated IGF-II to some cell membranes, one can identify the membrane-associated binding proteins. Whether these are specifically bound by membrane receptors for binding proteins or whether the RGD sequence allows an integrin class of receptors to attach the binding protein remains to be determined. How that attachment is involved in the transformation of cells is anybody's guess.

N. A. Samaan. You discussed protein binding of two peaks, the first of which disappeared on hypophysectomy. What would happen to the second peak on pancreatectomy?

R. G. Rosenfeld. You mean as the hypophysectomy was done?

N. A. Samaan. Hypophysectomy eliminated the first peak. If a pancreatectomy were also done, what would happen to the second peak?

R. G. Rosenfeld. I do not know if that experiment has been done. What is clear is that in animals and in the human situation of growth hormone deficiency, the high-molecular-weight binding protein, BP-3, virtually disappears, and all that remains is the low-molecular-weight form. This can be shown both on a peptide level and on a message level, but it would be interesting to see what would happen with pancreatectomy.

N. A. Samaan. When the nonsuppressible insulinlike activity (ILA) or the "atypical" ILA was first described by us in 1961, we showed that it markedly decreased with pancreatectomy. It disappeared completely in one animal and decreased to 25% in three animals. We were also the first to show that the nonsupressible ILA or atypical ILA was formed in the liver because after infusion of regular insulin in the liver its level increased, was very low in patients with hepatic cirrhosis, and was even lower in patients after portocaval shunts. We have to concentrate on the relationship of insulin to the phenomena you describe because others also present data that indicate that the somatomedins, which are the nonsuppressible ILA, come from growth hormone in the liver, but make no mention that insulin plays a major role. This confuses the issue and the literature. What is IGF-I? What is IGF-II? What is somatomedin? We must go back to the original work and specify that IGF-I and IGF-II come from the nonsuppressible ILA which is formed in the liver in the presence of insulin and that growth hormone has a synergistic effect. I was pleased that you discussed Baxter's work relating to the proteins binding to insulin. Actually, what you concluded about the possible function of the binding proteins is similar to what we said around 25 years ago: that this nonsuppressible ILA may be a form of a slow-release hormone.

R. G. Rosenfeld. I think your comments are absolutely correct. It has now been shown in *in vivo* studies that administration of pure IGF, especially intravenously, can result in profound hypoglycemia. As the peptide is bound by the binding proteins, the hypoglycemia resolves. Probably both the IGF peptide levels and the binding protein levels are regulated, either directly by insulin or by intracellular glucose concentrations, which appear to affect the expression of both the peptide and its binding protein.

R. S. Swerdloff. I would appreciate further clarification of the binding proteins. Are the affinities and capacities of these binding proteins in serum known? Have you studied differential tissue extraction of ligands from binding proteins? These questions result from studies by Pardridge on other hormones and their binding proteins, suggesting that certain tissues are able to extract ligands from binding proteins in a differential fashion, thus allowing some specificity of action.

R. G. Rosenfeld. The binding proteins, in fact, have turned out to be capable of binding both IGF-I and IGF-II with a greater affinity than the receptor . Some of the studies with purified binding proteins demonstrate K_ds of 10^{-10} as opposed to 10^{-9} for the classical receptors. All binding proteins identified to date, with the exception of the circulating truncated type 2 receptor, are capable of binding both IGF-I and IGF-II, although they vary in their relative affinities for each of those peptides. IGF-BP-2, for example, has a particularly high affinity for IGF-II compared with IGF-I. None of the binding proteins appears to have any affinity for insulin or for growth hormone, although there probably is a growth hormone-binding protein that Dr. Wood will discuss. In terms of the extraction of binding protein from tissues, the data have been difficult to interpret because of the hematogenesis contamination of the tissues because and of knowing whether the binding protein being extracted is, in fact, directly expressed by the tissue or whether what one is observing is serum contamination of the samples. There have been studies, however, which have confirmed in certain tissues that both message and peptide can be identified by immunohistochemical and *in situ* hybridization techniques. Thus, I believe that the tissue expression of these binding proteins will be defined much better in the next few years.

R. S. Swerdloff. Perhaps I did not word my question properly. I was interested in knowing whether there is evidence for certain tissues' being more capable of extracting and utilizing the ligand bound to the binding protein. Thus, the binding protein could enhance ligand action in targeted tissues instead of acting simply as a protective mechanism. In certain tissues, then, the binding protein would have an affinity for that cell and would then allow the ligand to stimulate a response.

R. G. Rosenfeld. I do not believe there are any data yet to really address that question or to even address the question of whether the transport of IGF from the serum into specific biological fluids is accompanied by the transport of any of the binding proteins, or whether the peptide is released by a serum-binding protein into the other fluid.

H. G. Friesen. Could you give us a brief synopsis of what is known about IGF-binding proteins in species other than humans or rats?

R. G. Rosenfeld. They have not been defined that well in most species. There are several articles now on porcine binding proteins, and it appears that the same three binding proteins which have been cloned in humans and observed in rats are also found in the porcine model. Ovine, bovine, and mouse binding proteins have all been identified. The one cloned rat binding protein, ICF-BP-2, shows about 85% amino acid homology between the rat and the human form, and, as we showed, antibodies against the human form can quite easily identify the rat binding protein. Thus, these BPs appear to be highly conserved across species.

H. G. Friesen. What about more primitive species, such as amphibians?

R. G. Rosenfeld.   I am not aware of data on them.

M. R. Walters.   I am interested in the presence of the IGF-II receptor in the choroid plexus. There is a report that there is a high concentration of insulin receptors there too. Do you think there is any correlation between those observations? I presume the antibodies are highly specific.

R. G. Rosenfeld.   There are studies showing the distribution of insulin, IGF-I, and IGF-II receptors in the brain. I do not know about the interrelationship between the insulin receptor there and the IGF-II receptor, except to point out that so far as I know, the IGF-II receptor is present in the highest concentrations of the three forms in the choroid plexus.

M. R. Walters.   I am also interested in the relationship between the IGF-II receptor and its target tissue. Do you think that the IGF-II receptor (in tissues in which IGF-II might be active) is present on the cell membrane, at least in part?

R. G. Rosenfeld.   There is no question that the IGF-II receptor is present on the cell membrane and typically comprises 10% of the total cellular content of that receptor. However, the receptor is present in such abundance that 10% actually represents quite high membrane concentrations.

M. R. Walters.   So in most of the tissues in which the receptor is found, a small percentage is on the membrane and a large percentage is internalized. Since a dichotomy is not observed in tissues in which there is a lot of receptor on the membrane and little in the cell, do you think or has it been shown that IGF-II and its receptor are internalized?

R. G. Rosenfeld.   It has been shown that there is a cycling of the receptor from the Golgi apparatus through the cytoplasm to the cell membrane and subsequent internalization. Although in the newborn the receptor appears to be shed from the cell surface in fair abundance, it is also internalized. The big question is what does that receptor do in terms of IGF-II action. Can all of the classic insulinlike and IGF-like activity of IGF-II be defined entirely by the interaction of IGF-II with the insulin and IGF-I receptors, or do we need to postulate some unique biological action for the IGF-II receptor? It appears now that that receptor may, in fact, be linked to diacyl glycerol and IP_3 production, and data from Japan suggest that it is also linked to G proteins and to calcium channels. However, what that means in terms of IGF-II action remains to be seen. We sent our antibody against the IGF-II receptor to Nishimoto in Japan. This group has shown that cells with IGF-II receptors could respond selectively to IGF-II by both a mitogenic action and by calcium flux. We sent them the antireceptor antibody to see if the antibody could block the effect of IGF-II. What it has turned out to do is to exactly mimic the action of IGF-II, much as has been described for some insulin receptor antibodies.

M. R. Walters.   In some ways that is reassuring.

R. G. Rosenfeld.   I think there is a growing body of data to suggest that this receptor may have some unique role for specific action by IGF-II, but what that action exactly is remains to be seen.

M. R. Walters.   Is it known whether all the newly synthesized receptors cycle out to the plasmalemma and then have to recycle back into the cell, or is there a divergent pathway?

R. G. Rosenfeld.   My understanding is that it is a portion of the receptor which cycles from the membrane to the circulation.

G. B. Cutler.   Can you comment on the role that the IGF-I binding proteins play in the developmental changes in circulating IGF in humans during childhood and puberty? Will new information on these proteins help improve the usefulness of measurements of IGF-I in the diagnosis of growth hormone deficiency?

R. G. Rosenfeld.   Those are both good questions. I will deal with the second issue first. There is no question in my mind that accurate assay of IGF-I and IGF-II requires rigorous removal of all binding proteins. Binding proteins will clearly interfere with radioimmunoassays, radioreceptor assays, and bioassays. We have been "burned" often enough to know that you have to account for the binding proteins in any assay. Thus, it is possible that as assay methods are improved to more rigorously observe "pure" IGF-I and IGF-II, these factors will prove to have better predictive value for responsiveness to growth hormone. For example, the data from some of the Genentech-sponsored studies indicate that the IGF assay that employs acid chromatography to remove binding protein has a statistically significant better predictive value than assays which do not use procedures that remove binding protein. In terms of your first question about what the role of these binding proteins might be in the regulation of growth, I haven't got a clue, other than to say that they clearly are very tightly ontogenically regulated and that the ontogeny appears to be somewhat differently regulated in species. One observation which we have just "stumbled" on recently is that BP-3, the large plasma-binding protein, which is far and away the major binding protein in adult plasma, virtually disappears during pregnancy, both in humans and in mice.

M. Ascoli.   In reference to the IGF-II receptor, which binds lysosomal enzymes as well as IGF-II, does the binding of one class of ligand affect the binding of the other class of ligand?

R. G. Rosenfeld.   There are some data to suggest that binding of mannose 6-phosphate or analogs of mannose 6-phosphate results in a modest increase in IGF-II binding, and by "modest," I mean a 50% increase. They are clearly binding to different moieties and do not compete with one another. It is possible, however, that if mannose 6-phosphate is attached to a particularly large glycoprotein and if that protein then binds to the mannose 6-phosphate receptor, it may sterically hinder IGF-II binding. This type of relationship is just beginning to be studied now. It may, in fact, turn out that rather than this receptor binding IGF-II to degrade the IGF-II, IGF-II may have some regulatory role in lysosomal function.

RECENT PROGRESS IN HORMONE RESEARCH, VOL. 46

Growth Hormone Receptor and Binding Protein

STEVEN A. SPENCER,* DAVID W. LEUNG,* PAUL J. GODOWSKI,*
R. GLENN HAMMONDS,* MICHAEL J. WATERS,† AND
WILLIAM I. WOOD*

*Department of Developmental Biology, Genentech, Inc., South San Francisco, California
94080, and †Department of Physiology and Pharmacology, University of Queensland, St. Lucia,
Queensland 4067, Australia

I. Introduction

The ability of growth hormone (GH) to promote whole-body growth has been amply demonstrated both clinically in the treatment of GH-deficient children and in animals. This response is in contrast to the *in vitro* actions of GH, which have been more difficult to demonstrate and often small in magnitude (Hughes and Friesen, 1985; Isaksson *et al.*, 1985). The lack of easily demonstrated GH effects in cell-based assay systems has led, in part, to the somatomedin hypothesis (Salmon and Daughaday, 1957; Rechler *et al.*, 1987), according to which GH produced by the pituitary acts on the liver to induce the synthesis and secretion into the circulation of insulinlike growth factor I (IGF-I). This IGF-I is then responsible for skeletal and tissue growth. Thus, according to this hypothesis, the actions of GH are mediated by circulating IGF-I. However, the presence of high-affinity GH-binding sites in tissues other than the liver (Hughes and Friesen, 1985; Isaksson *et al.*, 1985) and the demonstration of important direct effects of GH on cartilage *in vitro* (Lindahl *et al.*, 1986) and *in vivo* (Isaksson *et al.*, 1982, 1985; Nilsson *et al.*, 1986) suggest that the direct action of GH on specific tissues could have an important role in growth. In addition, GH stimulates the production of IGF-I in a number of tissues other than the liver, and thus growth could be induced by a paracrine or autocrine mechanism, rather than systemically (D'Ercole *et al.*, 1984).

To address these and other questions concerning the actions of GH, we have purified and characterized the GH receptor from rabbit liver (Spencer *et al.*, 1988). From this receptor preparation we have obtained amino acid sequence data that have allowed us to isolate cDNA clones for the rabbit receptor and to determine its full amino acid sequence (Leung *et al.*, 1987). Human GH receptor

165

cDNA clones were subsequently isolated by cross-hybridization. When these clones are transfected in mammalian tissue culture cells, high-affinity GH-binding sites are expressed. The cloning of these receptors will allow us to address the questions of tissue and developmental specificity of GH receptor expression, of whether more than one type of GH receptor exists (at least at the gene level), and of how GH transmits its signal within a cell.

A soluble GH-binding protein has also been identified in rabbit (Ymer and Herington, 1985) and human serum (Baumann et al., 1986; Herington et al., 1986). This protein has a high affinity for GH and shares several epitopes for monoclonal antibody binding with the membrane receptor (Barnard and Waters, 1986). We have purified the GH-binding protein from rabbit serum and have shown by direct amino acid sequence data that it is the extracellular hormone-binding domain of the GH receptor (Spencer et al., 1988).

In addition, we have isolated and characterized human genomic clones spanning the coding region of the GH receptor (Godowski et al., 1989). There are nine exons that encode the receptor and several exons in the 5'-untranslated region. We have used these data to characterize the GH receptor gene in Laron-type dwarfs, a population of growth-deficient individuals thought to be lacking a functional GH receptor. Examination of the DNA from nine of these patients showed that two have a large deletion in the GH receptor gene (Godowski et al., 1989).

II. Purification

Due to the lack of a functional assay for the GH receptor, we and previous workers have relied on specific high-affinity binding of the hormone as the receptor assay. Several groups have partially characterized receptors from rat hepatocytes (Donner, 1983), rat adipocytes (Carter-Su et al., 1984), mouse liver (Smith and Talamantes, 1987), rabbit liver (Waters and Friesen, 1979), and human IM-9 lymphocytes (Hughes et al., 1983; Asakawa et al., 1986). Molecular weight estimates based on the cross-linking of ^{125}I-GH have ranged from 50,000–80,000 for the receptor from rabbit liver (Hughes and Friesen, 1985; Waters and Friesen, 1979; Tsushima et al., 1982; Haeuptle et al., 1983) to 110,000 for IM-9 lymphocytes (Hughes et al., 1983; Asakawa et al., 1986). Previous work has also shown that rabbit liver is a good source for the receptor and that it can be solubilized in Triton X-100 with no loss in binding or affinity for GH (Waters and Friesen, 1979). One complication in using rabbit liver as the source for the GH receptor is that this tissue also contains prolactin receptors, which bind human GH (Waters and Friesen, 1979). However, the two receptors can be distinguished by the binding of bovine GH, which is selective for the GH receptor, and by the binding of ovine prolactin, which shows a strong preference for the prolactin receptor (Posner et al., 1974).

TABLE I

Liver GH Receptor Purification Summary[a]

Fraction	Total protein (mg)	High-affinity sites (pmol)	Specific activity (pmol/mg)	Purification (fold)	Yield (%)
Liver homogenate	40,000	—	—	—	—
14,000 g supernatant	19,000	970	0.051	1	100
142,000 g pellet	4,400	795	0.18	3.5	82
Affinity load	2,500	595	0.24	4.7	62
Urea eluate	0.14	110	790	15,500	11
MgCl$_2$ eluate	0.097	290	3000	59,000	30

[a]Values are for 220 g of liver as the starting material.

The GH receptor from rabbit liver was extracted from the membrane fraction with Triton X-100 and purified in one step on a GH affinity column (Spencer *et al.*, 1988) (Table I). This column was highly optimized and gave a 12,000-fold purification. The use of glycerol-controlled pore glass as the column support allowed the bound receptor to be washed with 4.5 M urea prior to elution with 4.5 M MgCl$_2$; this substantially improved the purity of the receptor. Sodium dodecyl sulfate (SDS) gel analysis of various steps of the purification is shown in Fig. 1. The final MgCl$_2$ eluate contained about 30% of the initial binding activity and showed a prominent band of 130 kDa on SDS gel analysis (Fig. 1A, lane 5). This band was identified as the receptor by immunoblotting with a monoclonal antibody to the receptor (Fig. 1B). The receptor was estimated to be at least 40% pure, based on the SDS gel analysis (Fig. 1) and on a maximum theoretical specific binding of 7700 pmol/mg, assuming one GH-binding site per 130-kDa receptor. The binding constant for the purified receptor is 10–30 nM^{-1}, about the same as that found for liver membranes (9 nM^{-1}).

Despite the use of several protease inhibitors throughout the purification, receptor isolated from frozen rather than fresh rabbit liver or the purified receptor stored at 4°C contained much less of the 130-kDa receptor band and more of a broad band at 50–60 kDa. This receptor degradation occurred with no loss in GH binding. The sensitivity to proteolysis probably accounts for the 50- to 80-kDa size reported previously for the rabbit liver GH receptor (Hughes and Friesen, 1985; Waters and Friesen, 1979; Tsushima *et al.*, 1982; Haeuptle *et al.*, 1983).

The GH-binding protein was purified from rabbit serum using a similar GH affinity column (Spencer *et al.*, 1988). This protein is soluble, and thus, detergent is unnecessary. A considerably greater degree of purification is required, however, because of the high protein concentration in the starting serum. An additional sizing step was added after the affinity column to give an overall purification of 400,000-fold with a 14% yield (Table II). SDS gel analysis of various steps of the purification is shown in Fig. 2A. The broad band centered at

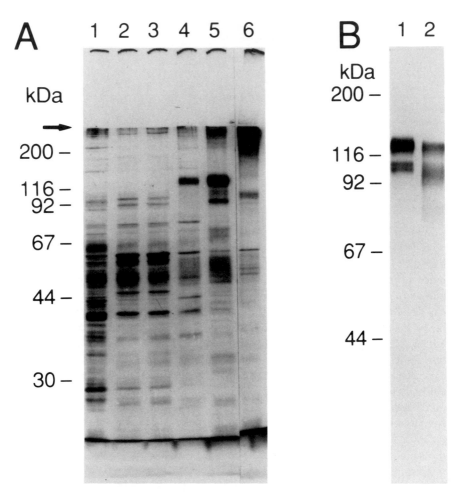

FIG. 1.   (A) Silver-stained 9.5% SDS–PAGE of the human GH affinity column fractions for the rabbit liver GH receptor. One microgram of total protein per lane, lanes 1–5 reduced: lane 1, affinity column load; lane 2, flow-through; lane 3, wash; lane 4, urea eluate; lane 5, $MgCl_2$ eluate; lane 6, $MgCl_2$ eluate nonreduced. The arrow indicates the top of the resolving gel. (B) Immunoblot with Mab 5 of the affinity column $MgCl_2$ eluate: lane 1, starting with fresh nonpregnant female rabbit liver; lane 2, starting with frozen (commercially obtained) pregnant rabbit liver. Both samples are reduced.

51 kDa was identified as the receptor by cross-linking to labeled GH (Fig. 2B) and by elution of binding activity from a nonreduced SDS gel. The final material was judged to be at least 70% pure, based on SDS gel analysis and a maximum theoretical binding of 20,000 pmol/mg, assuming one GH-binding site per 51 kDa of protein. The binding constant of the purified binding protein is 6 nM^{-1}.

TABLE II
GH-Binding Protein Purification Summary[a]

Fraction	Total protein (mg)	High-affinity sites (pmol)	Specific activity (pmol/mg)	Purification (fold)	Yield (%)
Affinity load	24,000	1200	0.050	1	100
Urea eluate	0.87	430	494	9900	36
MgCl$_2$ eluate	0.15	470	3130	63,000	39
S-300 pool	0.086	170	20,000	396,000	14

[a]Values are for 500 ml of serum as the starting material.

Amino-terminal amino acid sequence data were obtained from both the purified GH receptor and the serum-binding protein after elution from preparative SDS gels (Table III). The receptor gave a mixture of two sequences, one of which was ubiquitin at about 20–50% the level of the receptor sequence. The GH-binding protein gave a mixture of three sequences, which could be sorted into one sequence containing several proteolytic clips (Table III). These amino-terminal amino acid sequence data show that the receptor and the binding protein share the same sequence through the first 36 residues. Additional sequence data obtained from peptides of the rabbit-binding protein show that it is probably colinear with the receptor through the first 238 amino acids or nearly to the transmembrane domain (unpublished observations). These data provide a direct demonstration that the GH-binding protein is the extracellular hormone-binding domain of the receptor. Internal amino acid sequence data were also obtained from 10 tryptic and V8 protese peptides from the GH receptor (Table IV).

III. Isolation of cDNA Clones

Clones encoding the rabbit GH receptor were isolated by screening a λgt10 cDNA library with a 57-base oligonucleotide probe based on the amino acid sequence from one of the tryptic peptides (Leung *et al.*, 1987) (TIV, Table IV). From 100,000 oligo(dT)-primed and 100,000 random-primed clones, two and 27 positive clones were identified, respectively. Rescreening of these and specifically primed libraries with probes from the initial isolates gave a set of clones encompassing the entire coding and 3'-untranslated regions of the rabbit receptor (Fig. 3). Clones encoding the full-length human GH receptor were isolated by cross-hybridization to human liver cDNA libraries with probes based on the rabbit receptor (Fig. 3). Two independent clones were obtained and sequenced for all of the protein-coding regions.

The six human and three rabbit cDNA clones containing the 5'-untranslated region of the receptor mRNA diverge considerably. Beginning 12 bp 5' of the

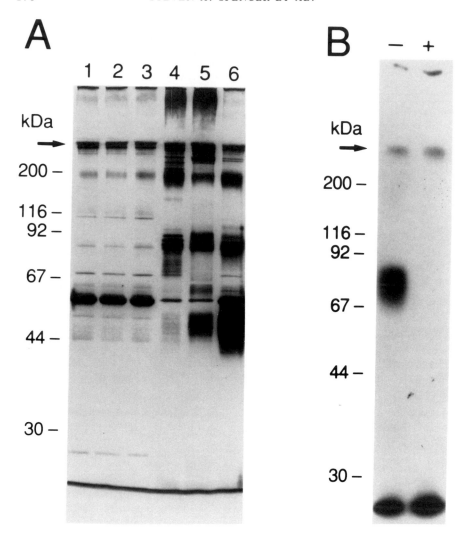

FIG. 2. (A) Silver-stained 9.5% SDS–PAGE of nonreduced fractions from the serum-binding protein purification. One microgram of total protein per lane: lane 1, affinity column load; lane 2, flow-through; lane 3, wash; lane 4, urea eluate; lane 5, MgCl$_2$ eluate; lane 6, S-300 pool. The arrow indicates the top of the resolving gel. (B) Autoradiogram for 48 hours at $-80°$C of ^{125}I-hGH cross-linked to the serum-binding protein MgCl$_2$ fraction in the absence ($-$) or presence ($+$) of excess unlabeled human GH. The arrow indicates the top of the resolving gel.

TABLE III
Amino-Terminal Amino Acid Sequences for the Rabbit Liver GH Receptor and Serum-Binding Protein[a]

```
                  5               10              15              20              25              30              35
GHR-N    F S G S E A (T) P A  T  L  G  R  A  S  E  [S  V  Q  R  V  H  P  G  L  G  T  N  S  S  G  K  P  K  F  T  K]
SBP-N1   X X X S E A  T  P A  T  L  G  R  A  S  E   S  V  Q  X  V  H  P
SBP-N2   — — — — — X  X  E(S) V  Q  R  V  H  P  G   L (G) T  X  X  S (S) G  K  P  K  F  T  X
SBP-N3   — — — — — —  —  X  X  P  X  L  X (T) X  X   S (S  G) K  P  K  F  X  K
```

[a] Sequences were determined by gas phase sequencer analysis of the electroeluted proteins. Brackets indicate residues determined from the cDNA sequence. X shows residues which could not be identified. Parentheses indicate uncertain residues. GHR-N, GH receptor amino-terminal sequence; SBP-N1–3, three simultaneous amino-terminal sequences found for the serum-binding protein.

TABLE IV

Tryptic and V8 Peptides from the 130-kDa Liver GH Receptor[a]

	Approximate initial yield (pmol)	cDNA sequence position	Repetitive yield (%)
Tryptic peptides			
T2.1 (L) [D] K E (Y) (E) V [R] ⎱ mixture	65	204–211	76
T2.2 (E) V [N] E (T) (Q) [W] K ⎰	98	180–187	
T3 (S) G T A E D A P G S E M P V P D Y	40	561–577	92
T4 V E P S F N Q E D I Y I T T E S L T T [T] (A)(E)	60	538–559	92
T5 [C] F [S] V E E I V Q P	29	122–131	68
T6.1 S P G S V (Q)(L)(F) Y I R ⎱ mixture	34	60–70	88
T6.2 T [S][C](Y)(E)(P)(D)(I)[L](E) N D F N A [S] D ⎰	19	369–385	
V8 peptides			
V3 [W] K [E][C] P (D)(Y) V [S](A)(G)(E)(N)[S][C](Y) F	—	80–96	—
V5.1 (S) T L Q A A P S Q L S N P N S L A N I D F Y ⎱ mixture	24	448–469	88
V5.2 (F) I E L D I D D ⎰	12	327–334	

[a]Parentheses indicate uncertain residues. Brackets indicate residues not called or incorrectly called, in which case, the residue shown is from the cDNA sequence.

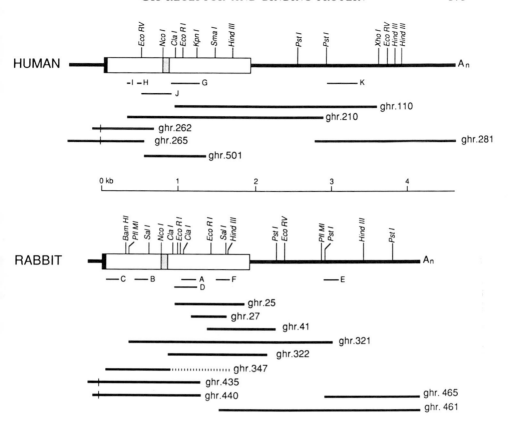

FIG. 3. Maps of the cloned cDNAs for the human and rabbit GH receptors. The coding region of the mRNA is shown as a box. The solid region is the signal sequence; the stippled part is the transmembrane domain. A–K, Probes and oligonucleotide primers used in the cDNA cloning. The individual cDNA clones are labeled ghr.25–501. The clones diverge 5' of the vertical bar shown on clones ghr.262, 265, 435, and 440. The 3' divergence of clone ghr.347 is shown by a dotted line.

initiating ATG, the nine clones have seven different sequences. Genomic cloning data (Section V) show that the point of divergence of these clones corresponds to an exon boundary, and thus, there must be considerable splicing variation in the 5'-untranslated region. The significance of this multiple splicing and whether these divergent regions are the result of different promoters have not yet been investigated.

Both the rabbit and human GH receptor clones contain an open reading frame of 638 amino acids (Fig. 4). The predicted rabbit and human amino acid sequences can be aligned without insertions or deletions and show 84% identity overall. All 11 of the amino acid sequences determined for the rabbit receptor (Tables III and IV) are found in the open reading frame. The amino-terminal

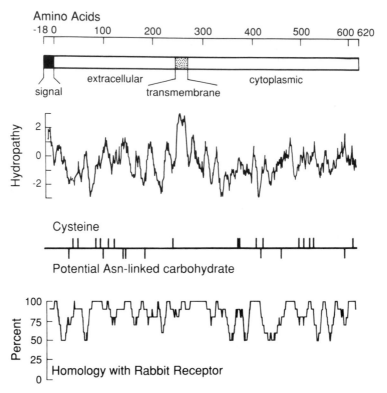

FIG. 4. The human GH receptor. The hydropathy plot is with a window of 10 residues; positive values indicate increasing hydrophobicity. The potential N-linked glycosylation sites are NXS/T. The similarity with the rabbit receptor is for exact matches over a window of 10 amino acids.

amino acid sequence of the receptor is preceded by an 18-amino-acid secretion signal sequence beginning with a methionine residue. Thus, the cDNA clones predict a mature full-length receptor of 620 amino acids. The predicted molecular weight of this protein would be 70,000, considerably smaller than the 130,000 found for the purified receptor. However, much of the apparent discrepancy can be accounted for by glycosylation (Spencer *et al.*, 1988) and the covalently bound ubiquitin.

A hydropathy plot (Fig. 4) indicates a single transmembrane domain in the middle of the receptor. In computer-assisted searches of several protein data bases, no substantial similarity was found between the GH receptor sequence and other known proteins (Leung *et al.*, 1987). Recently, however, clones encoding the rat prolactin receptor have been isolated (Boutin *et al.*, 1988), and this receptor has about 35% overall sequence identity (some regions as high as 70%) with the GH receptor. Thus, these two receptors define a new class of single transmembrane receptor proteins for which the signaling mechanism is currently unknown (Waters *et al.*, 1988).

Clear evidence suggesting that the GH-binding protein is transcribed from an alternatively spliced GH mRNA (at least in mice) has been recently provided by Talamantes and co-workers (Smith *et al.*, 1989). In the course of characterizing and cloning the mouse GH receptor, they have found and isolated clones from two receptor mRNA species from mouse liver. The larger of these is about 3.9 kb and corresponds to the full-length GH receptor clones we have isolated, while the smaller (1.2 kb) has the identical sequence for the 5' region, but diverges just before the transmembrane domain. The divergent sequence continues for 27 hydrophilic amino acids and thus should produce a soluble secreted GH-binding protein.

Although the 1.2-kb mRNA has been observed in mouse and rat tissues, it has not been observed in rabbit liver (Leung *et al.*, 1987) or human IM-9 mRNA preparations (data not shown). Because the isolated rabbit GH receptor is easily proteolyzed, we have speculated that the GH-binding protein might be derived from the receptor by proteolysis (Leung *et al.*, 1987). This possibility is supported by a recent report that in human IM-9 lymphocytes a protease can be activated by sulfhydryl modifying reagents that rapidly cleaves the high-molecular-weight receptor, releasing a form of the GH-binding protein (Trivedi and Daughaday, 1988). More work is needed to establish how the binding protein is produced in various species and to determine whether there are species-dependent mechanisms for generating it. In addition, no biological function has been demonstrated for the GH-binding protein.

IV. Expression

Expression of the rabbit GH receptor was achieved by assembling a full-length cDNA clone in a mammalian expression vector in which transcription is directed by a human cytomegalovirus promoter (Leung *et al.*, 1987). When this plasmid is transfected into COS-7 monkey kidney cells, high-level receptor expression is found on the cell membranes, as determined by GH binding (Fig. 5). An average of 200,000 copies of the receptor are expressed per cell. The binding constant for human GH is 10 nM^{-1}, comparable to that of the natural purified receptor.

Expression and secretion of a form of the human GH-binding protein have been achieved (Leung *et al.*, 1987). When the human receptor is engineered to place a stop codon at the start of the transmembrane domain and is transfected into COS-7 cells, high-affinity GH binding is found in the culture medium (Fig. 5). This secreted binding protein has a binding constant of 3 nM^{-1}. The hormone-binding specificities for the expressed rabbit receptor and human binding protein are as expected from the known species specificity of binding. The expressed rabbit receptor binds human and bovine GH, but binds ovine prolactin

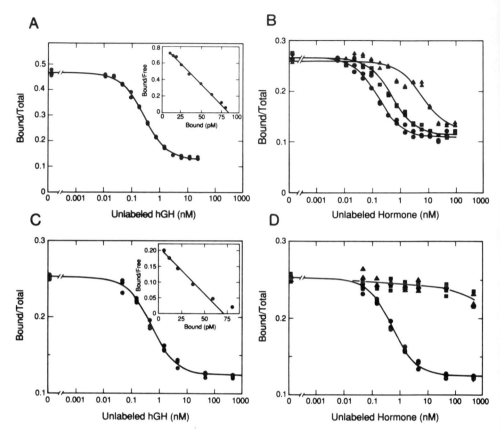

FIG. 5.   Expression of the rabbit and human GH receptor cDNA clones in COS-7 monkey kidney cells. Assays of expressed GH receptor and binding protein by competition with ^{125}I-hGH. (A) Competition assay with unlabeled human GH (hGH) of membranes from transfected cells expressing rabbit GH receptor. (Inset) Scatchard plot of the same data. (B) Competition assay with unlabeled hGH (●), bovine GH (■), or ovine prolactin (▲) of the rabbit receptor shown in (A). (C) Competition assay with unlabeled hGH of culture medium from transfected cells expressing human soluble binding protein. (Inset) Scatchard plot of the same data. (D) Competition assay with unlabeled hGH (●), bovine GH (■), or ovine prolactin (▲) of the human binding protein shown in (C).

only poorly, while the expressed human binding protein binds human GH, but not bovine GH or ovine prolactin (Fig. 5).

V.   Isolation of Genomic Clones

Six genomic clones were isolated from human λ libraries with cDNA probes from the cloned GH receptor (Godowski *et al.*, 1989) (Fig. 6). The hybridizing regions from these clones were sequenced to determine the exact extent of each

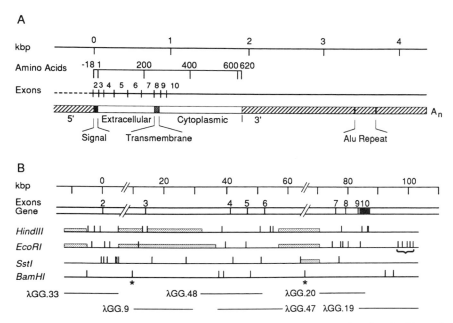

FIG. 6. (A) The human GH receptor mRNA and protein. Shown are scales of nucleotides and amino acids, the location of the exon boundaries, and the major features of the protein and the mRNA. (B) Map of the human GH receptor gene. Shown are a scale of nucleotides, location of the exons, restriction map for four enzymes, and location of six genomic clones. Two gaps in the map are shown at their minimum length. The length of the 3 to 4 intron is established only by the coincidence of genomic *Sst*I fragments in the region, and thus could be longer. The *Bam*HI sites indicated by asterisks might represent more than one site, separated by an unknown distance. The order of the bracketed *Eco*RI sites is unknown. The restriction map is unknown in the stippled regions.

exon. The sequence data show that the protein-coding region of the human GH receptor is encoded by nine exons numbered 2–10 (Fig. 6). Exons 2–9 range in size from 66 to 179 bp, while exon 10 is about 3400 bp, encoding nearly all of the cytoplasmic domain as well as the 3′-untranslated region. Exon 2 is nearly coincident with the secretion signal sequence; exon 8, with the transmembrane domain. The extracellular domain is encoded by exons 3–7. Most of the as yet uncharacterized 5′-untranslated region is present on a series of differentially spliced exons. The gene for the human receptor has been localized to chromosome 5p13.1–p12 by *in situ* hybridization (Barton *et al.*, 1989) and spans at least 87 kbp.

Characterization of the nine exons encoding the receptor has allowed us to assign the approximately 10 bands found for the receptor on genomic blots. Prior to this assignment it was unclear whether these multiple hybridizing bands were due to the cloned GH receptor or whether they represented a family of related receptor genes. Based on the assignment of all of the receptor bands, we conclude that these blots show no evidence for a family of GH receptors.

VI. Analysis of DNA from Laron-Type Dwarfs

Laron-type dwarfism (LTD) is a rare autosomal recessive growth disorder characterized by normal or elevated levels of circulating GH and low levels of IGF-I (Laron et al., 1966, 1968; Laron, 1984; McKusick, 1988). Some LTD patients have been shown to lack liver GH binding (Eshet et al., 1984) as well as GH-binding activity in their serum (Daughaday and Trivedi, 1987; Baumann et al., 1986; Laron et al., 1989). To establish directly that LTD can result from a defect in the GH receptor, we examined the receptor gene from nine individuals with LTD (Godowski et al., 1989). Blot hybridization of LTD DNA with a full-length human GH receptor cDNA probe showed that for seven of the DNA samples there was no clear alteration in the pattern of hybridizing bands (with the exception of one band from one individual that was the result of a DNA alteration outside the protein-coding region). Two of the nine patients showed alterations in the pattern of hybridizing bands with more than one restriction enzyme digest and were analyzed further. Exon-specific blot hybridization shows clearly that several exons were missing in both of these patients (Fig. 7). Normal-sized bands were found for exons 2 and 7–10 (Fig. 7; some data not shown); however, no bands were found for exons 3, 5, and 6, and an unusual band was found for exon 4. These data show that a large portion of the extracellular GH-binding domain of the receptor was missing in these two patients. Clearly, more than a simple deletion has occurred, because noncontiguous exons were missing. It is likely that this deletion of about one-half of the extracellular domain was responsible for the growth defect in these two individuals. Thus, we conclude that the GH receptor we have identified is required for proper growth. Clearly, however, LTD can also result from other defects in the receptor or from defects in additional proteins required for signaling.

VII. Conclusion

The purification and cloning of the GH receptor and the binding protein have contributed to our understanding of hormonally controlled growth in mammals (Leung et al., 1987; Spencer et al., 1988). The GH and prolactin receptors (and probably the as yet uncloned placental lactogen receptor) constitute a new family of signaling proteins with a single transmembrane domain (Boutin et al., 1988; Waters et al., 1988). It is hoped that availability of the cloned receptors will allow elucidation of the intracellular signaling mechanism for these hormones. Since the GH receptor was initially identified only by its binding activity, there

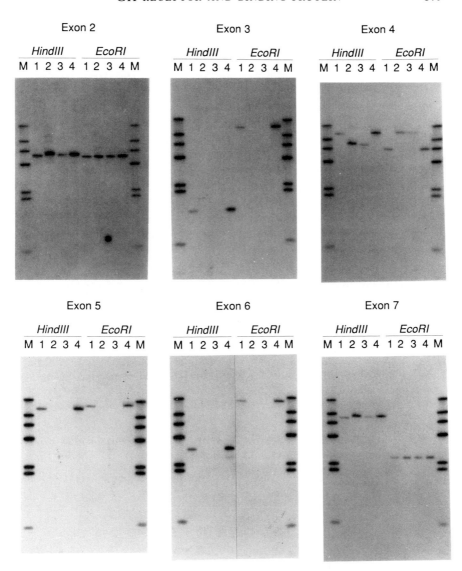

FIG. 7. Genomic blots hybridized with exon-specific probes. Blots containing DNA from two normal individuals (lanes 1 and 4) or LTD patients 147 (lane 2) or D1 (lane 3) were hybridized with exon-specific probes as indicated. Marker DNA (lane M) is ^{32}P-labeled λHindIII.

has been some concern that it might not be the receptor responsible for controlling growth. The demonstration of a deletion in the GH receptor gene in individuals with LTD provides strong evidence that this receptor plays a central role in growth (Godowski *et al.*, 1989).

In situ hybridization work in progress suggests that the GH receptor is widely distributed on many tissues, although it is most abundant in the liver. This wide distribution suggests that direct actions of GH could play a role in the growth process in addition to (or perhaps instead of) the indirect action suggested by the somatomedin hypothesis. Although a family of GH receptor genes has not been identified, subtypes of the receptor with different biological actions could exist, possibly the result of differential posttranslational modifications of the receptor. Different receptor-associated proteins might also regulate its action.

The availability of the GH receptor expressed by recombinant DNA techniques has already been useful in determining which amino acids in GH are required for binding to the receptor (Cunningham *et al.*, 1989; Cunningham and Wells, 1989). It is hoped that in the near future direct structural analysis will show in detail the interaction between GH and its receptor.

REFERENCES

Asakawa, K., Hedo, J. A., McElduff, A., Rouiller, D. G., Waters, M. J., and Gordon, P. (1986). *Biochem. J.* **238,** 379–386.

Barnard, R., and Waters, M. J. (1986). *Biochem. J.* **237,** 885–892.

Barton, D. E., Foellmer, B. E., Wood, W. I., and Francke, U. (1989). *Cytogenet. Cell Genet.* **50,** 137–141.

Baumann, G., Stolar, M. W., Amburn, K., Barsano, C. P., and DeVries, B. C. (1986). *J. Clin. Endocrinol. Metab.* **62,** 134–141.

Boutin, J.-M., Jolicoeur, C., Okamura, H., Gagnon, J., Edery, M., Shirota, M., Banville, D., Dusanter-Fourt, I., Djiane, J., and Kelly, P. A. (1988). *Cell (Cambridge, Mass.)* **53,** 69–77.

Carter-Su, C., Schwartz, J., and Kikuchi, G. (1984). *J. Biol. Chem.* **259,** 1099–1104.

Cunningham, B. C., and Wells, J. A. (1989). *Science* **244,** 1081–1085.

Cunningham, B. C., Jhurani, P., Ng, P., and Wells, J. A. (1989). *Science* **243,** 1330–1336.

Daughaday, W. H., and Trivedi, B. (1987). *Proc. Natl. Acad. Sci. U.S.A.* **84,** 4636–4640.

D'Ercole, A. J., Stiles, A. D., and Underwood, L. E. (1984). *Proc. Natl. Acad. Sci. U.S.A.* **81,** 935–939.

Donner, D. (1983). *J. Biol. Chem.* **258,** 2736–2743.

Eshet, R., Laron, Z., Pertzelan, A., Amon, R., and Dintzman, M. (1984). *Isr. J. Med. Sci.* **20,** 8–11.

Godowski, P. J., Leung, D. W., Meacham, L. R., Galgani, J. P., Hellmiss, R., Keret, R., Rotwein, P. S., Parks, J. S., Laron, Z., and Wood, W. I. (1989). *Proc. Natl. Acad. Sci. U.S.A.* **86,** 8083–8087.

Haeuptle, M.-T., Aubert, M. L., Djiane, J., and Kraehenbuhl, J.-P. (1983). *J. Biol. Chem.* **258,** 305–314.

Herington, A. C., Ymer, S. I., and Stevenson, J. L. (1986). *J. Clin. Invest.* **77,** 1817–1823.

Hughes, J. P., and Friesen, H. G. (1985). *Annu. Rev. Physiol.* **47,** 469–482.

Hughes, J. P., Simpson, J. S. A., and Friesen, H. G. (1983). *Endocrinology (Baltimore)* **112,** 1980–1985.

Isaksson, O. G. P., Jansson, J.-O., and Gause, I. A. M. (1982). *Science* **216,** 1237–1239.

Isaksson, O. G. P., Edén, S., and Jansson, J.-O. (1985). *Annu. Rev. Physiol.* **47,** 483–499.

Laron, Z. (1984). *In* "Advances in Internal Medicine and Pediatrics" (H. P. Frick, G. A. Harnack, K. Kochsiek, G. A. Martini, and A. Prader, eds.), pp. 117–150. Springer-Verlag, New York.

Laron, Z., Pertzelan, A., and Mannheimer, S. (1966). *Isr. J. Med. Sci.* **2,** 152–155.

Laron, Z., Pertzelan, A., and Karp, M. (1968). *Isr. J. Med. Sci.* **4,** 883–894.

Laron, Z., Klinger, B., Erster, B., and Silbergeld, A. (1989). *Acta Endocrinol. (Copenhagen)* **121,** 603–608.

Leung, D. W., Spencer, S. A., Cachianes, G., Hammonds, R. G., Collins, C., Henzel, W. J., Barnard, R., Waters, M. J., and Wood, W. I. (1987). *Nature (London)* **330,** 537–543.

Lindahl, A., Isgaard, J., Nilsson, A., and Isaksson, O. G. P. (1986). *Endocrinology (Baltimore)* **118,** 1843–1848.

McKusick, V. A. (1988). "Mendelian Inheritance in Man," 8th ed., pp. 1141–1142. Johns Hopkins Univ. Press, Baltimore, Maryland.

Nilsson, A., Isgaard, J., Lindahl, A., Dahlström, A., Skottner, A., and Isaksson, O. G. P. (1986). *Science* **233,** 571–574.

Posner, B. I., Kelly, P. A., Shiu, R. P. C., and Friesen, H. G. (1974). *Endocrinology (Baltimore)* **95,** 521–531.

Rechler, M. M., Nissley, S. P., and Roth, J. (1987). *N. Engl. J. Med.* **316,** 941–943.

Salmon, W. D., Jr., and Daughaday, W. H. (1957). *J. Lab. Clin. Invest.* **49,** 825–836.

Smith, W. C., and Talamantes, F. (1987). *J. Biol. Chem.* **262,** 2213–2219.

Smith, W. C., Linzer, D. I. H., and Talamantes, F. (1988). *Proc. Natl. Acad. Sci. U.S.A.* **85,** 9576–9579.

Smith, W. C., Kuniyoshi, J., and Talamantes, F. (1989). *Mol. Endocrinol.* **3,** 984–990.

Spencer, S. A., Hammonds, R. G., Henzel, W. J., Rodriguez, H., Waters, M. J., and Wood, W. I. (1988). *J. Biol. Chem.* **263,** 7862–7867.

Trivedi, B., and Daughaday, W. H. (1988). *Endocrinology (Baltimore)* **123,** 2201–2206.

Tsushima, T., Murakami, H., Wakai, K., Isozaki, O., Sato, Y., and Shizume, K. (1982). *FEBS Lett.* **147,** 49–53.

Waters, M. J., and Friesen, H. G. (1979). *J. Biol. Chem.* **254,** 6815–6825.

Waters, M. J., Barnard, R., Hamlin, G., Spencer, S. A., Hammonds, R. G., Leung, D. W., Henzel, W. J., Cachianes, G., and Wood, W. I. (1988). *In* "Progress in Endocrinology" (H. Imra, K. Shizume, and S. Yoshida, eds.), pp. 601–607. Elsevier, Amsterdam.

Ymer, S. I., and Herington, A. C. (1985). *Mol. Cell. Endocrinol.* **41,** 153–161.

DISCUSSION

H. G. Friesen. Can you tell whether osteoblasts or osteoclasts contain GH receptors?

W. I. Wood. We cannot.

R. S. Swerdloff. I am interested in the role of growth hormone in sexual maturation. Children who are growth hormone deficient have delayed sexual maturation. What role, if any, growth hormone has in that process is unclear. About 15 or so years ago Odell and I presented at a Laurentian Hormone Conference work on sexual maturation which indicated that in the hypophysectomized immature rat, FSH would induce LH receptors. In related studies that were also presented, we demonstrated that growth hormone also had an effect on the induction of LH receptors. It was not clear at that time how pure the GH preparations were, thus leaving some doubt about the interpretation of the results. There has been continued interest and some confusion in this field over the years. In order to help answer the question, have you had a chance to study growth hormone receptors in the gonads? If there are receptors in the testes, have you used *in situ* techniques to determine what cells have these receptors?

W. I. Wood.   Such studies have not yet been done.

W. F. Crowley.   You showed that the arcuate nucleus stains densely for the growth hormone receptor. Have you cross-stained these neurons for content, such as for GnRH, which may be of interest? What is the relationship of your GH receptor to the lower-molecular-weight binding protein for growth hormone described by Baumann?

W. I. Wood.   In answer to the first question, we have examined other brain sections, but the survey in brain is not complete. We have not attempted to study the Baumann protein chiefly because the binding constant is sufficiently low that little of the growth hormone that circulates normally would be bound to that protein.

M. New.   Although these children are very small and are dwarfs, they do grow, albeit very slowly, over a long period of time. I just wondered whether anyone has speculated as to how these children do grow in view of the gene deletion you have demonstrated.

W. I. Wood.   My speculation about that would be that growth hormone only provides a certain measure of the control and that there is a basal amount of growth in its absence.

C. M. Foster.   Can you comment on the fact that the group of Carter-Su has shown that there is phosphorylation on tyrosine residues of the growth hormone receptor in response to binding growth hormone in intact cells and has now shown similar results in a solubilized membrane system?

W. I. Wood.   We have collaborated with Christin Carter-Su, and have been very interested in data showing that there appears to be phosphorylation of a molecule of similar size. It probably is the same growth hormone receptor molecule. This work resulted from suggestions that perhaps the molecule would be a tyrosine kinase. We have attempted to determine whether or not our expressed growth hormone receptor could be phosphorylated. To date, the data from this study as I understand it, are equivocal. It does not rule out the possibility that this molecule is phosphorylated; some experiments suggest it might be. So I think there is still an outstanding question, the answer to which could be one of perhaps two obvious possibilities. One would be the unusual circumstance that the cytoplasmic region is a tyrosine kinase with a whole different sequence which we are not as yet aware of, or that in preparations made to date, there is an activated kinase which is a separate protein or perhaps an associated kinase about which we know nothing as yet which is able to phosphorylate the receptor and add some regulatory effect. We are very eager to try to sort out what the "story" really is.

R. Rosenfeld.   Concerning the role of growth hormone in reproductive and sexual maturation function, you do not really have to postulate the presence of growth hormone receptors in gonadal tissues, since it is clear that both the ovary and the testis have abundant IGF receptors and that IGF is known to be synergistic with FSH, for example, in some of the progesterone synthetic functions of the ovary. Interestingly, if you treat granulosa cell cultures or rats *in vivo* with FSH, you get a dramatic reduction in IGF-binding protein production by those cells, which would theoretically liberate free IGF for biological use. Are you assuming that the seven Laron dwarfs who apparently do not have the gene deletions have point mutations?

W. I. Wood.   In 100 patients we found two deletions and four point mutations. I would guess that typically there should be an equal or greater frequency of point mutations than deletions in these types of situations. So, yes, I am assuming that a number of these should have point mutations. On the other hand, I would not suggest that they all do. There clearly could be other steps beyond the receptor and between that and IGF production which could give exactly the same phenotype.

R. Rosenfeld.   Have those seven dwarfs been shown, in fact, to have reduced growth hormone-binding proteins?

W. I. Wood.   Yes, they all have. So the assumption is that it should be in the same protein. Of the Laron dwarfs who have been assayed, I do not know how many have been shown to actually have growth hormone-binding protein.

F. S. French.   My understanding is that Laron dwarfs have increased levels of growth hormone. Is this correct?

W. I. Wood. They do have elevated levels some of the time.

F. S. French.   In your *in situ* hybridizations, would the localization of growth hormone receptors either in the pituitary or in the hypothalamus suggest that growth hormone itself is feeding back to regulate the level of growth hormone production, or is this regulation due to some other mechanism, such as somatomedin or IGF-I?

W. I. Wood.   Based especially on the localization of the pituitary, I think we are going to have to consider all the possible loops. We are going to have to consider loops through growth hormone and the longer loop through IGF-I. I think it just stresses the fact that we are going to have to spend quite a bit of effort in determining the actual physiology of these situations.

S. I. Taylor.   Normally, the major pathway whereby insulin is cleared from the circulation is via receptor-mediated endocytosis, primarily in the liver. In patients with a decreased number of insulin receptors, this leads to impaired clearance of insulin and, consequently, to elevated levels of insulin in plasma. By analogy, it is possible that a decrease in the number of growth hormone receptors would decrease the clearance of growth hormone from plasma. Thus, it may be possible to explain the observed elevation of growth hormone levels without invoking an abnormality in growth hormone secretion.

W. I. Wood.   I would agree with that, and since there may also be quite a bit of growth hormone clearance through the kidney, we have several possibilities to examine there too.

S. M. Rosenthal.   We reported some data in 1986 showing there was some effect of exogenous growth hormone in blunting basal growth hormone secretion in pituitary cells in tissue culture which was species specific. This would be some evidence for GH feedback on its own secretion at the level of the pituitary.

W. I. Wood.   Yes it would.

J. H. Clark.   You casually mentioned that you had failed to be able to express the gene in transfected cells. You must have done some work with this. Would you elaborate?

W. I. Wood.   We have been able to express the growth hormone receptor in transfected cells. We get in a transient transfection 200,000 receptors per cell. What we failed to do is to demonstrate that this receptor does anything other than bind the hormone; thus, we have been unable to show that the receptor transduces a signal of any kind.

M. Rozakis.   I know that you have not been able to express the human growth hormone receptor cDNA. Have you been able to overcome this? If not, what seems to be the problem?

W. I. Wood.   I have glossed over one embarrassing little problem and that is that, in spite of our best molecular biological efforts, our efforts to assemble the two halves of the human cDNA clones into one clone have not worked. The problem is that there are two sequences which, when juxtaposed in *E. coli,* did not grow. So we have had problems making this DNA.

M. Rozakis.   Are you aware of the paper by Ailhaud that was published in *PNAS* in January 1989, in which quiescent committed Ob1771 preadipocytes showed severalfold stimulation of DAG and protein kinase C upon the addition of growth hormone and in which Ailhaud postulated a novel transmembrane signaling system that does not involve inositol phosphates but possibly involves phospholipid glycans?

W. I. Wood.   Yes, we are aware of his work and are following up on it now.

Mutations in the Insulin Receptor Gene in Genetic Forms of Insulin Resistance

Simeon I. Taylor, Takashi Kadowaki, Domenico Accili, Alessandro Cama, Hiroko Kadowaki, Catherine McKeon, Victoria Moncada, Bernice Marcus-Samuels, Charles Bevins, Kaie Ojamaa, Catherine Frapier, Laurie Beitz, Nicola Perrotti, Robert Rees-Jones, Ronald Margolis, Eiichi Imano, Sonia Najjar, Felicia Courtney, Richard Arakaki, Phillip Gorden, and Jesse Roth

Diabetes Branch, National Institute of Diabetes and Digestive and Kidney Diseases, National Institutes of Health, Bethesda, Maryland 20892

I. Introduction

The insulin receptor is a cell surface glycoprotein that mediates the action of insulin on target cells. The receptor was originally identified by its ability to bind the hormone (Freychet *et al.*, 1971a,b; Cuatrecasas, 1971). Over the past two decades considerable progress has been made in defining the structure of the receptor molecule (Kahn *et al.*, 1981; Ullrich *et al.*, 1985; Ebina *et al.*, 1985; Taylor, 1988) as well as the biochemical mechanism by which it mediates insulin action (Kasuga *et al.*, 1982a,b; Rosen, 1987). In addition, the insulin receptor has been identified as a target for pathological processes in human disease. For example, some patients develop autoantibodies directed against insulin receptors. These antireceptor antibodies can either cause hypoglycemia by mimicking insulin action (Kahn *et al.*, 1977; Taylor *et al.*, 1982a) or induce insulin resistance by inhibiting insulin binding and accelerating the rate of receptor degradation (Flier *et al.*, 1976; Taylor and Marcus-Samuels, 1984).

In this review we describe mutations in the insulin receptor gene that have been identified in patients with genetic forms of insulin resistance (Fig. 1, Table I). Two clinical features are commonly observed in patients with extreme insulin resistance, irrespective of the biochemical mechanism which causes the insulin resistance: (1) acanthosis nigricans, a hyperkeratotic hyperpigmented skin lesion and (2) hyperandrogenism, due to increased ovarian production of testosterone, a clinical sign that is commonly observed in premenopausal women with extreme

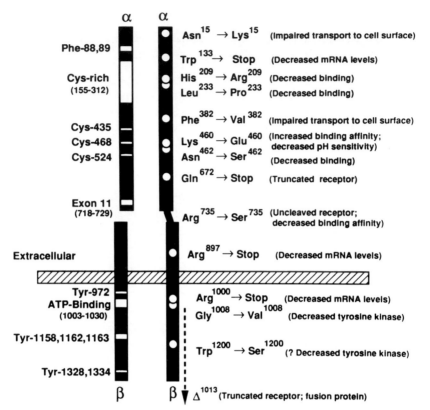

FIG. 1. Mutations in the insulin receptor gene in insulin-resistant patients. Key structural land-marks are identified on the left. Phe-88, Phe-89, and the cysteine-rich domain have all been implicated as playing a role in the insulin-binding domain. Cys-435, Cys-468, and Cys-524 are candidates to contribute sulfhydryl groups for the formation of the disulfide bonds between adjacent α subunits. Exon 11 has been described to undergo variable splicing. As described in the text, the five or six tyrosine residues which are sites of autophosphorylation are indicated. The consensus sequence for an ATP-binding domain is located between amino acid residues 1003–1030. The locations of all of the mutations reported to cause insulin resistance are noted on the right.

insulin resistance (Fig. 2). While all of the syndromes of extreme insulin resistance share some features in common, multiple distinct syndromes can be defined based on the presence or absence of specific clinical features (Table II). For example, type A extreme insulin resistance is defined by the triad of insulin resistance, acanthosis nigricans, and hyperandrogenism in the absence of obesity or lipoatrophy. In lipoatrophic diabetes there is atrophy of subcutaneous fat, hypertriglyceridemia, and fatty metamorphosis of the liver. Patients with leprechaunism have multiple abnormal features, including intrauterine growth retardation and fasting hypoglycemia. Rabson–Mendenhall syndrome is associated

TABLE I
Genetics of Insulin Resistance[a]

Mutation	Syndrome	Reference
Simple homozygotes (consanguineous kindred)		
Pro-233	Leprechaunism	Klinkhamer *et al.* (1989)
Arg-209	Leprechaunism	Kadowaki *et al.* (1990b)
Val-382	Type A insulin resistance	Accili *et al.* (1989)
Ser-735	Type A insulin resistance	Yoshimasa *et al.* (1988)
Compound heterozygotes		
Amber-672/Glu-460	Leprechaunism	Kadowaki *et al.* (1988)
Opal-897/low mRNA[b]	Leprechaunism	Kadowaki *et al.* (1990a)
Amber-133/Ser-462	Type A	Kadowaki *et al.* (1990b)
Opal-1000/Lys-15	Rabson–Mendenhall	Kadowaki *et al.* (1990b)
Presumed simple heterozygotes (dominant inheritance)		
Glu-460	Father of leprechaun	Kadowaki *et al.* (1988, 1990b)
Δ-1013	Type A insulin resistance	Taira *et al.* (1989)
Val-1008	Type A insulin resistance	Odawara *et al.* (1989)
Trp-1200	Type A insulin resistance	Moller and Flier (1988)

[a]Patients with genetic forms of extreme insulin resistance are classified with respect to whether they are simple homozygotes (i.e., homozygous for the same mutation), compound heterozygotes (i.e., heterozygous for two distinct mutations), or simple heterozygotes (i.e., heterozygous for one mutation). All of the simple homozygotes who have been described in the literature have resulted from consanguineous marriages. In some patients classified as simple heterozygotes, the allele which is presumed to be normal has not been completely sequenced, so it remains possible that there is a mutation which has not been identified. Thus, it is possible that some of these patients are actually compound heterozygotes (see footnote [b]).

[b]Leprechaun/Minn-1 is classified as a compound heterozygote, despite the fact that a mutation has not been directly identified in her maternal allele. Nevertheless, indirect data have been obtained supporting the conclusion that there is a mutation in this allele (see Section II,A).

with abnormalities of the teeth and nails and, reportedly, pineal hyperplasia.

In most of the patients with genetic forms of extreme insulin resistance, two mutant alleles of the insulin receptor gene have been identified (Table I). In the case of consanguineous kindreds, the affected patients are homozygous for the same mutation. However, in pedigrees in which there is no inbreeding, the affected individuals are compound heterozygotes, having inherited two different mutant alleles of the insulin receptor gene. In some patients mutations have been identified in only one allele of the insulin receptor gene, and the patients are thought to be simple heterozygotes. It has been proposed that these mutations cause insulin resistance in a dominant fashion. Nevertheless, it is important to remember that the second allele of the insulin receptor gene has been completely sequenced in only one of these presumed heterozygotes (father of leprechaun/Ark-1). Thus, it is possible that some of these patients are compound heterozygotes as well.

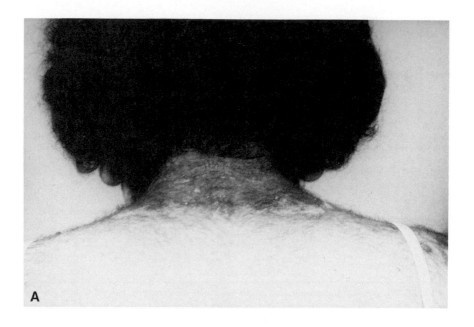

FIG. 2.   Patients with leprechaunism and Type A extreme insulin resistance. (A) Patient A-5 (Barnes *et al.*, 1974; Accili *et al.*, 1989), who has acanthosis nigricans on the back of her neck. The hirsutism noted on her back reflects the hyperandrogenism due to increased ovarian production of testosterone. (B) Leprechaun/Minn-1 (Taylor *et al.*, 1982), who was small for gestational age, weighing only 1.3 kg at birth. In addition, she had multiple phenotypic abnormalities, including low-set ears and a depressed nasal bridge.

II.   Defects in Insulin Receptor Biosynthesis

The pathway of insulin receptor biosynthesis is complex, involving transcription of the gene, translation of the mRNA, and multiple posttranslational modifications. After the completion of biosynthesis, the mature receptor molecule is transported to the cell surface for insertion into the plasma membrane. Defects have been described that impair many of these steps and thereby lead to a reduction in the number of insulin receptors on the cell surface.

A.   TRANSCRIPTION OF THE INSULIN RECEPTOR GENE

The insulin receptor is encoded by a single-copy gene which has been mapped to the short arm of chromosome 19 (bands p13.2 → p13.3) (Yang-Feng *et al.*, 1985). The gene spans at least 150 kbp of DNA and contains 22 exons (Seino *et*

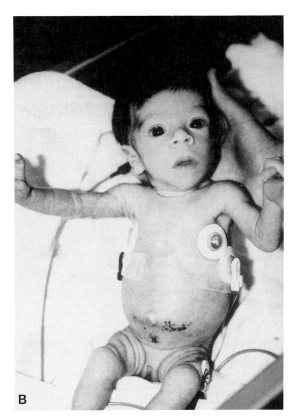

FIG. 2 B.

al., 1989). Typical of a "housekeeping" gene, the promoter lacks a TATA box. Instead, there appear to be multiple start sites for transcription located 300–600 bp upstream of the AUG codon encoding the amino-terminal methionine of the preproreceptor (Mamula *et al.*, 1988; Tewari *et al.*, 1989; McKeon *et al.*, 1990). Furthermore, there are at least five different species of insulin receptor mRNA, ranging in length from approximately 5 to 11 kb (Ullrich *et al.*, 1985; Ojamaa *et al.*, 1988; Tewari *et al.*, 1989) (Fig. 3). This size heterogeneity arises from the utilization of alternate polyadenylation signals in exon 22. The physiological significance of this size heterogeneity has not been elucidated.

We have studied an insulin-resistant patient with leprechaunism (leprechaun/Minn-1) (Fig. 2) in whose cells there is a 90% reduction of the number of insulin receptors (Taylor *et al.*, 1982b). This decrease in receptor number results from a 90% decrease in the level of insulin receptor mRNA in the patient's cells

TABLE II
Clinical Syndromes of Extreme Insulin Resistance

Syndrome	Acanthosis nigricans	Hyperandrogenism	Selected other features
Genetic			
Type A insulin resistance	+[a]	+[a]	
Lipoatrophic diabetes	+	+	Atrophy of subcutaneous adipose tissue
Leprechaunism	±	±	Intrauterine growth retardation
Rabson–Mendenhall	+	+	Dystrophic nails and teeth; pineal hyperplasia(?)
Autoimmune			
Type B insulin resistance	+[a]	±	Antireceptor antibodies; other autoimmune manifestations

[a]This feature is a part of the definition of the syndrome.

(Fig. 3C), which causes a proportionate reduction in the rate of receptor biosynthesis (Ojamaa *et al.*, 1988; Muller-Wieland *et al.*, 1989). A nonsense mutation has been identified in codon 897 of exon 14 of the allele of the insulin receptor gene inherited from the patient's father (Kadowaki *et al.*, 1990a). Similarly, nonsense mutations have been identified at codons 133 and 1000 in the insulin receptor genes of two other patients (Kadowaki *et al.*, 1990b). Like nonsense mutations in other genes (Atweh *et al.*, 1988; Fojo *et al.*, 1988; Urlaub *et al.*, 1989), these nonsense mutations lead to a 90% decrease in the level of the mRNA transcribed from the paternal allele of the insulin receptor gene. We have not yet identified a mutation in the maternal allele of the patient leprechaun/Minn-1. However, indirect data support the hypothesis that there a cisdominant mutation in the insulin receptor gene which does not alter the protein coding sequence. This conclusion is based on studies of the levels of transcripts derived from the two alleles of the insulin receptor gene in cells from the patient's mother.

We amplified insulin receptor cDNA from cells of leprechaun/Minn-1, the mother, and a control subject (Fig. 4). Both leprechaun/Minn-1 and the mother had silent polymorphisms at codon 234 in exon 3 (Asp–GAC versus Asp–GAT) (Fig. 4, upper panels). This silent polymorphism at nucleotide 831 provided a marker that allowed us to differentiate the two alleles in both leprechaun/Minn-1 and her mother. In leprechaun/Minn-1 the allele with the nonsense mutation has cytosine at nucleotide 831 (C-831 allele). Therefore, the presence of thymine at

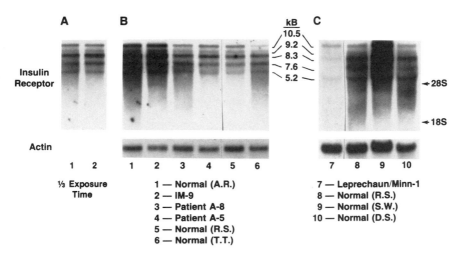

FIG. 3. Northern blot analysis of insulin receptor mRNA levels in cells from patients with decreased numbers of insulin receptors on the cell surface. Polyadenylated RNA from EBV-transformed lymphoblasts was analyzed by Northern blotting. The blots were probed with either human insulin receptor (upper panels) or chicken β-actin (lower panels) probes (Ojamaa *et al.*, 1988). (B) Cells from patients A-5 and A-8 (lanes 3 and 4), which have normal levels of insulin receptor mRNA. [(A) Autoradiograph of lanes 1 and 2, with the exposure time reduced from 3 days to 1 day to allow for better visualization of the insulin receptor mRNA bands]. (C) Marked reduction in insulin receptor mRNA in leprechaun/Minn-1 (lane 7) as compared to the normal subjects (lanes 8–10).

nucleotide 831 provides a marker for the allele which leprechaun/Minn-1 inherited from the mother (T-831 allele). As expected, when amplified cDNA from a control subject who was homozygous for cytosine at nucleotide 831 was analyzed, only the sequence containing cytosine at nucleotide 831 was detected (Fig. 4, lower panels). However, with amplified cDNA from leprechaun/Minn-1 and her mother, sequences containing both cytosine and thymine were detected (Fig. 4). In leprechaun/Minn-1 both transcripts were present in approximately equally low levels. However, in cells from the patient's mother, the level of the transcript from the T-831 allele was approximately 10-fold lower than the level of the transcript from the C-831 allele (Fig. 4, lower panels). As a methodological control, we confirmed that the alleles containing cytosine and thymine were present in a ratio of approximately 1:1 in amplified genomic DNA (Fig. 4, upper panels).

If the low level of expression of the mother's T-831 allele were caused by a trans-acting dominant mutation, then one would predict that the levels of transcripts derived from both alleles would be reduced symmetrically. However, there is a selective reduction in the level of the transcript derived from the T-831 allele. Thus, we conclude that there is a cis-dominant mutation in this T-831

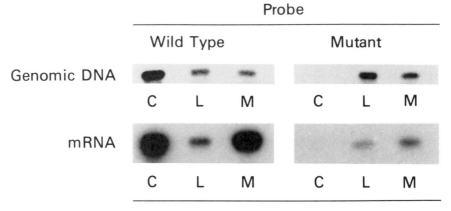

FIG. 4. Allele-specific oligonucleotide hybridization of amplified cDNA from lep-
rechaun/Minn-1 and her mother. Genomic DNA, including exon 3 of the insulin receptor gene, was
amplified by polymerase chain reaction (PCR). A 378-bp fragment of cDNA spanning the region
including nucleotide 831 was amplified from the total cellular RNA (2.5 μg) by reverse-transcriptase
PCR. Thereafter, amplified genomic DNA (~20 ng of DNA; upper panels) and amplified cDNA
(approximately one-tenth of the total product obtained; lower panels) were analyzed by agarose gel
electrophoresis followed by Southern blotting. Blots were hybridized with oligonucleotides specific
for either the C-831 allele (left-hand panels) or the T-831 allele (right-hand panels). Amplified
genomic DNA and cDNA were derived either from leprechaun/Minn-1 (L), her mother (M), or a
control subject (C) whose genomic DNA had been sequenced and was determined to be homozygous
for cytosine at nucleotide 831 (patient RM-1) (Kadowaki *et al.*, 1990a). Both leprechaun/Minn-1 and
her mother are heterozygous for cytosine and thymine at nucleotide 831. The T-831 allele is the allele
which leprechaun/Minn-1 inherited from her mother. The presence of cytosine at nucleotide 831 is a
marker for the allele with the nonsense mutation in leprechaun/Minn-1, but a marker for the normal
allele in the mother.

allele in the mother's cells. Importantly, it is this T-831 allele which lepre-
chaun/Minn-1 inherited from her mother. We have analyzed the entire protein-
coding sequence of the maternal T-831 allele as well as the sequence of the
intron–exon boundaries for all 22 exons (data not shown), but have not yet
detected the presumed mutation. Because the mutation might be located anywhere in the gene which spans in excess of 150 kbp of genomic DNA (Seino *et
al.*, 1989), it might be difficult to identify this mutation directly. In principle, the
mutation might either decrease the rate at which insulin receptor mRNA is
synthesized or, alternatively, decrease the stability of insulin receptor mRNA
(Kadowaki *et al.*, 1990a).

Thus, leprechaun/Minn-1 is a compound heterozygote having inherited two
distinct mutations in the insulin receptor gene (Table I). There is a nonsense
mutation in the paternal allele, which leads to a decrease in the level of insulin
receptor mRNA. Although we have not yet directly identified a mutation in the
maternal allele, there is strong evidence to suggest the existence of such a

mutation. Importantly, in the mother this presumed mutation is associated with a 50% reduction in the level of insulin receptors on the surface of her circulating monocytes (Taylor, 1985).

B.   TRANSLATION OF INSULIN RECEPTOR mRNA

As with other integral membrane proteins, insulin receptor mRNA is translated by ribosomes associated with the rough endoplasmic reticulum. Several mutations have been identified which result in premature chain termination, thereby terminating translation of the mRNA prior to completion of the full-length insulin receptor protein. In addition to the nonsense mutation identified in one allele of the insulin receptor gene in leprechaun/Minn-1, we have identified a nonsense mutation of codon 672 in another patient with leprechaunism (leprechaun/Ark-1) (Taylor *et al.*, 1981; Kadowaki *et al.*, 1988) (Fig. 1). Interestingly, the nonsense mutation in leprechaun/Ark-1 does not appear to lead to a decreased level of insulin receptor mRNA. Nevertheless, this allele with a nonsense mutation at codon 672 encodes a truncated receptor that lacks a transmembrane domain and appears not to be expressed on the cell surface (Cama and Taylor, 1987). Although investigations of mutations in other genes have demonstrated that most premature chain-termination mutations lead to reduced levels of mRNA, it has been observed that some nonsense mutations do not decrease mRNA levels (Urlaub *et al.*, 1989). It is not understood why some nonsense mutations reduce mRNA levels while other do not.

In the patient leprechaun/Ark-1, the allele of the insulin receptor gene with the nonsense mutation is paired with an allele containing a different mutation (Kadowaki *et al.*, 1988) (see Section II,C; Table I). However, the patient's father is heterozygous for the allele with the nonsense mutation and is also insulin resistant, although not as severely insulin resistant as his daughter (Taylor *et al.*, 1986; Kadowaki *et al.*, 1988) (Table I). We have shown that the nucleotide sequences of all 22 exons of the father's second allele of the insulin receptor gene are normal (Kadowaki *et al.*, 1990b). Thus it is likely that the phenotype of insulin resistance caused by this nonsense mutation is inherited in a co-dominant fashion (Taylor *et al.*, 1986).

Consistent with this conclusion, there is a 60–70% decrease in [^{125}I]insulin binding to the father's circulating monocytes (Fig. 5). This suggests that the normal allele of the insulin receptor gene does not increase the level of expression to compensate for the nonsense mutation. In fact, because the father is hyperinsulinemic, with plasma insulin levels elevated 5- to 10-fold above the normal range (Taylor *et al.*, 1986; Elders *et al.*, 1982), it is likely that his receptors become down-regulated *in vivo*, thus exacerbating the decrease in the number of insulin receptors on the surface of his cells. In fact, when the contribution due to down-regulation is eliminated by cultivating Epstein–Barr virus

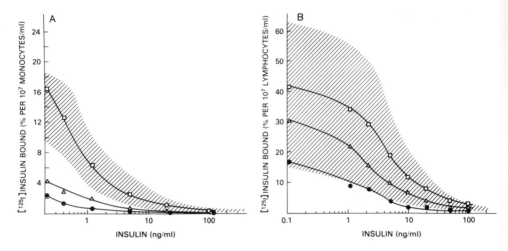

FIG. 5.   Decreased [^{125}I]insulin binding to circulating monocytes of leprechaun/Ark-1 and her father. (A) Circulating monocytes and (B) EBV-transformed lymphoblasts were incubated with [^{125}I]insulin (0.1 ng/ml) plus varying concentrations of unlabeled insulin. The percentage of [^{125}I]insulin bound specifically is plotted as a function of the insulin concentration. The hatched areas are the range of binding observed in normal subjects (Taylor *et al.*, 1986). □, Mother; △, father; ●, leprechaun/Ark-1.

(EBV)-transformed lymphoblasts in the absence of insulin, the number of insulin receptors on the cell surface is normal—albeit in the lower half of the range (Fig. 5).

Taira *et al.* (1989) described two patients (a mother and her daughter) with a deletion of the portion of the insulin receptor gene encoding most of the intracellular domain of the receptor β subunit (Fig. 1, Table I). Based on the nucleotide sequence, they predict that the mRNA would encode a fusion protein which has an open reading frame for 65 amino acids after the deletion break point at codon 1012. Thus, this deletion could result in premature chain termination and the production of a receptor with a truncated intracellular domain. However, this type of deletion could lower receptor mRNA levels by interfering with the splicing of the RNA transcript or by destabilizing the mRNA. Data were not presented to indicate whether it is possible to detect either the mRNA transcribed from the mutant allele or the fusion protein which it would encode (Taira *et al.*, 1989).

C.   POSTTRANSLATION MODIFICATION AND TRANSPORT TO THE PLASMA MEMBRANE

The insulin receptor undergoes cotranslational N-linked glycosylation in the endoplasmic reticulum (Hedo *et al.*, 1981, 1983). Thereafter, the proreceptor undergoes proteolytic cleavage into two separate subunits (pre-α and pre-β) (Hedo *et al.*, 1983; Deutsch *et al.*, 1983; Jacobs *et al.*, 1983; Ronnett *et al.*, 1983). Subsequently, the high-mannose forms of the N-linked oligosaccharides are processed to complex carbohydrate (Hedo *et al.*, 1981, 1983), presumably in the Golgi apparatus. At some point the receptor undergoes other posttranslational modifications, including O-linked glycosylation (Herzberg *et al.*, 1985; Collier and Gorden, 1989) and fatty acylation (Hedo *et al.*, 1987). Finally, the mature insulin receptor is transported to the cell surface, where it is inserted into the plasma membrane.

Two mutations have been described which interfere with posttranslational processing of the insulin receptor. These are discussed below.

1. Defect in Proteolytic Cleavage

Two sisters with type A extreme insulin resistance have been described who are homozygous for a mutation substituting serine for arginine at position 735, the last amino acid in the tetrabasic amino acid sequence (Arg–Lys–Arg–Arg) in the proteolytic processing site (Fig. 1, Table I). This mutation, initially reported by Yoshimasa *et al.* (1988) and subsequently confirmed by Kobayashi *et al.* (1988b), prevents proteolytic processing of the receptor precursor into two subunits. As shown in studies of the patients' cultured cells, the uncleaved receptor has a decreased affinity to bind insulin (Kakehi *et al.*, 1988; Kobayashi *et al.*, 1988a). Presumably, it is the failure of cleavage into subunits which causes the reduction in the binding affinity.

2. Defect in Intracellular Transport of Receptors to Plasma Membrane

We have studied two sisters with type A extreme insulin resistance (patients A-5 and A-8) in whom there is an 80–90% decrease in the number of insulin receptors on the cell surface (Barnes *et al.*, 1974; Accili *et al.*, 1989) (Figs. 2 and 6). However, unlike what was observed in leprechaun/Minn-1 (see Section II,A), we detected normal levels of insulin receptor mRNA in EBV-transformed lymphoblasts from patients A-5 and A-8 (Ojamaa *et al.*, 1988) (Fig. 3B). Moreover, the rate of receptor biosynthesis is normal (Hedo *et al.*, 1985). Why, then, is the number of receptors on the cell surface decreased? This does not result from an accelerated rate of receptor degradation. When receptors on the surface of EBV-transformed lymphoblasts from patient A-5 were labeled by lactoperoxidase-catalyzed radioiodination and the rate of receptor degradation was measured, the half-life of the patient's receptors was within normal limits ($t_{1/2}$ = 4.8 hours; normal range, 6.5 $\pm$ 2.4 hours, mean $\pm$ 2 SD) (McElduff *et al.*, 1984). This led to the hypothesis that there is a defect in the transport of insulin receptors to the plasma membrane. We have described a similar biochemical phenotype in an insulin-resistant patient with Rabson–Mendenhall syndrome (Moncada *et al.*, 1986).

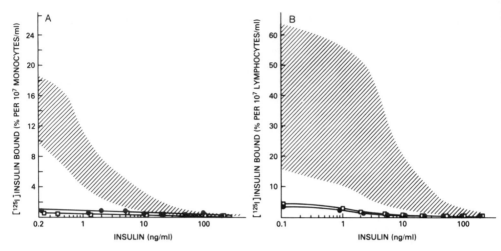

FIG. 6. Decreased insulin binding to the surface of cells from two sisters [patients A-5 (●) and A-8 (□)] with Type A extreme insulin resistance. (A) Circulating monocytes and (B) EBV-transformed lymphoblasts were incubated with [125I]insulin (0.1 ng/ml) plus varying concentrations of unlabeled insulin. The percentage of [125I]insulin bound specifically is plotted as a function of the insulin concentration. The hatched areas are the range of binding observed in normal subjects (Taylor, 1987).

A defect in the transport of receptors to the cell surface has also been described with low-density lipoprotein (LDL) receptors in the Watanabe heritable hyperlipidemic rabbit and some patients with familial hypercholesterolemia (Yamamoto *et al.*, 1986; Hobbs *et al.*, 1986). In these cases mutations were detected in the structural gene encoding the LDL receptor. The mutant LDL receptors were impaired in their ability to be transported to the cell surface. Therefore, the abnormal phenotype observed in insulin receptors from patients A-5 and A-8 could result either from an intrinsic defect in the receptor or, alternatively, from a defect in some other component of the cellular machinery required for transporting plasma membrane proteins to the cell surface. To distinguish between these two possibilities, we inquired whether the disease genetically cosegregated with restriction fragment-length polymorphisms (RFLPs) at the insulin receptor locus.

Genotypes were determined at each of seven known RFLPs in the insulin receptor locus (Accili *et al.*, 1989). Under the assumption that there was no crossing-over within the insulin receptor locus in the meioses producing the children, these observations enabled us to identify three haplotypes in the family: *A, B,* and *C* (see Fig. 7 legend for definition of the alleles). The two affected sisters had genotype *A/A;* the mother and the brother had genotype *A/C;* the father and the unaffected sisters had genotype *A/B* (Fig. 8).

The mode of inheritance of the disease is almost certainly autosomal recessive, inasmuch as the parents are first cousins and the phenotype was not observed in earlier generations. We used the method of homozygosity mapping (Lander and Botstein, 1987) to analyze these linkage data. The underlying principle is as follows: In a consanguineous marriage such as this, it is predicted that one of the patients' great-grandparents was a carrier for a mutant allele of the insulin receptor gene. Furthermore, it is predicted that this mutant allele would be inherited by both of the patients' parents, and that the two patients should be homozygous by descent for this mutant allele. The observed data were consistent with all of these predictions. The probability of these observations arising as a result of random chance is approximately 1:100 to 1:200. According to the method of homozygosity mapping, based on our estimate of the frequency of the allele A haplotype, this corresponds to a logarithm of the odds ratio (LOD) score for the family of approximately 2.0–2.3. This LOD score exceeds the threshold for declaring linkage when studying a single candidate locus.

Having established that the patients' mutation was genetically linked to the insulin receptor gene, we cloned insulin receptor cDNA from patient A-8 and identified a single amino acid substitution in the patient's insulin receptor: substitution of valine for phenylalanine at position 382 in the α subunit (Accili *et al.*, 1989) (Fig. 1). Both insulin-resistant sisters are homozygous for this mutation (Fig. 8). The parents and the four unaffected siblings are all heterozygous carriers of the mutation. In contrast, we did not detect this mutation in any of 160 alleles of the insulin receptor gene in 80 normal individuals (Fig. 9). These studies support the conclusion that the two sisters are homozygous for an extremely rare allele of the insulin receptor gene. Thus, as we had previously concluded on the basis of the genetic linkage studies (see above), the patients have almost certainly inherited both copies of the mutant allele from the same great-grandparent (i.e., homozygosity by descent).

To evaluate the significance of the substitution of valine for phenylalanine at position 382, the mutant form of the insulin receptor cDNA was expressed by transfection in cultured cells. These demonstrate that the Val-382 mutation impairs posttranslational processing of the receptor precursor and thereby decreases the number of receptors on the cell surface (Accili *et al.*, 1989). Posttranslational processing of the 190-kDa precursor to the mature receptor was investigated in NIH-3T3 cells transfected with cDNA encoding either normal insulin receptors (WT-8) or insulin receptors with the Val-382 mutation (V382-2). The transfected cells were pulse-labeled with [^{35}S]methionine for 3 hours, followed by a chase period of 1.5 or 4 hours (Fig. 10). These pulse–chase studies provide clear evidence for a defect in the posttranslational processing of the mutant receptor. In the cells transfected with wild-type cDNA, two bands (of 130 and 100 kDa) were seen in the regions of the α and β subunits. In the cells transfected with mutant cDNA, four bands were seen: two bands (of 120 and 130 kDa) were seen in the region of the α subunit, and two bands (of 90 and 100 kDa) were seen in the

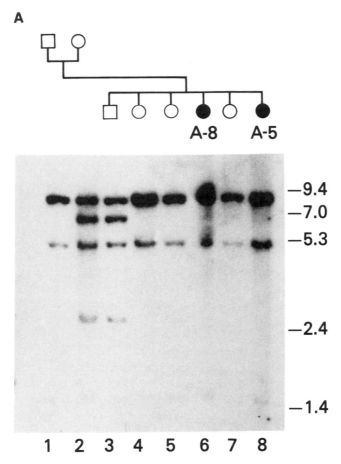

FIG. 7. Restriction fragment-length polymorphisms (RFLPs) of the insulin receptor gene in the family of patients A-5 and A-8. Genomic DNA was digested with either *Sac*I (A) or *Eco*RI (B), and the Southern blots were hybridized with either a *Pst*I fragment (nucleotides 2742–4341) or a *Bgl*I fragment (nucleotides 1599–2961) of insulin receptor cDNA, respectively (Accili *et al.*, 1989). The lanes are identified by the symbols from the pedigree. The three alleles in the kindred (Fig. 7) can be identified by these two RFLPs as shown in the tabulation:

Allele	*Sac*I polymorphism		*Eco*RI polymorphism	
	9.4-kb Band	7.0 + 2.4-kb Bands	5.5-kb Band	5.8-kb Band
A	+		+	
B	+			+
C		+		+

All three alleles were identical with respect to five additional restriction fragment-length polymorphisms defined by the enzymes *Sac*I, *Rsa*I, *Bgl*II, *Hin*dIII, and *Eco*RI (Accili *et al.*, 1989).

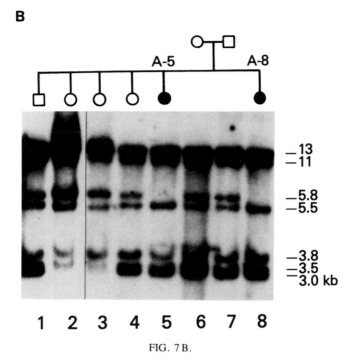

FIG. 7 B.

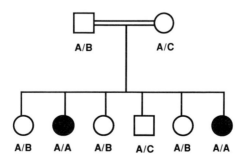

FIG. 8. Pedigree of consanguineous kindred of two insulin-resistant sisters (A-5 and A-8). The parents of patients A-5 and A-8 are first cousins (Barnes *et al.*, 1974). Solid circles represent the two affected sisters. Open circles represent the unaffected family members. Allele A is the allele with the Phe-382 mutation. Alleles B and C are the normal alleles observed in the father and the mother, respectively.

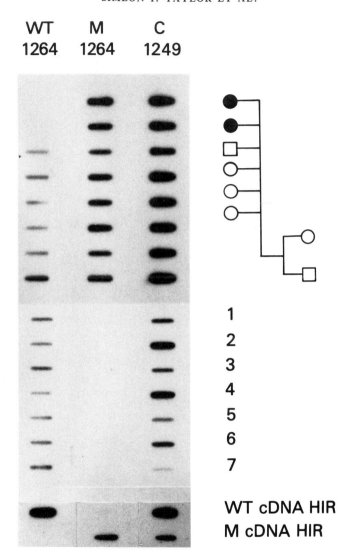

FIG. 9.   Inheritance of the Val-382 mutation as detected by allele-specific oligonucleotide hybrid-ization of amplified genomic DNA. The 134-bp fragment of genomic DNA corresponding to nu-cleotides 1172–1306 of insulin receptor cDNA was amplified with *Taq* DNA polymerase (Accili *et al.*, 1989). Thereafter, amplified DNA was applied to a nitrocellulose filter using a slot-blot apparat-us. The blot was hybridized to sequence-specific oligonucleotides corresponding to nucleotides 1264–1281 of either the wild-type sequence (WT 1264), the mutant sequence (M 1264), or a control sequence (nucleotides 1249–1266) located upstream from the mutation (C 1249). Amplified genomic DNA from the family members is located in the upper eight rows, denoted by the symbols of the pedigree. Rows 1–7 represent amplified DNA from seven representative normal individuals. Seven-ty-three additional normal individuals were studied (not shown). As a methodological control, hy-bridization to clones containing either the wild-type (WT) or mutant (M) sequences is shown in the bottom two rows.

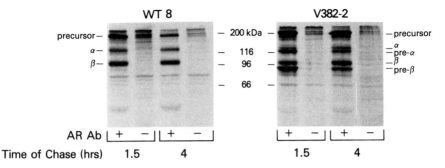

FIG. 10. The Val-382 mutation impairs posttranslational processing of the insulin receptor. Transfected cells expressing either wild-type insulin receptor cDNA (WT 8) or mutant receptor cDNA (V382-2) were pulse-labeled with [^{35}S]methionine for 3 hours, followed by a chase with unlabeled methionine for either 1.5 or 4 hours (Accili *et al.*, 1989). The cells were solubilized and the receptors were immunoprecipitated. Fluorographs of the SDS–PAGEs are shown. The M_r of the receptor precursor (190,000) and the mature receptor α and β subunits (130,000 and 100,000, respectively) together with the molecular weight size markers are indicated on the left. The M_r of the pre-α and pre-β precursor (120,000 and 90,000, respectively) are indicated on the right. AR Ab, anti-receptor antibody.

region of the β subunit. Previous studies had suggested that proteolytic cleavage of the receptor precedes maturation of the N-linked carbohydrate moieties (Hedo *et al*, 1983; Ronnett *et al.*, 1983). Therefore, it seems likely that the low-molecular-weight forms of the α and β subunits represent precursors in which the N-linked oligosaccharides had not undergone final processing in the Golgi apparatus.

As has been suggested previously, the kinetics of labeling are consistent with the 90- and 120-kDa bands' being precursors of the 100- and 130-kDa bands, respectively. Specifically, the ratio of the mature α and β subunits (130 and 100 kDa, respectively) to the lower-molecular-weight precursor forms (120 and 90 kDa, respectively) increases as a function of time during the chase period. Thus, the posttranslational processing of the 190-kDa proreceptor is less efficient in the cells transfected with mutant cDNA.

Is the defect in posttranslational processing associated with impaired transport of the mutant receptor to the cell surface? To address this question, three transfected cell lines which expressed similar levels of insulin receptor mRNA were studied: two cell lines expressing normal insulin receptor cDNA (WT-2 and WT-8) and one cell line expressing Val-382 mutant insulin receptor cDNA (V382-1). As demonstrated by the Scatchard plots of [^{125}I]iodoinsulin binding (Accili *et al.*, 1989) (Fig. 11), cells transfected with wild-type insulin receptor cDNA (WT-2 and WT-8) express approximately 5- to 10-fold more insulin receptors on their cell surface than do the cells transfected with Val-382 mutant insulin receptor cDNA (V382-1). Similarly, missense mutations that impair post-translational processing and transport to the cell surface have been identified in

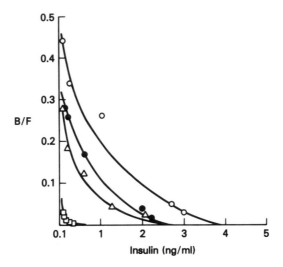

FIG. 11. The Val-382 mutation decreases the number of insulin receptors on the cell surface. Shown is a Scatchard plot of [^{125}I]insulin binding to transfected cells expressing wild-type ($\triangle$ and $\bigcirc$) or mutant ($\square$ and ●) insulin receptor cDNA (Accili *et al.*, 1989). Three cell lines ($\triangle$, $\bigcirc$, and $\square$) express approximately 2000 insulin receptor mRNA molecules per cell; one cell line (●) expresses approximately 20,000 insulin receptor mRNA molecules per cell. B/F, ratio of bound to free [^{125}I]insulin.

two other patients (Kadowaki *et al.*, 1990b). In a patient with the Rabson–Mendenhall syndrome, one allele of the insulin receptor gene had a mutation substituting lysine for Asn-15. Another patient (leprechaun/Winnipeg), who was a member of a consanguineous pedigree, was homozygous for a mutation substituting arginine for His-209.

III. Defects in Insulin Receptor Function

A. DEFECTS IN INSULIN BINDING

All of the mutations described above cause insulin resistance by decreasing insulin binding—by decreasing the number of insulin receptors on the cell surface (Kadowaki *et al.*, 1988, 1990a,b; Accili *et al.*, 1989) and/or by decreasing the affinity of the receptor to bind insulin (Yoshimasa *et al.*, 1988; Kakehi *et al.*, 1988; Kobayashi *et al.*, 1988a,b). Recently, another mutation has been identified in the insulin receptor of leprechaun/Geldermalsen: substitution of proline for leucine at position 233 in the β subunit (Klinkhamer *et al.*, 1989). The patient, who is part of a consanguineous pedigree, is homozygous for the Pro-233 mutation (Table I, Fig. 1). The mutation is associated with a marked decrease in insulin binding to the surface of the patient's cultured skin fibroblasts. However, when the receptors were solubilized in detergent, the solubilized receptor was observed to bind insulin normally. It is possible that the effect of the detergent is to solubilize intracellular insulin receptors, and that the Pro-233 mutation decreases insulin binding by preventing transport of the receptors to the cell surface (cf. patients A-5 and A-8; see Section II,C.) Alternatively, it is possible that the mutation causes a decrease in the binding affinity when the receptor is on the cell surface, but that solubilization with detergent somehow restores the binding affinity to normal. Expression of the mutant receptor cDNA will enable investigations to answer these questions.

B.   DEFECTS IN TYROSINE KINASE ACTIVITY

The intracellular domain of the insulin receptor possesses tyrosine-specific protein kinase activity (Kasuga *et al.*, 1982a,b; Rosen, 1987). When insulin binds to the extracellular domain of its receptor, this activates the tyrosine kinase activity. A growing body of evidence supports the hypothesis that activation of the tyrosine kinase plays a necessary role in mediating insulin action on the target cell (Rosen, 1987). Nevertheless, the precise mechanism by which the tyrosine kinase mediates insulin action has not been elucidated. When insulin binds to the receptor, this causes autophosphorylation of tyrosine residues in the receptor (Kasuga *et al.*, 1982a,b; Tornqvist *et al.*, 1988; White *et al.*, 1988). Receptor autophosphorylation stimulates the activity of the tyrosine kinase to phosphorylate other protein substrates (Rosen, 1987). For example, we have identified a 120-kDa glycoprotein in plasma membranes of hepatocytes (pp120) which is phosphorylated on tyrosine residues by the insulin receptor in a cell-free system and in intact cells (Rees-Jones and Taylor, 1985; Perrotti *et al.*, 1987; Margolis *et al.*, 1988) (Fig. 12). Recent data (Margolis *et al.*, 1990) have suggested that pp120 is identical to a membrane-associated ATPase which has been extensively investigated in another context (Lin and Guidotti, 1989). It is not known whether protein phosphorylation regulates the ATPase activity of pp120, nor whether the protein plays a role in mediating insulin action. Other protein substrates for tyrosine-specific phosphorylation by the insulin receptor have been identified (White *et al.*, 1985; Bernier *et al.*, 1987), although the enzymatic functions of these proteins have generally not been identified.

Consistent with the hypothesis that activation of the tyrosine-specific protein kinase is necessary to mediate insulin action, several patients have been described in whom insulin resistance is caused by defects in the insulin receptor tyrosine kinase activity (Grunberger *et al.*, 1984; Grigorescu *et al.*, 1984). In collaboration with Kasuga and colleagues, we have cloned insulin receptor cDNA from one such patient (Odawara *et al.*, 1989). In this patient we identified a missense mutation which encodes substitution of valine for Gly-1008, the third

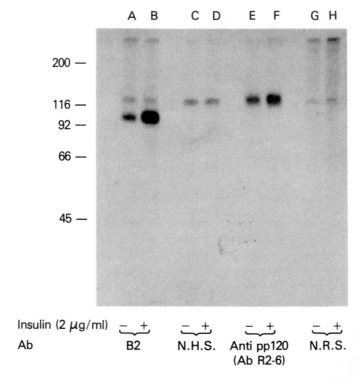

FIG. 12. Insulin stimulates phosphorylation of tyrosine residues in pp120 (membrane-associated ecto-ATPase) in H35 cells. H35 cells were loaded with [³²P]phosphate. Thereafter, cells were incubated in the presence or absence of insulin. Cell proteins were extracted with detergent and immunoprecipitated with antiinsulin receptor antibody (lanes A and B), normal human serum (N.H.S.) (lanes C and D), anti-pp120 antibody (lanes E and F), or normal rabbit serum (N.R.S.) (lanes G and H). The immunoprecipitates were analyzed by SDS–PAGE followed by autoradiography (Perrotti *et al.*, 1987).

glycine in the Gly–X–Gly–X–X–Gly motif which is part of the putative ATP-binding site (Fig. 1). By transfecting mutant insulin receptor cDNA into Chinese hamster ovary cells, we have shown that the Val-1008 mutation essentially abolishes tyrosine kinase activity (Odawara *et al.*, 1989) (Fig. 13). The patient's other allele of the insulin receptor gene has the normal sequence in this region, so that the patient is heterozygous for the Val-1008 mutation (Table I). Because the patient's other allele has not been fully sequenced, we do not know whether it is normal or has a second mutation. Thus, it is not known whether the Val-1008 mutation is dominant or recessive.

Nevertheless, the oligomeric structure of the insulin receptor suggests a mechanism by which insulin resistance due to a mutation in the tyrosine kinase domain might be inherited in a dominant fashion. If a mutant insulin receptor hetero-

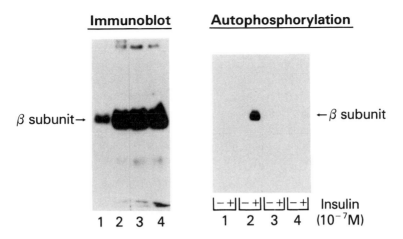

FIG. 13. Expression of the normal and mutant human insulin receptor cDNA in Chinese hamster ovary (CHO) cells. CHO cells were stably transfected with either normal insulin receptor cDNA or cDNA encoding the Val-1008 mutant form of the receptor. (Left) Protein blotting of partially purified insulin receptors (Odawara *et al.*, 1989). A site-specific antibody (Ab-IRC) directed against the COOH terminus of the human insulin receptor β subunit was used to quantitate the number of insulin receptors in the cells: (lane 1) nontransfected cells; (lane 2) cells transfected with normal human insulin receptor cDNA (Gly-1008); (lanes 3 and 4) two cell lines transfected with mutant insulin receptor cDNA (Val-1008). Based on insulin-binding studies, we estimate that the transfected cell lines have 30,000–50,000 receptors per cell. In contrast, the nontransfected cells have approximately 1500 receptors per cell. (Right) Autophosphorylation of partially purified insulin receptors from nontransfected cells, cells transfected with normal human insulin receptor cDNA (Gly-1008), or cells transfected with Val-1008 mutant insulin receptor cDNA. CHO cells were solubilized in the presence of Triton X-100, and the receptors were partially purified over wheat germ agglutinin–agarose. After incubation in the absence (−) or presence (+) of 10^{-7} M insulin, partially purified receptors (10 μg per lane) were phosphorylated in the presence of 50 μM [γ-^{32}P]ATP and 4 mM MnCl$_2$. After immunoprecipitation with Ab-IRC, receptors were analyzed by SDS–PAGE, followed by autoradiography (Odawara *et al.*, 1989).

dimer (α–β_m) associated with a wild-type insulin receptor heterodimer (α–β_{wt}), then it is possible that the hybrid heterotetramer (α_2–β_m–β_{wt}) might be impaired in its tyrosine kinase activity. Indeed, if the hybrid molecule were totally inactive as a tyrosine kinase, then a mutation in a single allele might lead to a 75% reduction in insulin receptor tyrosine kinase activity. The identification of a mutation in the tyrosine kinase domain of the insulin receptor from an insulin-resistant patient demonstrates that a defect in the tyrosine kinase can interfere with insulin action *in vivo* and strongly supports the hypothesis that the insulin receptor tyrosine kinase is necessary to mediate the physiological actions of insulin *in vivo*.

Moller and Flier (1988) have described a variant sequence in which serine is substituted for Trp-1200 in the β subunit (Fig. 1). This mutation is found in only one allele of the patient's insulin receptor gene; the other allele is normal in this region (Table I). The Ser-1200 mutation impairs receptor-associated tyrosine kinase activity. Similarly, the same Val-382 mutation that impairs the transport of the receptor to the cell surface also impairs the ability of insulin to activate the receptor tyrosine kinase. Presumably, the mutation causes the receptor to misfold and to assume an abnormal conformation. This abnormal conformation causes two functional defects: (1) a decreased number of insulin receptors on the cell surface by inhibiting the transport of receptors through the endoplasmic reticulum and the Golgi apparatus and (2) impaired transmembrane signaling by inhibiting insulin-induced activation of the tyrosine kinase (Accili *et al.*, 1989, 1990).

C.   RECEPTOR INTERNALIZATION, RECYCLING, AND DEGRADATION

After insulin binds to its receptor, the ligand–receptor complex is internalized into endosomes (Fig. 14). These endosomes possess proton pumps in their membranes and thereby generate an acidic pH within their lumina. This acidic pH plays a crucial role in dissociating the ligand from its receptor. Subsequent to internalization at least two distinct pathways are available to the receptor; recycling to the cell surface for reutilization or degradation within the lysosomes.

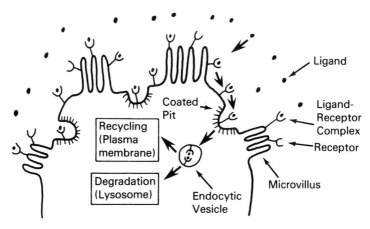

FIG. 14.   Pathway of receptor-mediated endocytosis and receptor recycling. After insulin binds to its receptor, the hormone–receptor complex undergoes endocytosis. Because of the presence of proton pumps in their membranes, the endosomes acquire an acidic pH in their lumina. Once within the cell two alternative fates are available to the ligand and its receptor. They can be targeted to the lysosome, where they will be degraded. Alternatively, the receptor can be recycled back to the plasma membrane for reutilization. If the ligand escapes degradation, it can be retroendocytosed intact into the extracellular fluid.

Studies with a site-directed mutant of the LDL receptor suggest that failure of the ligand to dissociate could inhibit the pathway of receptor recycling (Davis *et al.*, 1987). In these studies a mutant LDL receptor was constructed in which there was a deletion of the portion of the extracellular domain of the LDL receptor homologous to the epidermal growth factor precursor molecule. This deletion did not interfere with LDL binding at neutral pH, but rendered LDL binding insensitive to changes in pH. Desensitization to changes in pH was associated with inhibition of the recycling pathway and hypersensitivity to ligand-induced downregulation. After binding to the receptor at the cell surface, the ligand was not dissociated from the receptor in the endocytic vesicle, and the receptor was targeted preferentially for degradation within the lysosome (Davis *et al.*, 1987).

We have identified a mutation (substitution of glutamic acid for Lys-460, Fig. 1) in the insulin receptor which impairs dissociation of insulin from its receptor in the endosome. This Glu-460 mutation was found in leprechaun/Ark-1 in the allele of the insulin receptor gene inherited from the patient's mother (Taylor *et al.*, 1981; Kadowaki *et al.*, 1988). [This is the same patient whose paternal allele had a nonsense mutation (Table I) and therefore encoded a nonfunctional receptor (see Section II,B) (Kadowaki *et al.*, 1988).] The Glu-460 mutation increases the affinity of the receptor to bind insulin (Taylor *et al.*, 1981; Taylor and Leventhal, 1983). Interestingly, the Glu-460 mutation does not inhibit the tyrosine kinase activity of the insulin receptor (Whittaker *et al.*, 1985; Cama and Taylor, 1987). Thus, it seems likely that this mutant insulin receptor would be competent to mediate insulin action if it remained on the cell surface.

However, the mutation renders the insulin receptor less sensitive to changes in pH (Kadowaki *et al.*, 1988; Taylor *et al.*, 1981) (Fig. 15). With normal insulin receptors (e.g., Lys-460), decreasing the pH from 7.8 to 6.0 causes a 10 fold acceleration in the rate at which [^{125}I]insulin dissociates from its receptor. The effect of acid pH to accelerate [^{125}I]insulin dissociation is markedly blunted with the Glu-460 mutant receptor (Fig. 15). Thus, the Glu-460 mutant insulin receptor resembles the deletion mutant of the LDL receptor described above (Davis *et al.*, 1987). Both mutant receptors are desensitized to the effect of acid pH to dissociate the ligand from its receptor. In analogy to the mutant form of the LDL receptor, the Glu-460 mutation in the insulin receptor appears to inhibit receptor recycling and to accelerate the rate of receptor degradation.

According to this hypothesis, the cause of insulin resistance is a decrease in the number of insulin receptors on the surface of target cells, which results from an accelerated rate of receptor degradation. Two observations support this hypothesis. (1) Insulin receptors on the surface of EBV-transformed lymphoblasts of leprechaun/Ark-1 are degraded almost twice as fast as receptors on the surface of cells from normal individuals ($t_{1/2}$ = 3.5 hours; normal range, 6.5 ± 2.4 hours, mean ± 2 SD) (McElduff *et al.*, 1984). (2) The number of insulin receptors on the surface of the patient's circulating monocytes is decreased by

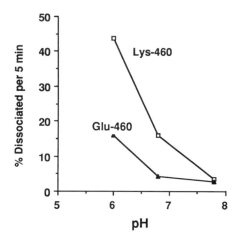

FIG. 15.   The Glu-460 mutation decreases the sensitivity of insulin receptors to changes in pH. NIH-3T3 cells transfected with either wild-type insulin receptor cDNA (Lys-460) or mutant insulin receptor (Glu-460) cDNA were incubated with [^{125}I]insulin. Thereafter, unbound [^{125}I]insulin was removed by washing the cells at 4°C. Fresh media with varying pH (6.0, 6.8, or 7.8) were added, and the rate at which [^{125}I]insulin dissociated was measured (Kadowaki *et al.*, 1988).

80–85% below the normal range (Taylor *et al.*, 1986). Interestingly, we have recently identified a mutation that causes a similar phenotype in a different patient (A-1). This patient is a compound heterozygote with one allele with a nonsense mutation and the second allele with a missense mutation substituting serine for Asn-462 (Kadowaki et al., 1990b).

Mutations in the insulin receptor gene have the potential to provide insights into structure–function relationships of the insulin receptor. Therefore, it is interesting to inquire where Lys-460 is located in the three-dimensional structure of the insulin receptor molecule. Because substitution of glutamic acid at position 460 increases the affinity of insulin binding, it is tempting to speculate that this residue might be located in the insulin-binding domain. However, we think that it is more likely that Lys-460 is located at the interface between adjacent α subunits in the oligomeric receptor molecule. This tentative conclusion is based on several lines of evidence: (1) Substitution of other amino acids for lysine at position 460 inhibits the ability of disuccinimidyl suberate (DSS) to cross-link adjacent α subunits (Cama and Taylor, 1987; Kadowaki *et al.*, 1989a,b). This suggests the possibility that Lys-460 actually contributes the amino groups with which DSS reacts to cross-link the two adjacent α subunits. (2) The Glu-460 mutation impairs site–site interaction among insulin-binding sites, as evidenced by the impairment of positive cooperativity (Taylor and Leventhal, 1983; Kadowaki *et al.*, 1989b). Similarly, the Arg-460 substitution impairs negative cooperativity (Kadowaki *et al.*, 1989b). (3) Lys-460 is located near the cysteines which have been proposed to form the disulfide bonds between adjacent α subunits: Cys-435, Cys-468, or Cys-524 (Frias and Waugh, 1989).

IV. Insulin Receptors in Patients with Non-Insulin-Dependent Diabetes Mellitus

In light of the central role of insulin resistance in predisposing to the development of non-insulin-dependent diabetes mellitus (NIDDM) (Reaven, 1988; DeFronzo, 1988), it is reasonable to inquire whether patients with NIDDM might have mutations in the insulin receptor gene. In favor of this hypothesis, some patients with extreme insulin resistance have had relatives in whom heterozygosity for mutations in the insulin receptor gene is associated with a moderate degree of insulin resistance. For example, the father of leprechaun/Ark-1, who is heterozygous for a nonsense mutation in the insulin receptor gene, has a moderate degree of insulin resistance comparable to what is observed in patients with NIDDM (Taylor et al., 1986; Kadowaki et al., 1988, 1990b). Furthermore, the mutations detected thus far in the insulin receptor gene have all caused major defects in the function of the insulin receptor. It is possible that patients with a milder degree of insulin resistance might have mutations which cause less severe disruption of the function of the insulin receptor.

Analysis of RFLPs has yielded equivocal results (reviewed by Taylor et al., 1990). However, there are many reasons that this approach might fail to detect association of the disease with the insulin receptor gene. For example, there could be more than one mutation causing insulin resistance in the diabetic population, and these mutations might not all be in linkage disequilibrium with the same RFLP. If this were true, population studies would not detect strong association of NIDDM with a particular RFLP. Furthermore, even in studies of the inheritance of RFLPs in families, it might be difficult to demonstrate linkage of NIDDM to a particular gene. For example, if the development of NIDDM requires simultaneous mutations at more than one locus, linkage might be difficult to detect, unless all of the relevant loci are analyzed simultaneously.

Accordingly, we have embarked on a more direct approach—to determine the nucleotide sequence of the insulin receptor gene in diabetic patients. Thus far, we have studied one insulin-resistant Pima Indian in a family with a high prevalence of NIDDM (Cama et al., 1990). Both alleles of his insulin receptor gene encode a normal amino acid sequence. Moller and Flier (1989) have reached a similar conclusion in studies of two diabetic Pima Indians. Of course, even if there are no mutations in the structural gene, it remains possible that there is a mutation in a regulatory domain of the gene. However, the regulatory domains of the gene has not been clearly delineated, so it is difficult to address this question at the present time.

The mechanism by which insulin elicits its multiple biological responses in target cells is extremely complex. Furthermore, insulin has multiple effects on multiple different target cells. For target cells to respond to insulin requires the function of many proteins encoded by many genes. At least in theory, each of these genes is a candidate to be the locus of a mutation causing insulin resistance in NIDDM. As progress is made in the identification of cloning of all of the many genes required for the normal response to insulin, it will become possible to identify the loci of the mutations which cause insulin resistance in NIDDM.

V. Conclusion

Studies of mutations in the insulin receptor gene have begun to provide insight into structure–function relationships of the insulin receptor. Especially when combined in the future with physical methods to define the three-dimensional structure of the receptor, mutational analysis of the receptor should provide major insights into the mechanisms by which the receptor accomplishes its task of transmembrane signaling. In addition, the identification of mutations in the insulin receptor gene in patients with syndromes associated with insulin resistance has clarified the primary cause of these diseases. In light of the pleiotypic manifestations of these syndromes (e.g., the developmental abnormalities in leprechaunism), this emphasizes the important role of the insulin receptor in fetal development. In the future it will be interesting to attempt to understand how the fundamental defect—a mutation in the insulin receptor gene—causes all of the phenotypic abnormalities observed in these patients. Finally, study of these syndromes provides a paradigm for the utility of molecular biology in elucidating genetic factors which cause hormonal resistance. It should be possible to obtain great insights into the causes of insulin resistance in patients with NIDDM by applying a similar approach to analyze the insulin receptor gene as well as other genes required for insulin action.

ACKNOWLEDGMENTS

We gratefully acknowledge the support received throughout the course of this work from the Intramural Research Program of the National Institute of Diabetes and Digestive and Kidney Diseases as well as the Juvenile Diabetes Foundation and the American Diabetes Association. In addition, we are grateful to Dr. Axel Ullrich for collaboration in some of the studies and for contributing the insulin receptor cDNA. These studies would not have been possible without the collaboration of several physicians who identified the patients we have studied: Drs. M. Joycelyn Elders, Emilio Ramos, Rolf Engel, Manuel Serrano-Rios, Yuhei Mikami, and Nobuo Matsuura. The patient with the mutation in the ATP-binding site was studied in collaboration with Drs. Masato Kasuga, Masato Odawara, Ritsuko Yamamoto, and colleagues at Tokyo University School of Medicine. Finally, we wish to acknowledge the studies of insulin receptor biosynthesis in these patients carried out by the late Dr. José Hedo. He was a good friend and colleague. We wish to dedicate this review to his memory, in recognition of his many important contributions to the understanding of the insulin receptor.

REFERENCES

Accili, D., Frapier, C., Mosthaf, L., McKeon, C., Elbein, S., Permutt, M. A., Ramos, E., Lander, E., Ullrich, A., and Taylor, S. I. (1989). *EMBO J.* **8,** 2509–2517.

Accili, D., Mosthaf, L., Ullrich, A., and Taylor, S. I. (1990). *Diabetes* **39** (Suppl. 1), 113A (Abstr. 451).

Atweh, G. F., Brickner, H. E., Zhu, X.-X., Kazazian, H. H., Jr., and Forget, B. G. (1988). *J. Clin. Invest.* **82,** 557–561.

Barnes, N. D., Palumbo, P. J., Hayles, A. B., and Folgar, H. (1974). *Diabetologia* **10,** 285–289.

Bernier, M., Laird, D. M., and Lane, M. D. (1987). *Proc. Natl. Acad. Sci. U.S.A.* **84,** 1844–1848.

Cama, A., and Taylor, S. I. (1987). *Diabetologia* **30,** 631–637.

Cama, A., Patterson, A., Kadowaki, T., Siegel, G., Lillioja, S., Roth, J., and Taylor, S. I. (1990). *J. Clin. Endocrinol. Metab.* **70,** 1155–1161.

Collier, E., and Gorden, P. (1989). *Diabetes* **38** (Suppl. 2), 178A (Abstr. 686).

Cuatrecasas, P. (1971). *Proc. Natl. Acad. Sci. U.S.A.* **68,** 1264–1268.

Davis, C. G., Goldstein, J. L., Sudhof, T. C., Anderson, R. G., Russell, D. W., and Brown, M. S. (1987). *Nature (London)* **326,** 760–765.

DeFronzo, R. A. (1988). *Diabetes* **37,** 667–687.

Deutsch, P. J., Wan, C. F., Rosen, O. M., and Rubin, C. S. (1983). *Proc. Natl. Acad. Sci. U.S.A.* **80,** 133–136.

Ebina, Y., Ellis, L., Jarnagin, K., Edery, M., Graf, L., Clauser, E., Ou, J. H., Masiarz, F., Kan, Y. W., Goldfine, I. D., Roth, R. A., and Rutter, W. J. (1985). *Cell (Cambridge, Mass.)* **40,** 747–758.

Elders, M. J., Schedewie, H. K., Olefsky, J., Givens, B., Char, F., Bier, D. M., Baldwin, D., Fiser, R. H., Seyedabadi, S., and Rubenstein, A. (1982). *J. Natl. Med. Assoc.* **74,** 1195–1210.

Flier, J. S., Kahn, C. R., Jarrett, D. B., and Roth, J. (1976). *J. Clin. Invest.* **58,** 1442–1449.

Fojo, S. S., Stalenhoef, A. F. H., Marr, K., Gregg, R. E., Ross, R. S., and Brewer, H. B., Jr. (1988). *J. Biol. Chem.* **263,** 17913–17916.

Freychet, P., Roth, J., and Neville, D. M., Jr. (1971a). *Biochem. Biophys. Res. Commun.* **43,** 400–408.

Freychet, P., Roth, J., and Neville, D. M., Jr. (1971b). *Proc. Natl. Acad. Sci. U.S.A.* **68,** 1833–1877.

Frias, I., and Waugh, S. M. (1989) *Diabetes* **38** (Suppl. 2), 60A (Abstr. 238).

Grigorescu, F., Flier, J. S., and Kahn, C. R. (1984). *J. Biol. Chem.* **259,** 15003–15006.

Grunberger, G., Zick, Y., and Gorden, P. (1984). *Science* **223,** 932–934.

Hedo, J. A., Kasuga, M., Van Obberghen, E., Roth, J., and Kahn, C. R. (1981). *Proc. Natl. Acad. Sci. U.S.A.* **78,** 4791–4795.

Hedo, J. A., Kahn, C. R., Hayashi, M., Yamada, K. M., and Kasuga, M. (1983). *J. Biol. Chem.* **258,** 10020–10026.

Hedo, J. A., Moncada, V. Y., and Taylor, S. I. (1985). *J. Clin. Invest.* **76,** 2355–2361.

Hedo, J. A., Collier, E., and Watkinson, A. (1987). *J. Biol. Chem.* **262,** 954–957.

Herzberg, V. L., Grigorescu, F., Edge, A. S., Spiro, R. G., and Kahn, C. R. (1985). *Biochem. Biophys. Res. Commun.* **129,** 789–796.

Hobbs, H. H., Brown, M. S., Goldstein, J. L., and Russell, D. W. (1986). *J. Biol. Chem.* **261,** 13114–13120.

Jacobs, S. J., Kull, F. C. J., and Cuatrecasas, P. (1983). *Proc. Natl. Acad. Sci. U.S.A.* **80,** 1228–1231.

Kadowaki, H., Kadowaki, T., and Taylor, S. I. (1989a). *Diabetes* **38** (Suppl. 2), 2A (Abstr. 8).

Kadowaki, H., Kadowaki, T., and Taylor, S. I. (1989b). *Gene* **76,** 161–166.

Kadowaki, T., Bevins, C. L., Cama, A., Ojamaa, K., Marcus-Samuels, B., Kadowaki, H., Beitz, L., McKeon, C., and Taylor, S. I. (1988). *Science* **240,** 787–790.

Kadowaki, T., Kadowaki, H., and Taylor, S. I. (1990a). *Proc. Natl. Acad. Sci. U.S.A.* **87,** 658–662.

Kadowaki, T., Kadowaki, H., Rechler, M. M., Serrano-Rios, M., Roth, J., Gorden, P., and Taylor, S. I. (1990b). *J. Clin. Invest.* **86,** 254–264.

Kahn, C. R., Baird, K., Flier, J. S., and Jarrett, D. B. (1977). *J. Clin. Invest.* **60,** 1094–1106.

Kahn, C. R., Baird, K. L., Flier, J. S., Grunfeld, C., Harmon, J. T., Harrison, L. C., Karlsson, F. A., Kasuga, M., King, G. L., Lang, U. C., Podskalny, J. M., and Van Obberghen, E. (1981). *Recent Prog. Horm. Res.* **37,** 477–538.

Kakehi, T., Hisatomi, A., Kuzuya, H., Yoshimasa, Y., Okamoto, M., Yamada, K., Nishimura, H., Kosaki, A., Nawata, H., Umeda, F., Ibayashi, H., and Imura, H. (1988). *J. Clin. Invest.* **81,** 2020–2022.

Kasuga, M., Karlsson, F. A., and Kahn, C. R. (1982a). *Science* **215,** 185–187.

Kasuga, M., Zick, Y., Blithe, D. L., Crettaz, M., and Kahn, C. R. (1982b). *Nature (London)* **298,** 667–669.

Klinkhamer, M., Groen, N. A., van der Zon, G. C. M., Lindhout, D., Sandkuyl, L. A., Krans, H. M., Möller, W., and Maassen, J. A. (1989). *EMBO J.* **8,** 2503–2507.

Kobayashi, M., Sasaoka, T., Takata, Y., Hisatomi, A., and Shigeta, Y. (1988a). *Diabetes* **37,** 653–656.

Kobayashi, M., Sasaoka, T., Takata, Y., Ishibashi, O., Sugibayashi, M., Shigeta, Y., Hisatomi, A., Nakamura, E., Tamaki, M., and Teraoka, H. (1988b). *Biochem. Biophys. Res. Commun.* **153,** 657–663.

Lander, E. S., and Botstein, D. (1987). *Science* **236,** 1567–1570.

Lin, S., and Guidotti, G. (1989). *J. Biol. Chem.* **264,** 14408–14414.

Mamula, P. W., Wong, K. Y., Maddux, B. A., MacDonald, A. R., and Goldfine, I. D. (1988). *Diabetes* **37,** 1241–1246.

Margolis, R. N., Taylor, S. I., Seminara, D., and Hubbard, A. L. (1988). *Proc. Natl. Acad. Sci. U.S.A.* **85,** 7256–7259.

Margolis, R. N., Schell, M. J., Taylor, S. I., and Hubbard, A. L. (1990) *Biochem. Biophys. Res. Commun.* **166,** 562–566.

McElduff, A., Hedo, J. A., Taylor, S. I., Roth, J., and Gorden, P. (1984). *J. Clin. Invest.* **74,** 1366–1374.

McKeon, C., Moncada, V., Pham, T., Salvatore, P., Kadowaki, T., Accili, D., and Taylor, S. I. (1990). *Mol. Endocrinol.* **4,** 647–656.

Moller, D. E., and Flier, J. S. (1988). *N. Engl. J. Med.* **319,** 1526–1529.

Moncada, V. Y., Hedo, J. A., Serrano-Rios, M., and Taylor, S. I. (1986). *Diabetes* **35,** 802–807.

Muller-Wieland, D., Taub, R., Tewari, D. S., Kriauciunas, K. M., Sethu, S., Reddy, K., and Kahn, C. R. (1989). *Diabetes* **38,** 31–38.

Odawara, M., Kadowaki, T., Yamamoto, R., Shibasaki, Y., Tobe, K., Accili, D., Bevins, C., Mikami, Y., Matsuura, N., Akanuma, Y., Takaku, F., Taylor, S. I., and Kasuga, M. (1989). *Science* **245,** 66–68.

Ojamaa, K., Hedo, J. A., Roberts, C. T., Jr., Moncada, V. Y., Gorden, P., Ullrich, A., and Taylor, S. I. (1988). *Mol. Endocrinol.* **2,** 242–247.

Perrotti, N., Accili, D., Marcus-Samuels, B., Rees-Jones, R. W., and Taylor, S. I. (1987). *Proc. Natl. Acad. Sci. U.S.A.* **84,** 3137–3140.

Reaven, G. M. (1988). *Diabetes* **37,** 1595–1607.

Rees-Jones, R. W., and Taylor, S. I. (1985). *J. Biol. Chem.* **260,** 4461–4467.

Ronnett, G. V., Tennekoon, G., Knutson, V. P., and Lane, M. D. (1983). *J. Biol. Chem.* **258,** 283–290.

Rosen, O. M. (1987). *Science* **237,** 1452–1458.

Seino, S., Seino, M., Nishi, S., and Bell, G. I. (1989). *Proc. Natl. Acad. Sci. U.S.A.* **86,** 114–118.

Taira, M., Taira, M., Hashimoto, N., Shimada, F., Suzuki, Y., Kanatsuka, A., Nakamura, F., Ebina, Y., Tatibana, M., Makino, H., and Yoshida, S. (1989). *Science* **245,** 63–66.

Taylor, S. I. (1985). *Diabetes/Metab. Rev.* **1**, 171–202.

Taylor, S. I. (1987). *Clin. Res.* **35**, 459–467.

Taylor, S. I. (1988). *In* "The Liver: Biology and Pathobiology" (I. M. Arias, W. B. Jakoby, H. Popper, D. Schachter, and D. A. Shafritz, eds.), pp. 753–767. Raven, New York.

Taylor, S. I., and Leventhal, S. (1983). *J. Clin. Invest.* **71**, 1676–1685.

Taylor, S. I., and Marcus-Samuels, B. (1984) *J. Clin. Endocrinol. Metab.* **58**, 182–186.

Taylor, S. I., Roth, J., Blizzard, R. M., and Elders, M. J. (1981). *Proc. Natl. Acad. Sci. U.S.A.* **78**, 7157–7161.

Taylor, S. I., Grunberger, G., Marcus-Samuels, B., Underhill, L. H., Dons, R. F., Ryan, J., Roddam, R. F., Rupe, C. E., and Gorden, P. (1982a). *N. Engl. J. Med.* **307**, 1422–1426.

Taylor, S. I., Samuels, B., Roth, J., Kasuga, M., Hedo, J. A., Gorden, P., Brasel, D. E., Pokora, T., and Engel, R. R. (1982b). *J. Clin. Endocrinol. Metab.* **54**, 919–930.

Taylor, S. I., Marcus-Samuels, B., Ryan-Young, J., Leventhal, S., and Elders, M. J. (1986). *J. Clin. Endocrinol. Metab.* **62**, 1130–1135.

Taylor, S. I., Kadowaki, T., Kadowaki, H., Accili, D., Cama, A., and McKeon, C. (1990). *Diabetes Care* **13**, 257–279.

Tewari, D. S., Cook, D. M., and Taub, R. (1989). *J. Biol. Chem.* **264**, 16238–16245.

Tornqvist, H. E., Gunsalus, J. R., Nemenoff, R. A., Frackelton, H. R., Pierce, M. W., and Avruch, J. (1988). *J. Biol. Chem.* **263**, 350–359.

Ullrich, A., Bell, J. R., Chen, E. Y., Herrera, R., Petruzzelli, L. M., Dull, T. J., Gray, A., Coussens, L., Liao, Y. C., Tsubokawa, M., Mason, A., Seeburg, P. H., Grunfeld, C., Rosen, O. M., and Ramachandran, J. (1985). *Nature (London)* **313**, 756–761.

Urlaub, G., Mitchell, P. J., Ciudad, C. J., and Chasin, L. A. (1989). *Mol. Cell. Biol.* **9**, 2868–2880.

White, M. F., Maron, R., and Kahn, C. R. (1985). *Nature (London)* **318**, 183–186.

White, M. F., Shoelson, S. E., Keutmann, H., and Kahn, C. R. (1988). *J. Biol. Chem.* **263**, 2969–2980.

Whittaker, J., Zick, Y., Roth, J., and Taylor, S. I. (1985). *J. Clin. Endocrinol. Metab.* **60**, 381–386.

Yamamoto, T., Bishop, R. W., Brown, M. S., Goldstein, J. L., and Russell, D. W. (1986). *Science* **232**, 1230–1237.

Yang-Feng, T. L., Francke, U., and Ullrich, A. (1985). *Science* **228**, 728–731.

Yoshimasa, Y., Seino, S., Whittaker, J., Kakehi, T., Kosaki, A., Kuzuya, H., Imura, I., Bell, G. I., and Steiner, D. F. (1988). *Science* **240**, 784–787.

DISCUSSION

W. Vale. What about the Pima Indians? Is there any indication of what the mutation might be in that population?

S. I. Taylor. As many of you know, certain populations have an enormous increase in the prevalence of non-insulin-dependent diabetes mellitus (NIDDM). Among them, the Pima Indians have the highest reported prevalence of NIDDM, in excess of 50% in appropriate age groups. We have determined the nucleotide sequence of the insulin receptor cDNA in an insulin-resistant Pima Indian. Both alleles of the patient's receptor genes encode a receptor with a normal predicted amino acid sequence. Because the regulatory domains of the insulin receptor gene have not been completely elucidated, it is not possible to rule out that there may be mutations in regulatory domains of the gene. However, suffice it to say that there is really no evidence that the primary mutation in diabetic Pima Indians is in the insulin receptor gene. Furthermore, this is the only gene which has been investigated in detail in this population. It remains an important unanswered question to map the mutations which predispose Pima Indians to develop insulin resistance and diabetes.

J. Kirkland. Have you had the opportunity to investigate children with maturity-onset diabetes of youth (MODY) with the techniques you have just described?

S. I. Taylor. We have not done this. However, at least two laboratories have conducted studies to determine whether the mutation causing MODY is linked to the insulin receptor gene (Elbein *et al.*, 1987; O'Rahilly *et al.*, 1988). Their data suggested that the disease-causing gene was not linked to the insulin receptor locus, at least in the small number of families which were investigated.

C. Grunfeld. The Val-1008 mutation is going to be an interesting one to study in transfected cells in terms of biological activity. I am certain you know that there are monoclonal antibodies that have biological activity which have been reported to lack tyrosine kinase stimulatory activity. Have you had a chance to try those monoclonal antibodies in cells transfected with receptor containing this mutation in the tyrosine kinase domain?

S. I. Taylor. We have not done exactly that. However, let me briefly review the relevant work in the literature. Several antibodies to the insulin receptor have been reported to mimic insulin action without activating the tyrosine kinase: both polyclonal antibodies derived from patients with autoimmune forms of insulin resistance (Simpson and Hedo, 1984; Zick *et al.*, 1984) and monoclonal antibodies (Forsayeth *et al.*, 1987; Soos *et al,.* 1989). However, these antibodies fail to mimic insulin action in cells transfected with mutant insulin receptors lacking tyrosine kinase activity—for example, mutants in which Lys-1030 in the ATP-binding site has been replaced by another amino acid (Ebina *et al.*, 1987; Gherzi *et al.*, 1987). These studies suggest that tyrosine kinase activity is required for receptors to mediate the biological action of both antireceptor antibodies and insulin. However, it is important to emphasize that only some, but not all, of the antibodies have been investigated in this way. How can one explain this controversy? It is important to remember that there are spare receptors for insulin in most target cells. Insulin elicits a maximal biological response when only 10% of the receptors are occupied. Similarly, a submaximal ($\sim$10%) activation of receptor tyrosine kinase may be sufficient to elicit a maximal biological response. It is possible that the controversy arises from the fact that it is hard to detect such small activations of the tyrosine kinase. For example, one of the polyclonal antireceptor antibodies originally reported not to activate receptor tyrosine kinase (Simpson and Hedo, 1984; Zick *et al.*, 1984) was subsequently reinvestigated with more sensitive techniques (Gherzi *et al.*, 1987). In these later studies it was possible to demonstrate that the antibodies did activate the receptor tyrosine kinase (Gherzi *et al.*, 1987).

C. Grunfeld. I agree with you on the ambiguity, and that is the reason why the experiment crossing the mutant insulin receptor with the putative kinase incompetent antibodies is so critical.

S. I. Taylor. These are very important experiments. However, one must remember that a mutation which inactivates the tyrosine kinase might also alter the receptor conformation in such a way as to impair other putative functions of the receptor. For example, in studies in which Lys-1030 has been mutated, the mutation was introduced into this position because it was already known that this amino acid residue is necessary for protein kinase activity (Ebina *et al.*, 1987; Chou *et al.*, 1987). Of course it was reassuring that this mutation eliminated the ability of the receptor to mediate insulin action. However, this conclusion is greatly strengthened by the identification of spontaneous mutations in insulin-resistant patients (Moller and Flier, 1988; Odawara *et al.*, 1989). In this case the only selection was for a phenotype of insulin resistance. The mutations were not intentionally directed to a site which was known in advance to be necessary for tyrosine kinase activity. Nevertheless, the fact that these mutations turned out to impair tyrosine kinase activity strongly supports the hypothesis that tyrosine kinase is necessary for the receptor to mediate insulin action. Unfortunately, it may not be possible to be entirely comfortable with this conclusion until we understand the mechanism whereby the tyrosine kinase mediates insulin action.

M. R. Walters. When you grew the lymphocytes from the Type A patients, did you encounter problems in culturing them because of their insulin resistance?

S. I. Taylor. In general we have not had problems cultivating Epstein–Barr virus (EBV)-transformed lymphoblasts from patients with Type A extreme insulin resistance. In addition, these patients grow at a normal rate and achieve normal adult height. Thus, they do not appear to have a defect of "growth factors" either *in vitro* or *in vivo*. However, interestingly, we have the impression that EBV-transformed lymphoblasts from patients with leprechaunism do grow slowly in tissue culture. Similarly, the clinical syndrome is characterized by intrauterine growth retardation. It is noteworthy that the patients with leprechaunism appear to be more severely insulin resistant than the patients with Type A extreme insulin resistance. It is a very interesting, although unanswered, question as to how insulin functions as a growth factor in fetal life.

M. R. Walters. I was surprised that in the Type A family there were no members who were homozygous for the wild-type receptor. I would have thought that with the numbers you studied you would have come up with homozygotes.

S. I. Taylor. The two parents were obligate heterozygotes, and the two affected sisters were homozygous for the mutant allele. Of the four unaffected children, one would have expected one-third to be homozygous normal and two-thirds to be heterozygous carriers of the mutant allele. Thus, the number of homozygous normal children expected in this family is 1.33, which is not statistically different from the number which we observed (i.e., zero). This was just the "luck of the draw."

G. B. Cutler. Have any of the types of studies you have done been carried out on the closely related IGF-I receptor? Do you think we have the same kind of family of mutations awaiting discovery among our pediatric patients with unexplained growth failure? What is known about the IGF-I receptor and its genetics?

S. I. Taylor. In some patients with leprechaunism, there have been reports of parallel decreases in the binding of both insulin and IGF-I (Van Obberghen-Schilling *et al.*, 1981). In addition, there have been reports of children with short stature in association with decreased IGF-I binding (Heath-Monnig *et al.*, 1987). However, to the best of my knowledge, there are no reports of direct demonstrations of mutations in the IGF-I receptor gene. Furthermore, recent work from Rosen's laboratory has suggested the existence of two different IGF-I receptor proteins, possibly encoded by two distinct genes. If this were so, it could provide redundancy in the system. For example, it might be necessary to have mutations in both alleles at both loci to cause resistance to IGF-I. Thus, this type of redundancy might protect against the development of genetic forms of resistance to the biological action of IGF-I.

G. B. Cutler. In patients with leprechaunism, is it your assumption that their intrauterine growth retardation is related to the insulin receptor or is there a likelihood that there are other genes that are abnormal in these patients?

S. I. Taylor. Yes, it is my assumption that intrauterine growth retardation in leprechaunism is caused by a mutation in the insulin receptor gene. Of course, even if this were true, I do not know whether the effect is direct or indirect. The evidence in favor of this hypothesis is based on the observation that all of the patients with leprechaunism whose insulin receptor genes have been investigated in detail have turned out to have mutations in that gene. It seems unlikely that this is a coincidence. It also seems unlikely that the patients have mutations at other genes also, although we cannot entirely rule out this possibility.

G. B. Cutler. Do you think the normal growth of all the other insulin-resistant patients is simply due to the lesser severity of their insulin resistance?

S. I. Taylor. That is my hypothesis, but whether it is right or not, I do not know.

M. New. You discussed a family in which the father carried a nonsense mutation and the mother, a missense mutation, and the index case was a compound heterozygote. Are there any patients that are homozygous for the missense mutation in any other families?

S. I. Taylor. We have never studied anyone with the Glu-460 mutation besides leprechaun/Ark-1 and her mother. We hope to screen other family members to determine whether other individuals have this mutation and, if so, whether they are insulin resistant. I agree that it would be interesting to determine the phenotype associated with homozygosity for the Glu-460 mutation. I predict that such an individual would be insulin resistant, although probably not as severely insulin resistant as leprechaun/Ark-1. We have no data on the prevalence of the Glu-460 mutation in the gene pool, so it is not possible to estimate the probability of finding a homozygous individual.

M. New. In Type A patients with extreme insulin resistance, I understand that through genetic linkage studies and transfection studies an abnormality in the function of the insulin receptor can be demonstrated. Do you think this is the cause of their disease? Is the hyperandrogenization, the obesity, the acanthosis due to the genetic defect?

S. I. Taylor. Yes, I believe that the mutations in the insulin receptor gene are the cause of the hyperandrogenism and acanthosis nigricans in the patients we studied. Of course, this does not imply that all patients with insulin resistance, hyperandrogenism, and acanthosis nigricans have mutations in their insulin receptor genes. We plan to study additional patients to determine what fraction of the patients with this syndrome have mutations in their insulin receptor gene. Thus far, we have not studied any of the patients in whom insulin resistance, acanthosis nigricans, and hyperandrogenism are associated with obesity. This group will be especially interesting because weight loss has been reported to improve insulin sensitivity in these patients. Thus, if these patients have mutation in their insulin receptor genes, these investigations may provide insight into the interactions between obesity and genetic factors which predispose to insulin resistance.

M. New. I guess that without unethical breeding experiments in humans, one could find patients who are androgenized and not obese and not acanthotic.

S. I. Taylor. We are planning to do such studies. Until very recently, studying each patient has represented a major commitment of resources. Now, with the advent of PCR technology and techniques to facilitate nucleotide sequencing and identification of mutants, studying larger numbers of patients is more feasible.

H. G. Friesen. Do the patients with the insulin receptor mutations you have studied exhibit common complications of diabetes, nephropathy, retinopathy, and neuropathy, or are these complications separately inherited entities?

S. I. Taylor. Because patients with leprechaunism generally die within the first year of life, they do not live long enough to develop chronic complications of diabetes. However, some of the patients with Type A extreme insulin resistance have developed diabetic complications. For example, one patient (A-1) is blind as the result of proliferative retinopathy and requires treatment with dialysis for chronic renal failure. In addition, she has neuropathy and has had strokes as a result of cerebrovascular disease. In summary, she has developed both the microvascular and macrovascular complications associated with diabetes. This is consistent with the view that chronic complications are caused by the metabolic abnormalities (e.g., hyperglycemia) associated with diabetes, irrespective of the molecular mechanisms which cause diabetes. Clearly, in patient A-1 diabetes is caused by mechanisms which are totally distinct from the factors which predispose to autoimmune destruction of pancreatic β cells in patients with insulin-dependent diabetes mellitus.

H. G. Friesen. Would you comment on the mutations that affect protein tyrosine kinase or tyrosine kinase activation? Are these cells insulin sensitive or responsive, or is there simply a quantitative difference in activation of tyrosine kinase?

S. I. Taylor. In the patient we studied (Odawara *et al.*, 1989) one allele of the insulin receptor gene had a mutation in the ATP-binding site. The other allele did not have this mutation. Thus, it seems likely that most of the residual tyrosine kinase activity was caused by the receptor with the normal amino acid sequence in the ATP-binding site. Under the conditions of our *in vitro* assay, the receptor with the Val-1008 substitution in the ATP-binding site did not have detectable tyrosine kinase. Of course, we cannot entirely rule out the possibility that there is some small residual enzymatic activity.

H. G. Friesen. In the patients you studied with mutations that affected tyrosine kinase, was this a partial defect of tyrosine kinase? Is this why they were still insulin responsive?

S. I. Taylor. The patients with the Val-1008 and Ser-1200 mutations were heterozygous. Because their other alleles encoded a receptor with normal tyrosine kinase activity, the patients could respond to insulin to some extent. Although the two sisters with the Val-382 mutation were homozygous, this mutation caused a partial defect in receptor tyrosine kinase activity.

W. Vale. Have you found the same mutation in different families?

S. I. Taylor. We have never yet found the same mutation in unrelated individuals. There may be many different mutations in insulin receptor genes of different patients.

DISCUSSION REFERENCES

Chou, C. K., Dull, T. J., Russell, D. S., Ghrezi, R., Lebwohl, D., Ullrich, A., and Rosen, O. M. (1987). *J. Biol. Chem.* **262,** 1842–1847.

Ebina, Y., Araki, E., Taira, M., Shimada, F., Mori, M., Craik, C. S., Siddle, K., Pierce, S. B., Roth, R. A., and Rutter, W. J. (1987). *Proc. Natl. Acad. Sci. U.S.A.* **84,** 704–708.

Elbein, S. C., Borecki, I., Corsetti, L., Fajans, S. S., Hansen, A. T., Nerup, J., Province, M., and Permutt, M. A. (1987). *Diabetologia* **30,** 641.

Forsayeth, J. R., Caro, J. F., Sinha, M. K., Maddux, B. A., and Goldfine, I. D. (1987). *Proc. Natl. Acad. Sci. U.S.A.* **84,** 3448–3451.

Gherzi, R., Russell, D. S., Taylor, S. I., and Rosen, O. M. (1987). *J. Biol. Chem.* **262,** 16900–16905.

Heath-Monnig, E., Wohltmann, H. J., Mills-Dunlap, B., and Daughaday, W. H. (1987). *J. Clin. Endocrinol. Metab.* **64,** 501–507.

Moller, D. E., and Flier, J. S. (1988). *N. Engl. J. Med.* **319,** 1526–1529.

Odawara, M., Kadowaki, T., Yamamoto, R., Shibasaki, Y., Tobe, K., Accili, D., Bevins, C., Mikami, Y., Matsuura, N., Akanuma, Y., Takaku, F., Taylor, S. I., and Kasuga, M. (1989). *Science* **245,** 66–68.

O'Rahilly, S., Trembath, R. C., Patel, P., Galton, D. J., Turner, R. C., and Wainscoat, J. S. (1988). *Diabetologia* **31,** 192–197.

Simpson, I. A., and Hedo, J. A. (1984). *Science* **233,** 1301–1304.

Soos, M. A., O'Brien, R. M., Brindle, N. P., Stigter, J. M., Okamoto, A. K., Whittaker, J., and Siddle, K. (1989). *Proc. Natl. Acad. Sci. U.S.A.* **86,** 5217–5221.

Van Obberghen-Schilling, E. E., Rechler, M. M., Romanus, J. A., Knight, A. B., Nissley, S. P., and Humbel, R. E. (1981). *J. Clin. Invest.* **68,** 1356–1365.

Zick, Y., Rees-Jones, R. W., Taylor, S. I., Gorden, P., and Roth, J. (1984). *J. Biol. Chem.* **259,** 4396–4400.

Characteristics of the cAMP Response Unit

Marc R. Montminy, Gustavo A. Gonzalez, and
Karen K. Yamamoto

*The Clayton Foundation Laboratories for Peptide Biology, The Salk Institute,
La Jolla, California 92037*

cAMP regulates a striking number of physiological processes, including intermediary metabolism, cellular proliferation, and neuronal signaling, by altering basic patterns of gene expression. In the liver, for example, cAMP stimulates glucose production in part by inducing the transcription of the gene for phosphoenolpyruvate carboxykinase (PEPCK), a rate-limiting gluconeogenic enzyme, more than 15-fold (Lamers *et al.,* 1982; Sasaki *et al.,* 1984). The transcriptional induction by cAMP is rapid, peaking at 30 minutes and declining gradually over 24 hours. This burst in transcription does not depend on new protein synthesis and suggests, therefore, that transcriptional modulation by cAMP involves the covalent modification of a preexisting nuclear factor. Since all of the known cellular effects of cAMP occur via cAMP-dependent protein kinase, it appears that phosphorylation is the most likely mechanism by which cAMP would regulate gene expression.

In the process of characterizing cis-acting sequences underlying cAMP responsiveness of the somatostatin gene, we (Montminy *et al.,* 1986) and others (Comb *et al.,* 1986; Short *et al.,* 1986) observed a short palindromic core motif 5′–TGACGTCA–3′ which was highly conserved among several cAMP-inducible promoters, including those for c-*fos,* somatostatin, tyrosine hydroxylase, vasoactive intestinal polypeptide, proenkephalin, and PEPCK (Fig. 1). The cAMP response element (CRE) displayed properties of a classical enhancer sequence, stimulating transcription in a distance, and orientation-independent manner. The CRE also conferred cAMP inducibility when placed upstream of a nonresponsive gene, moreover, indicating that CRE binding factors could interact with components of the transcriptional machinery (e.g., TATA factors) which were not specific to cAMP-inducible promoters. As expected, transcriptional regulation by cAMP appears to be mediated by cAMP-dependent protein kinase (kinase A). Kinase A-deficient cell lines, for example, are unable to

219

Gene	Sequence
Somatostatin*	CTGGGGGCGCCTCCTTGGCTGACGTCAGAGAGAGAG (−32)
PEPCK*	TGATCCAAAGGCCGGCCCCTTACGTCAGAGGCGAGC (−74)
VIP*	TCCCATGGCCGTCATACTGTGACGTCTTTCAGAGCA (−60)
Parathyroid hormone	GGGAGTGACGTCATCT (−65)
Proenkephalin*	GGGCCTGCGTCAGC (−87)
α-Chorionic gonadotropin	AAAATTGACGTCATGG (−113)
c-fos*	CCGCCCAGTGACGTAGGA (−57)
Cytomegalovirus enhancer	CCACCCCATTGACGTCAATGGGAGTT (−124)
BLV LTR	ACCAGACAGAGACGTCAGCTGCCAGA (−144)
HTLV-II LTR	CCACGGCCCTGACGTCCCTCCCCCCC (−162)
Intracisternal A particle	CCTCTCCCGTGACGTCATCTGGGG (−86)

FIG. 1. A short palindromic sequence 5′-TGACGTCA-3′ is conserved among cAMP-responsive genes. Asterisks indicate genes known to be transcriptionally regulated by cAMP. Boldface type indicates palindromic sequences. The position of the 3′-most nucleotide is indicated in parentheses next to each sequence. PEPCK, Phosphoenolpyruvate carboxykinase; VIP, vasoactive intestinal polypeptide; BLV, bovine leukemia virus; LTR, long terminal repeat; HTLV-II, human T-lymphotropic virus type II.

support somatostatin transcription in response to forskolin (Montminy *et al.*, 1986; Grove *et al.*, 1987). Microinjection of catalytic subunit into cells, furthermore, can directly activate CRE-dependent transcription without the simultaneous addition of cAMP (Riabowol *et al.*, 1988).

The observation that CRE sequences are highly conserved prompted us to ask whether these elements would recognize a common nuclear factor. Using a DNase I protection assay, we were able to detect CRE-binding (CREB) activity in nuclear extracts of PC12 cells (Montminy and Bilezikjian, 1987). By using DNA sequence-specific affinity chromatography, we purified a 43-kDa protein to apparent homogeneity from PC12 cells and brain tissue (Montminy and Bilezikjian, 1987; Yamamoto *et al.*, 1988) (Fig. 2). When added to nuclear extracts, purified CREB specifically stimulated transcription of CRE-containing genes such as somatostatin, suggesting that CREB was a transcription factor as well as a DNA-binding protein. Further biochemical experiments have revealed that CREB stimulates transcription of these genes by binding to DNA as a dimer. Moreover, the transcriptional efficacy of CREB is regulated by protein kinase A phosphorylation (Yamamoto *et al.*, 1988).

Experiments showing that the dimerization and transcriptional efficacy of CREB are each stimulated by phosphorylation at distinct sites suggest that this activity is regulated by multiple kinases *in vivo*. Nuclear extracts prepared from cAMP-treated PC12 cells appear to be identical to untreated cells in both DNA-binding and transcriptional activity; however, the absence of detectable changes in these parameters might arise from (1) the liberation of kinases during extract preparation, which causes extensive phosphorylation of CREB and subsequently "deregulates" the extract or (2) the loss of other nuclear factors which are required for transcriptional regulation by cAMP. These experiments demonstrate

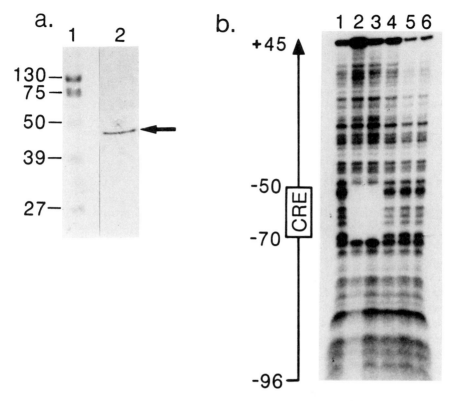

FIG. 2.   Purification of a 43-kDa nuclear protein with CRE-binding activity. (a) SDS–PAGE showing CREB from rat brain after purification over a CRE oligonucleotide affinity column (lane 2). The arrow indicates purified CREB. Lane 1, markers (in kilodaltons). (b) DNase I protection assay using a ^{32}P-labeled c-*fos* probe extending from −96 to +45. The position of the CRE sequence is shown. After incubating the DNA probe with protein fractions, samples were digested with DNase I. Products of digestion were resolved on urea–PAGE. Lane 1, no protein; lane 2, purified CREB; lanes 3–6, protein fractions eluted and renatured from the SDS–PAGE shown in (a). Only lane 3, which contains the 43-kDa protein, shows CRE-binding activity.

the inherent limitations of transcription studies without purified components which have been thoroughly characterized.

We have recently isolated a cDNA clone for CREB using amino acid sequence information from purified CREB protein (Gonzalez *et al.*, 1989) (Fig. 3). When expressed in *Escherichia coli,* the protein encoded by this cDNA possesses CREB activity which is identical to that of purified CREB. Sequence analysis of the CREB cDNA predicts a cluster of protein kinase A, protein kinase C, and casein kinase II consensus recognition sites near the amino terminus of the protein. The close proximity of these sites to one another suggests that they might interact to regulate CREB activity. A stretch of regularly spaced leucine

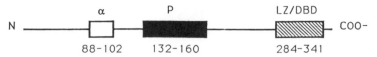

FIG. 3. CREB protein as predicted from a cDNA clone obtained from rat PC12 mRNA. The open box with "α" above it indicates an alternately spliced trans-activating region (amino acids 88–102). The solid box with "P" above it (amino acids 132–160) indicates the position of phosphorylation sites for kinase C, kinase A, and casein kinase II. The hatched box with LZ/DBD above it (amino acids 284–341) indicates the position of the leucine-zipper and DNA-binding dimerization domains.

residues, characteristic of a potential "leucine-zipper" dimerization domain (Landshulz *et al.*, 1988), is located near the carboxy terminus of the CREB molecule. CREB shares substantial homology in this region with other leucine-zipper proteins, including c-*fos*, c-*myc*, and c-*jun*. The prevalence of such dimerization domains among nuclear factors illustrates the potential for combinatorial regulation through the formation of heterodimers with factors such as CREB. Another laboratory has also characterized a CREB cDNA clone by screening a λgt11 cDNA expression library from human placenta with a CRE oligonucleotide (Hoefler *et al.*, 1988).

The isolation of a cDNA encoding CREB, the production of a bacterial CREB fusion protein, and the characterization of antisera which immunoprecipitate this factor have allowed us to examine the interaction of CREB with other proteins which are necessary to form a cAMP-responsive transcription complex. The presence of two domains—the phosphorylation and dimerization domains—in the CREB molecule offers two different, though not mutually exclusive, conceptual models for regulation by cAMP.

In model I cAMP stimulates phosphorylation of CREB, thereby causing it to undergo a conformational change which exposes the transcriptional-activating domain of the molecule to its target protein (Fig. 4). Current evidence supports the notion that such activating domains are usually acidic in character, and they have been termed "negative noodles" (Ma and Ptashne, 1987; Ptashne, 1988). The six glutamate residues carboxy terminal to the kinase A domain would constitute such a potential structure. Based on the ability of CREB to trans-activate promoters not normally regulated by cAMP, the target protein for this activating domain would presumably be a nonspecific TATA factor such as Transcription Factor IID (TFIID) or an RNA polymerase II-associated protein. In fact, CREB [also referred to as ATF (Lee and Green, 1987)] has been shown to interact with TFIID, forming a preinitiation complex, and to increase the affinity of TFIID for its recognition site (Horikoshi *et al.*, 1988).

Model II suggests that, by analogy with transcription factor AP-1, CREB regulates transcription primarily through interactions (possibly at its dimerization domain) with other nuclear factors. This model might be particularly ap-

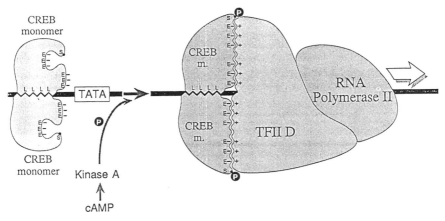

FIG. 4. The induction of eukaryotic genes by cAMP. CREB is shown bound to DNA as a dimer. L, Leucine residues which form the leucine-zipper dimerization domain; E−, negatively charged glutamate residues thought to be critical for the trans-activating potential of CREB. S, the single serine residue which is phosphorylated by the C subunit *in vitro*. Following hormonal stimulation, cAMP levels increase, leading to the release of active C subunit from inactive kinase A holoenzyme. C subunit is directly transported to the nucleus, where it phosphorylates CREB. Phosphorylation causes a change in the conformation of the CREB molecule, allowing the putative CREB trans-activating domain (glutamate residues) to interact with its target protein TFIID. As a result of this CREB–TFIID interaction, TFIID can bind to the TATA box and stimulate gene transcription.

plicable to the tissue-specific regulation of genes such as chorionic gonadotropin and somatostatin. The chorionic gonadotropin gene promoter, for example, contains a tissue-specific element flanked by two consensus CRE motifs (Delegeane *et al.*, 1987; Jameson *et al.*, 1986). Deletion of these CREs completely inactivates tissue-specific expression. As with TFIID, the tissue-specific factor can only bind to its cognate sequence when CREB is present. Recent studies showing that the tissue-specific expression of the somatostatin gene is also dependent on the CRE sequence (Andrisani *et al.*, 1987) suggest that CREB might perform a more general function, serving perhaps as an anchor for tissue-specific factors.

To support the hypothesis that CREB is regulated by kinase A, we have examined the phosphorylation of CREB in PC12 cells in response to forskolin treatment (Gonzalez and Montminy, 1989). PC12 cells were incubated in inorganic ^{32}P for 5 hours and then treated with forskolin (10 mM) or an ethanol vehicle for 30 minutes. Cells were then harvested in sodium dodecyl sulfate (SDS) lysis buffer, and immunoprecipitates were prepared using CREB antiserum 219. After SDS–polyacrylamide gel electrophoresis (PAGE) the 43-kDa ^{32}P-labeled bands representing the CREB protein were identified and excised. Two-dimensional tryptic maps (Fig. 5A) revealed a single spot which migrated at the same position as the kinase A phosphorylated CREB peptide. Phosphorylation of this site was enhanced approximately 6-fold in samples treated with

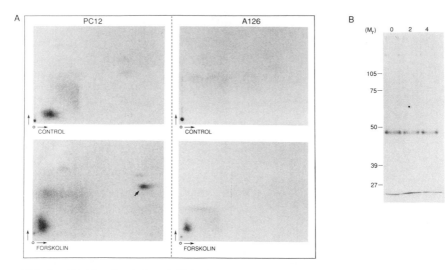

FIG. 5. (A) Phosphorylation of CREB in response to forskolin treatment of PC12 and A126 cells. Two-dimensional phosphotryptic maps of ^{32}P-labeled CREB protein after immunoprecipitation with W39 CREB antiserum. The arrow indicates the ^{32}P-labeled spot which migrates at the same position as W51 CREB peptide. (B) Biosynthesis of CREB in PC12 cells in response to forskolin. 0, 2, 4, Hours of forskolin treatment. The arrow indicates ^{35}S-labeled CREB. M_r, Relative molecular mass (in kilodaltons). Cells were treated with forskolin (10 μM) for the times indicated and then labeled with [^{35}S]methionine (0.1 mCi/ml) for 15 minutes. Cell extracts were immunoprecipitated with affinity-purified W39 CREB antiserum. Samples were then resolved by SDS–PAGE.

forskolin. PC12 cells labeled with [^{35}S]methionine showed no increase in immunoprecipitable CREB over the same period, indicating that the increase in phosphorylation which we observed was independent of new protein synthesis (Fig. 5B). In contrast, using A126–1B2 cells, which are deficient in kinase A activity, we observed no increase in forskolin-stimulated CREB phosphorylation (Fig. 5A). In light of previous work showing that A126 cells are also incapable of supporting somatostatin transcription in response to cAMP (Montminy *et al.*, 1986), these results provide compelling evidence to support the kinase A-mediated activation of CREB.

To show that CREB *directly* participates in transcriptional regulation, we constructed a CREB expression vector and cotransfected this plasmid into PC12 cells with the somatostatin CRE–chloramphenicol acetyltransferase (CAT) reporter gene (Fig. 6). Having observed that the Rous sarcoma virus (RSV) promoter is particularly active in PC12 cells (Montminy *et al.*, 1986), we inserted the CREB cDNA into a plasmid containing the RSV long terminal repeat. When transfected into PC12 cells, RSV–CREB stimulated CRE–CAT activity approximately 4-fold over the baseline level. Not surprisingly, the ability of RSV–CREB to induce CRE–CAT activity was dependent on cAMP stimulation. RSV–

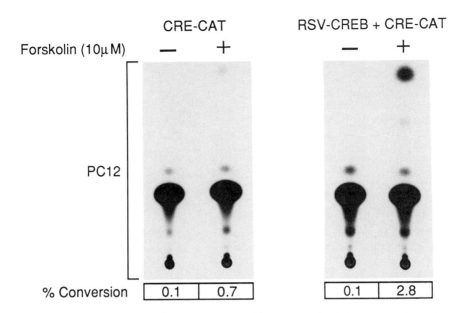

Forskolin (10μM)

CRE-CAT

RSV-CREB + CRE-CAT

PC12

% Conversion   0.1   0.7   0.1   2.8

FIG. 6.   Effect of CREB on Δ(−71) CAT expression in PC12 cells. Cells were transfected with either Δ(−71) CAT (CRE–CAT) or Δ(−71) CAT plus CREB (RSV–CREB) expression plasmids. −, +, Control (ethanol vehicle) or forskolin (10 μM) treatment, respectively. CAT activity is expressed as the percentage of conversion, shown below each.

CREB was unable to stimulate transcription in forskolin-stimulated A126 cells (not shown), further emphasizing the requirement for kinase A activity.

To demonstrate that cells regulate CREB bioactivity by reversible phosphorylation in response to kinase A, we have constructed several mutants in the kinase A site of CREB (Fig. 7). Mutant M1 contains a conservative serine-to-valine substitution at position 133. This mutant would not be phosphorylated by kinase A and therefore should not trans-activate CRE–CAT in response to cAMP. Mutant M2, containing a serine-to-aspartate substitution, was designed to provide the negative charge otherwise incurred by phosphorylation at this site. If phosphorylation stimulates transcription simply by making this region more acidic, we predict that M2 will be constitutively up-regulated but unresponsive to cAMP. Mutant M3 was designed to test whether phosphorylation by kinase C at Ser-133 was important for activity. We therefore substituted the carboxy-terminal basic residues Arg-135, Lys-136 with Met-135, Glu-136. Should kinase C be critical to cAMP induction, this mutant would be completely inactive.

To assess the activity of each CREB mutant, we used the murine teratocarcinoma cell line F9 (Fig. 8). In the absence of retinoic acid-induced differentiation, these cells are largely unresponsive to cAMP. Cotransfection of eukaryotic expression plasmids encoding either CREB or the catalytic subunit (C subunit)

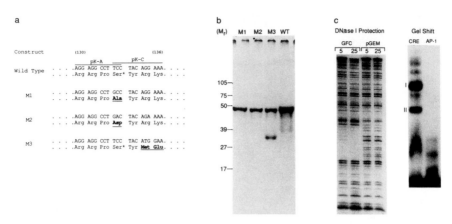

FIG. 7.   Characterization of CREB point mutants. (a) Nucleotide and corresponding amino acid sequence of point mutants M1, M2, and M3 compared to wild-type (WT) CREB cDNA near the Ser-133 phosphoacceptor site. Consensus protein kinase A (pK-A) and protein kinase C (pK-C) phosphorylation sites are overlined and labeled. The positions of the amino acids are shown in parentheses. The serine phosphoacceptor is indicated by asterisks. Mutated residues are underlined and shown in boldface type. (b) Immunoprecipitation of ^{35}S-labeled wild-type and mutant CREB proteins expressed *in vitro*. M_r, molecular mass standard (in kilodaltons); M1, M2, M3, WT, lanes corresponding to mutant and wild-type CREB proteins. (c) Effect of C-subunit phosphorylation on CREB activity of the bacterial CREB fusion protein *in vitro*. Gel shift assay of extract using ^{32}P-labeled double-stranded CRE oligonucleotide probes. I and II, Putative dimer and monomer forms of CREB, respectively.

had only modest effects on CRE–CAT reporter activity. When both CREB and C-subunit plasmids were introduced, however, CRE–CAT activity was induced 200-fold. This effect was specific for the CRE, as neither CREB nor C-subunit plasmids had any inductive effect on an RSV–CAT reporter (which lacks a CRE and is unresponsive to cAMP).

Mutants M1, M2, and M3 were evaluated in F9 cells by cotransfection with the C-subunit and CRE–CAT reporter plasmids (Fig. 9). When compared to wild-type CREB, mutant M1 (Ser-133 to Ala-133) was completely inactive. These results suggest that the Ser-133 phosphoacceptor is indeed critical for transcriptional induction by cAMP. Furthermore, mutant M2 (Ser-133 to Asp-133) was also inactive, indicating that phosphorylation allows CREB to stimulate transcription by a mechanism other than simply providing negative charge. Mutant M3, in which the kinase C phosphorylation component is removed, nevertheless maintains wild-type activity, demonstrating that the kinase A component alone is sufficient for induction.

All of the mutants were expressed at levels comparable to wild-type CREB and were appropriately targeted to nuclei of transfected cells. Moreover, M1, M2,

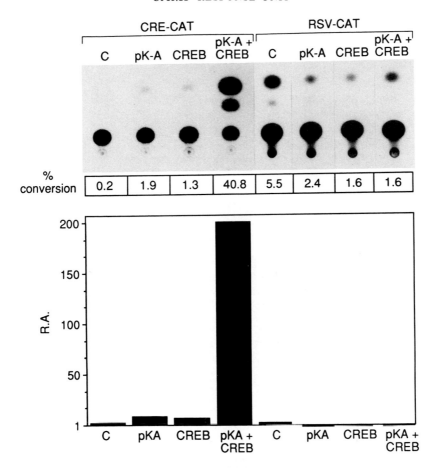

FIG. 8. Effect of CREB and protein kinase A on Δ(−71) CAT and RSV–CAT expression in undifferentiated F9 teratocarcinoma cells. Cells were transfected with either Δ(−71) CAT or RSV–CAT reporter genes plus C-subunit (pK-A), CREB, or both expression plasmids. Control (C), F9 cells transfected with reporter gene alone. CAT activity is expressed as the percentage of conversion, shown below each. The relative activities (R.A.) of Δ(−71) CAT and RSV–CAT fusion genes when cotransfected with the expression plasmids shown above are depicted graphically as n-fold stimulation over the control.

and M3 had DNA-binding activity which was indistinguishable from the wild-type protein. Together, these results indicate that phosphorylation of CREB specifically alters the trans-activation domain so as to render the protein transcriptionally active. Future studies will focus on other structural determinants of the CREB protein which are critical for induction by cAMP.

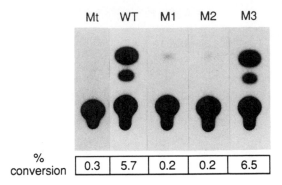

	Mt	WT	M1	M2	M3
% conversion	0.3	5.7	0.2	0.2	6.5

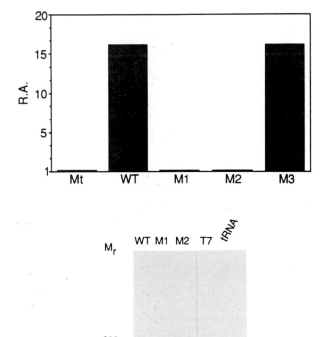

FIG. 9. Analysis of wild-type and mutant CREB proteins by transient expression assay. Representative CAT assays of F9 cells transfected with wild-type (WT) or mutant (Mt, M1, M2, M3) RSV–CREB plasmids. The mutant Mt, which contains a nonsense mutation at residue 131 and does not express immunoprecipitable CREB protein, was used to control for nonspecific effects of the RSV–CREB plasmid on transcription. Each CREB plasmid was cotransfected with $\Delta(-71)$ CAT reporter, C-subunit vector MtC, and RSV–β-galactosidase as described in Fig. 2. The percentages of conversion are indicated, and the relative activities (R.A.) are shown graphically below. Assays were normalized for β-galactosidase activity. Each mutant was tested in at least three separate assays.

ACKNOWLEDGMENTS

The authors wish to thank Joan Vaughan, Dr. Wylie Vale, and Dr. Jean Rivier for synthetic peptides and antisera, and Patricia Menzel for expert technical assistance. This work was funded by National Institutes of Health grant GM37828 NCI grant CA-14195, and was conducted in part by the Clayton Foundation for Research, California Division. M.R.M. is a Clayton Foundation Investigator.

REFERENCES

Andrisani, O. M., Hayes, T. E., Roos, B., and Dixon, J. E. (1987). *Nucleic Acids Res.* **15**, 5715–5728.

Comb, M., Birnberg, N. C., Seasholtz, A., Herbert, E., and Goodman, H. M. (1986). *Nature (London)* **323**, 353–356.

Delegeane, A. M., Ferland, L. H., and Mellon, P. L. (1987). *Mol. Cell. Biol.* **7**, 3994–4002.

Gonzalez, G. A., and Montminy, M. R. (1989). *Cell (Cambridge, Mass.)* **59**, 675–680.

Gonzalez, G. A., Yamamoto, K. K., Fischer, W. H., Karr, D., Menzel, P., Biggs, W., III, Vale, W. W., and Montminy, M. R. (1989). *Nature (London)* **337**, 749–752.

Grove, J. R., Price, D. J., Goodman, H. M., and Avruch, J. (1987). *Science* **238**, 530–533.

Hoefler, J. P., Meyer, T. E., Yum, Y., Jameson, J. L., and Habener, J. F. (1988). *Science* **242**, 1430–1432.

Horikoshi, M., Hai, T., Lin, Y., Green, M. R., and Roeder, R. G. (1988). *Cell (Cambridge, Mass.)* **54**, 1033–1042.

Jameson, J. L., Jaffe, R. C., Gleason, S. L., and Habener, J. F. (1986). *Endocrinology (Baltimore)* **119**, 2560–2567.

Lamers, W. H., Hanson, R. W., and Meisner, H. M. (1982). *Proc. Natl. Acad. Sci. U.S.A.* **79**, 5137–5141.

Landshulz, W. H., Johnson, P. F., and McKnight, S. L. (1988). *Science* **240**, 1759–1763.

Lee, K. A., and Green, M. R. (1987). *EMBO J.* **6**, 1345–1353.

Ma, J., and Ptashne, M. (1987). *Cell (Cambridge, Mass.)* **51**, 113–119.

Montminy, M. R., and Bilezikjian, L. M. (1987). *Nature (London)* **328**, 175–178.

Montminy, M. R., Sevarino, K. A., Wagner, J. A., Mandel, G., and Goodman, R. H. (1986). *Proc. Natl. Acad. Sci. U.S.A.* **83**, 6682–6686.

Ptashne, M. (1988). *Nature (London)* **335**, 683–689.

Riabowol, K. T., Fink, J. S., Gilman, M. Z., Walsh, D. A., Goodman, R. H., and Feramisco, J. R. (1988). *Nature (London)* **328**, 83–86.

Sasaki, K., Cripe, T. P., Koch, S. R., Andreone, T. L., Peterson, D. D., Beale, E. B., and Granner, D. K. (1984). *J. Biol. Chem.* **259**, 15242–15251.

Short, J. M., Wynshaw-Boris, A., Short, H. P., and Hanson, R. W. (1986). *J. Biol. Chem.* **261**, 9721–9726.

Yamamoto, K. K., Gonzalez, G. A., Biggs, W. H., III, and Montminy, M. R. (1988). *Nature (London)* **334**, 494–498.

DISCUSSION

W. Vale.   What do you think the function of the delta CREB might be?

M. R. Montminy.   I think from our preliminary studies that the delta CREB protein is actually a little more abundant than the activated CREB protein. It could be, however, that this protein has some promoter-specific effects.

W. Vale.   Are there only these two CREBs?

M. R. Montminy. It appears that there is a good assortment of them. They seem to be less closely related than the two I have discussed. The CREBP1 that binds to CRE sequence, but is not related by primary structure at all, has been characterized in Japan. It appears to form a heterodimer with *fos*; however, its effects on transcription have not been studied yet.

W. Vale. What about differential expression in tissues of these different CREBs?

M. R. Montminy. For the two that I have described, it appears to be ubiquitous.

W. Vale. You mentioned that you thought there might be mutual negative regulation by the C kinase and A kinase sites. In the somatostatin gene both A and C turn on expression. But there are other systems in which they are mutually inhibitory. Do you have any evidence for this mutual regulation?

M. R. Montminy. I believe I was referring to C kinase 2 regulation. I do not know how C kinase fits into the system. We have observed that the protein is well phosphorylated and that, in fact, if you examine the bacterially expressed forms of CREB, you will note that the binding activity of CREB goes up. So it may be that C kinase has some subtle, as yet uncharacterized, effects on transcription.

J. L. Vaitukaitis. If a cell has two separate populations of receptors for polypeptide hormone and both receptors operate through an A kinase system, how does the cell confer specificity of hormone response if the effects of both are mediated through the catalytic subunits of cAMP-dependent protein kinase?

M. R. Montminy. I am not aware of an example of their both having the same effect.

J. L. Vaitukaitis. Many cells have two or more receptors which mediate their effects through A kinase—for instance, a cell that has FSH and LH receptors. FSH induces responses which differ from those for LH or hCG. How would the cell know which specific hormone-dependent process to turn on?

M. R. Montminy. I cannot answer that.

M. Ascoli. Your assay involved cotransfection with the catalytic subunit of the A kinase. So it is not really surprising to find that the M3 mutant (mutated on the kinase C site) was active when you cotransfected with the catalytic subunit of the A kinase. Is my interpretation correct?

M. R. Montminy. We wanted to test whether through some other mechanisms C kinase would be necessary for the activation of the protein, or if this residue was all important in the activity of the protein. So you are absolutely correct. It should make perfect sense if it is a kinase A substrate.

M. Ascoli. But that mutant then is inactive if you activate the pathway with an activator of the C kinase.

M. R. Montminy. If we treat cells with TPA, we see no phosphorylation protein at all. There is no induced phosphorylation, and the protein is unable to stimulate transcription in response to TPA.

S. Shenolikar. When you introduced the catalytic subunit of cAMP-dependent protein kinase you even noted some increase in the amount of CAT activity produced with the minus CRE construct. Is this evidence that perhaps even basal expression might be altered by cAMP, and, if so, does this occur through the CREB protein?

M. R. Montminy. I think that the basal activity is probably CREB dependent in those cells also.

S. Shenolikar. You mentioned that there was inhibition of CREB activity by delta CREB in coexpression studies. Do you know whether delta CREB binds to the same region (i.e., has the same sequence specificity and is as efficiently phosphorylated *in vivo*)? How do you think this inhibition occurs?

M. R. Montminy. We have not examined phosphorylation yet. We know that when the product is expressed in bacterial cells, it has normal binding activity and dimerization potential. Also, it appears to form heterodimers perfectly normally with CREBs, so it does not have any preference for its own form.

S. P. Bottari. From your experiments showing phosphorylation of CREB when stimulated with forskolin, you assume that protein kinase A translocates from the membrane to the nucleus. Have you ever tried to incubate purified isolated nuclei with forskolin?

M. R. Montminy. No, we have not. It would be an interesting experiment.

Inhibin: Role and Secretion in the Rat

CATHERINE RIVIER,* HELENE MEUNIER,† VERONICA ROBERTS,‡ AND
WYLIE VALE*

*The Clayton Foundation Laboratories for Peptide Biology and ‡Laboratory for Neural Structure
and Function, The Salk Institute, La Jolla, California 92037, and the †Division of
Endocrinology, Research Institute, The Hospital for Sick Children, Toronto, Canada M5G 1X8

I. Introduction

The presently known mechanisms controlling luteinizing hormone (LH) and follicle-stimulating hormone (FSH) secretion include gonadotropin-releasing hormone (GnRH), sex steroids, opiates, various neurotransmitters and peptides, inhibin, activin, and follistatin. Among these different secretagogues, a compound which would specifically inhibit FSH release, originally called inhibin to distinguish it from the steroidal substance androtin (later known as androgen), was proposed as early as 1932 (McCullagh, 1932). However, despite numerous attempts at is purification and characterization, the structure of inhibin has remained elusive until recently. Due, in particular, to improvements in chromatography, protein sequence, and molecular cloning, in 1986 a 32-kDa protein was finally isolated and characterized from ovine and bovine follicular fluids which has the biological activities expected of inhibin (reviewed by DeJong, 1988; Rivier et al., 1988b; Vale et al., 1988). A number of questions could then be answered, regarding, in particular, the physiological role played by inhibin in modulating FSH secretion, a possible differential effect of inhibin on FSH and LH release, the relationship between inhibin and FSH secretory patterns, and the site(s) of action of inhibin. This chapter describes and discusses experiments performed with specific radioimmunoassays (RIAs), polyclonal antisera directed against inhibin, and *in situ* hybridization techniques using ^{35}S-labeled mRNA probes, which were designed to answer some of the above questions.

II. Secretion and Expression of Inhibin

Several RIAs have been developed to measure inhibin levels in the blood or the culture medium of granulosa and Sertoli cells, using antibodies raised either

231

against the entire 32-kDa molecule (Gonzales *et al.*, 1989; Hasegawa *et al.*, 1988; McLachlan *et al.*, 1986b) or against the amino-terminal portion of the α chain of inhibin (Rivier *et al.*, 1986; Vaughan *et al.*, 1988). In this chapter inhibin levels measured with antibodies raised against porcine inhibin-α-(1-26) or -(1-25) are referred to as immunoreactive inhibin α (irIα). In many instances results obtained with both types of RIAs have shown good agreement not only between themselves, but also with data previously obtained with inhibin bio-assays. However, there is increasing evidence that forms other than the 32-kDa molecule (Grootenhuis *et al.*, 1989), including the α chain itself or its aggregates and/or its precursor, are present in follicular fluid (Robertson *et al.*, 1989; Sugino *et al.*, 1989) and can be secreted (Bicsak *et al.*, 1988; Gonzales *et al.*, 1989; Knight *et al.*, 1989), therefore leaving open the possibility of disagreement of results obtained with different RIAs. It should be noted, however, that al-though, as mentioned above, the α chain has been observed in the culture medium of gonadal cells, its presence in the circulation and its possible physio-logical role remain unknown.

A. FEMALE

1. *Basal Release*

The concept of the existence of inhibin, that is, that a molecule existed (ini-tially studied as charcoal-extracted follicular fluid) which would specifically interfere with FSH secretion and that FSH, in turn, would stimulate inhibin release, deemed that there be a functional inverse relationship between the cir-culating levels of the protein and those of FSH (Channing *et al.*, 1985). Indeed, using bioassays to measure inhibin levels, several investigators had demonstrated such a relationship during at least parts of the estrous cycle (DePaolo *et al.*, 1979a; Fujii *et al.*, 1983; Tsukamoto *et al.*, 1986), as well as during periods of sexual maturation (Meijs-Roelofs *et al.*, 1983; Sander *et al.*, 1985, 1986). The temporal correlations between plasma inhibin and FSH levels, on the one hand, and the observation that changes in circulating inhibin values appeared to be linked to changes in ovarian follicular maturation, on the other, had suggested, first, that FSH might alter inhibin production and, second, that inhibin secretion might be related to follicular development.

In the developing female rat the possible functional relationship between in-hibin and FSH was subsequently exemplified by our finding that irIα levels remained low in the female rat until day 17, then showed an abrupt rise, which coincided with a dramatic fall in plasma FSH levels (Rivier and Vale, 1987b). Because of the intense follicular development which takes place during this stage of sexual maturation (Ojeda *et al.*, 1980; Uilenbroek *et al.*, 1976), our results also supported the hypothesis of a relationship between follicle growth and inhibin production.

In the adult cycling female rat the phenomena of follicle maturation, ovulation, and formation of the corpus luteum, as well as the periodic changes in sex steroids which accompany the maturation of the granulosa cells and the appearance of luteal cells, have been extensively described (reviewed by Schwartz, 1969). The role of both sex steroids and GnRH (as well as the mechanisms which lead to changes in GnRH secretion) in controlling the primary (proestrous) and secondary (estrous) surges of gonadotropins has also been studied in detail. While the role, in particular, of endogenous GnRH is well established and accepted (Blake and Kelch, 1981; Condon et al., 1984; Hasegawa et al., 1981), the possible effect of endogenous inhibin had been suggested (DePaolo et al., 1979b; Rush et al., 1981; Schwartz and Talley, 1978; Shander et al., 1980), but not demonstrated. The main question which we and other investigators therefore attempted to answer was this: Is endogenous inhibin involved in modulating the estrus rise of FSH? Several approaches were used to investigate this question, including measurements of circulating inhibin levels during the estrous cycle, removal of endogenous inhibin by immunoneutralization, and studies of the changes in inhibin expression within the ovary.

The demonstration that inhibin is primarily produced by the granulosa cells (Bicsak et al., 1986; Sander et al., 1984; Suzuki et al., 1987; Zhang et al., 1988; Zhiwen et al., 1987a,b), had suggested that plasma inhibin levels vary during follicular growth. Indeed, we have observed that during the estrous cycle irIα levels, which were low during diestrus-1 and -2, increased shortly after the primary proestrous gonadotropin (Gn) surge (Rivier et al., 1989). Plasma irIα values then showed an abrupt decline, reaching a nadir between 2 and 4 A.M. on estrus. This decline preceded the secondary FSH surge observed in the early part of estrus (Fig. 1). No measurable pattern of circulating irIα was observed during any other part of the 4-day cycle.

Similar results have been obtained by Hasegawa et al. (1989), using antibodies raised against porcine 32-kDa inhibin. Good correlation between changes in ovarian function and inhibin production has also been demonstrated in species other than the rat. In the pig the amount of inhibin has been shown to increase from the late luteal phase to the early follicular phase, then to decrease; these changes were not related to estradiol production, but showed a consistent inverse relationship with circulating FSH values (Hasegawa et al., 1988). During the breeding season ewes also show an increase in inhibin release during the follicular phase (a time at which inhibin and FSH levels are inversely related), followed by a decrease (Findlay et al., 1990). These results, as well as those of other investigators (Mann et al., 1989), suggested that, as observed in other species, the large ovine antral follicles represent a major source of peripheral inhibin.

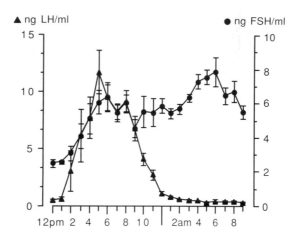

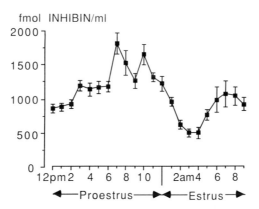

FIG. 1.   Plasma levels of LH, FSH, and irlα during proestrus and estrus. Each point represents the mean ± SEM of six animals. [Reprinted by permission from *Endocrinology* **125,** 152 (1989).]

The pattern of hormonal secretion is somewhat different during the human menstrual cycle, in which inhibin levels rise in parallel with estradiol during the late follicular phase (McLachlan *et al.,* 1987b). In humans the inverse correlation between inhibin and FSH was only observed during the mid- and late follicular phase, but not at the time of the midcycle Gn surges, when inhibin values also increased. Similarly, inhibin concentrations were reported to be low during the follicular phase of the macaque monkey, then to rise after ovulation (Fraser *et al.,* 1989). These results indicate that, as we had seen at the time of the proestrus Gn surge of the rat, the midcycle period of the human menstrual cycle represents a time when there is a loss of the normal inhibitory effect of inhibin on FSH release. These findings also confirm the earlier hypothesis that inhibin represents a product of the maturing follicle.

Apart from being present in developing follicles, there is also evidence that at least the α subunit can be found in newly formed luteal tissue of rats (Meunier *et al.*, 1988a,b), sheep (Tsonis *et al.*, 1988), cattle (Rodgers *et al.*, 1989), and humans (McLachlan *et al.*, 1987a). In the macaque suppression of luteal function with a GnRH antagonist caused a marked decrease in plasma progesterone and immunoreactive inhibin, as measured with antibodies raised against the bovine 31-kDa protein (Basseti *et al.*, 1990; Fraser *et al.*, 1989; Woodruff *et al.*, 1988). Similar results were obtained in women (Roseff *et al.*, 1989). These results supported the hypothesis that the corpus luteum represents an important source of inhibin secreted during the luteal phase.

Measurement of inhibin gene expression and mRNA levels showed excellent agreement with the secretion studies. Using *in situ* hybridization techniques and immunochemistry, we (Meunier *et al.*, 1988b) and others (Rodgers *et al.*, 1989; Torney *et al.*, 1989; Woodruff *et al.*, 1988, 1989) have studied the distribution of the inhibin chains in different ovarian compartments in cycling rats or in cattle. In our laboratory (Meunier *et al.*, 1988b) mRNA for the inhibin α subunit was detected in the granulosa cells of follicles at all stages of maturation, as well as in the theca interna, interstitial gland cells, and luteal cells. In contrast, Woodruff *et al.* (1988) only found the inhibin α subunit in the granulosa cells of healthy follicles. β Subunits were detected exclusively in the granulosa cells of healthy tertiary follicles. We further observed that the changes in inhibin expression were more pronounced during the follicular phase of the cycle, with the inhibin α subunit reaching its highest level in granulosa cells, theca interna, and interstitial gland cells a few hours after the primary Gn surge. At that time the β subunits decreased dramatically in the granulosa cells of mature follicles. Immediately before ovulation the α subunit sharply declined in preovulatory follicles and was mainly present in granulosa cells from nonovulatory follicles at various stages of maturation. Similar changes were reported by Woodruff *et al.* (1988).

Comparison between the pattern of expression and secretion of inhibin, on the one hand, and that of FSH production, on the other, suggested that a decrease in inhibin production might be responsible for the secondary FSH surge. We had proposed the existence of dynamic changes in the ratios of activin/inhibin production, in which the levels of β subunits would decrease first, followed by a drop in the levels of α subunit and a resurgence of activin A produced by the granulosa cells of large tertiary follicles (Meunier *et al.*, 1988b). This hypothesis has been recently supported by experiments (described in Section III) which examined the pattern of inhibin secretion under conditions of experimental manipulations of Gn release (Rivier *et al.*, 1989).

2. *Influence of Gn's, Sex Steroids, and GnRH*

As discussed above, the pattern of inhibin expression and release changes with the stages of the cycle. A logical hypothesis was that these changes were modulated by Gn's, sex steroids, and/or GnRH, according to interactions which

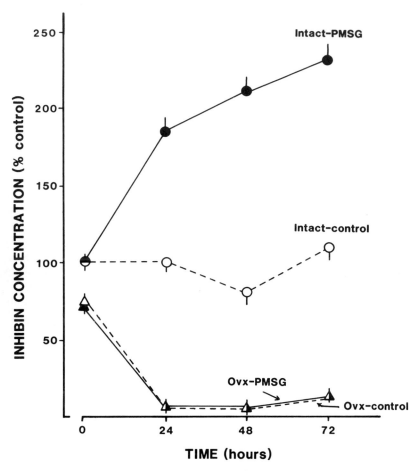

FIG. 2.   Effect of the intravenous injection of the vehicle (control) or 10 IU of pregnant mare serum gonadotropins (PMSG) on inhibin secretion by intact or ovariectomized (Ovx) female rats. Results are expressed as the percentage of preinjection values. Each point represents the mean ± SEM of five animals.

remained to be determined. A number of early experiments had indicated that Gn's (in particular, FSH) had a stimulatory influence on inhibin secretion (Au *et al.*, 1985; Kimura *et al.*, 1983; Lee *et al.*, 1981, 1982). These results were later confirmed by measurement of inhibin mRNA levels or immunoreactive inhibin values in the blood and the culture medium of gonadal cells. In both the immature (Rivier *et al.*, 1987) (Fig. 2) and the mature (Rivier *et al.*, 1986) female rat, as well as in cultured granulosa cells (Bicsak *et al.*, 1986; Hillier *et al.*, 1989; Zhang *et al.*, 1988), FSH strongly increased inhibin release. Inhibin gene expression was similarly enhanced by FSH or FSH-like molecules in ovarian cells

(Davis *et al.*, 1986, 1988; Meunier *et al.*, 1988c,d; Woodruff *et al.*, 1987). Treatment of women with Gn's also markedly augmented the levels of circulating inhibin (Buckler *et al.*, 1988, 1989; Healy *et al.*, 1988; McLachlan *et al.*, 1986a, 1987a). Conversely, removal of FSH by hypophysectomy, known from earlier studies to cause a decrease in bioassayable gonadal inhibin content (Au *et al.*, 1985; Kaneko *et al.*, 1987), was recently shown to dramatically reduce plasma irIα (Rivier and Vale, 1989b) and ovarian inhibin gene expression (Davis *et al.*, 1988).

The observation of intense signals for α-subunit mRNA in recruited follicles after the endogenous Gn surge (Meunier *et al.*, 1988a) further suggested that Gn's might represent a physiological signal for the changes measured in the circulating levels of inhibin during the estrous cycle. The possible role of the primary Gn surges in regulating inhibin secretion had originally been proposed on the basis of experiments showing that exogenous LH or FSH restored the estrous release of FSH in pentobarbital-blocked rats, thereby suggesting that Gn might induce FSH secretion through changes in inhibin secretion (Schwartz and Talley, 1978). Both our group (Rivier *et al.*, 1989) and Schwartz's group (Woodruff *et al.*, 1989) reexamined this question with the use of RIA for inhibin and *in situ* hybridization techniques, and observed that blockade of the primary Gn surge by a GnRH antagonist prevented the decrease in irIα (Rivier *et al.*, 1989) or inhibin mRNA (Rivier *et al.*, 1989; Woodruff *et al.*, 1989) normally measured in late proestrus. Administration of exogenous LH (Rivier *et al.*, 1989; Woodruff *et al.*,1989) or FSH (Woodruff *et al.*, 1989) to antagonist-treated proestrous female rats inhibited the decrease in plasma irIα or inhibin mRNA levels. Interestingly, administration of LH also restored the secondary FSH surge, which had been reduced by the antagonist (Rivier *et al.*, 1989). These results confirmed Schwartz and Talley's (1978) hypothesis that the proestrous surge of LH mediates the estrous rise in plasma FSH levels. It should be also noted that a similar interaction between LH- and FSH-like molecules on inhibin expression has been reported in pregnant mare serum Gn's (PMSG)-primed immature female rats (Davis *et al.*, 1989; Meunier *et al.*, 1989).

Apart from Gn's, sex steroids and GnRH also modulate the expression and secretion of inhibin. Estrogenlike compounds exert powerful stimulatory effects on inhibin expression (Meunier *et al.*, 1988c; Turner *et al.*, 1989) and plasma irIα levels (Rivier and Vale, 1989b). The influence and the role of GnRH, a peptide known to exert direct gonadal effects (Hsueh and Jones, 1981), were demonstrated in hypophysectomized rats. In this model GnRH was capable of inhibiting both spontaneous and PMSG-induced inhibin secretion, while a GnRH antagonist augmented the stimulatory effect of PMSG (Rivier and Vale, 1989b) (Fig. 3).

It therefore becomes increasingly evident that inhibin release is under the modulating influence of a number of the factors known to influence reproductive

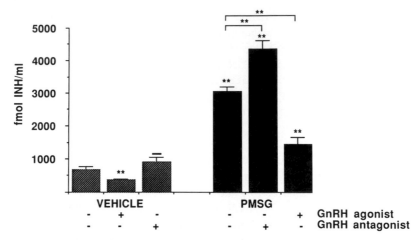

FIG. 3. Interaction among pregnant mare serum gonadotropins (PMSG), a GnRH antagonist, and a GnRH agonist on inhibin secretion by immature hypophysectomized female rats. Blood samples were obtained 48 hours after treatment. Each bar represents the mean ± SEM of six animals. —, $p > 0.5$; ∗∗, $p \leq 0.01$. [Reprinted by permission from *Endocrinology* **124**, 195 (1989).]

functions in general. While some of them, such as Gn's sex steroids, and GnRH, have been demonstrated to alter circulating levels of irIα, others such as activin and inhibin-related proteins, have only been studied in *in vitro* experiments (Tsafriri *et al.*, 1989; Vale *et al.*, 1989).

B. MALE

The circulating levels of androgens and Gn's undergo marked changes during sexual maturation (Odell and Swerdloff, 1976). In the male rat plasma LH levels fall between 10 and 20 days of age, then increase again. FSH secretion, on the other hand, increases between days 10 and 40, then slightly decreases as mature sperm become detectable in the tubules. This increase in FSH levels and the increase in LH values after day 20 are compatible with a decreasing feedback sensitivity of the male hypothalamic-pituitary axis to gonadal steroids.

A question which had been asked repeatedly, but not answered satisfactorily, concerned the possible role of inhibin, alone or in conjunction with the other known secretagogues, in mediating some of the events related to the onset of puberty. Among the lines of evidence for the role of inhibin, the observations that castration done at different ages exerted markedly different effects on FSH secretion by male rats (Swerdloff *et al.*, 1971), that gonadectomy had divergent effects on LH and FSH secretion (Fig. 4) (Hermans *et al.*, 1980), and that androgen replacement was not always effective in reversing castration-induced FSH release (Negro-Vilar *et al.*, 1973), suggested that a factor other than differential pituitary and brain sensitivities to sex steroid removal was at play.

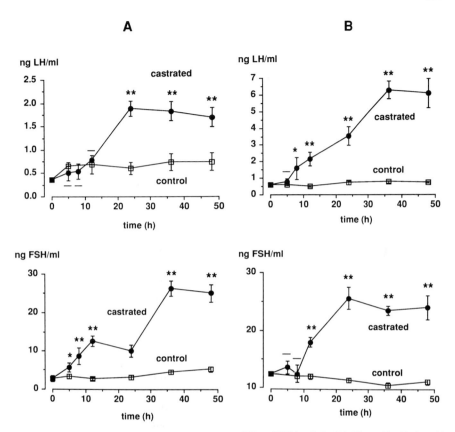

FIG. 4.   Effect of bilateral castration on plasma LH or FSH levels in (A) 15- or (B) 40-day-old male rats. Each point represents the mean ± SEM of six animals.—, $p > 0.5$; *, $p \leq 0.5$; **, $p \leq 0.01$.

Despite the fact that the initial hypothesis of the existence of inhibin was obtained in the male rat (McCullagh, 1932), studies of the secretory pattern and the possible role of inhibin in this sex have been significantly more difficult than those performed on the female. In particular, circumstances have been described under which both inhibin and FSH levels appeared elevated (Tsatsoulis *et al.*, 1988), an observation which did not support the original inhibin concept.

Some of the earlier series of experiments, including the effects of castration (mentioned above) and those of cryptorchidism or damage to the testicular germinal epithelium (Main *et al.*, 1978), had suggested that the pattern of male inhibin secretion might be age related. However, there was no consensus as to how sexual maturation modified inhibin release. Using bioassays to measure inhibin levels, Au *et al.* (1986) reported increases in the levels of testicular inhibin content. In contrast, Ultee-VanGessel and DeJong (1987) measured a decrease in inhibin production after 14 days of age. Because these measurements could not take into account the putative influence of the blood–testis barrier, the increasing volume of blood into which inhibin was released, changes in the number and function of the Sertoli cells, and the possible existence of cycles in the pattern of inhibin release, a better understanding of the importance of age and stages of sexual development in the secretion and role of inhibin had to await the availability of, in particular, *in situ* hybridization techniques.

In the male the testes represent the main source of inhibin (Bhasin *et al.*, 1989; Lincoln and McNeilly, 1989; McNeilly and Baird, 1989; Rivier *et al.*, 1987; Sharpe *et al.*, 1988), and there is increasing evidence that inhibin is secreted by both Sertoli and Leydig cells (Maddocks and Sharpe, 1990; Risbridger *et al.*, 1989a,b; Roberts *et al.*, 1989; Shaha *et al.*, 1989; Veeramachaneni *et al.*, 1989). Despite our finding that tissues other than the gonads contain inhibin subunit mRNAs (Meunier *et al.*, 1988c), removal of the gonads is accompanied by a rapid decline in plasma irIα (Fig. 5). As in the case of granulosa cells, FSH stimulates inhibin expression (Toebosch *et al.*, 1988) and production (Bardin *et al.*, 1987, 1989; Bicsak *et al.*, 1987; Klaij *et al.*, 1990; Morris *et al.*, 1988; Risbridger *et al.*, 1989b; Toebosch *et al.*, 1989) by cultured Sertoli cells, while hypophysectomy is reported to decrease testicular inhibin α-subunit mRNA levels (Keinan *et al.*, 1989), and to increase the expression of the βB subunit (Feng *et al.*, 1989).

While we were unsuccessful in establishing a stimulatory effect of FSH on inhibin secretion by intact male rats (C. Rivier, unpublished observations), Keinan *et al.* (1989) observed that FSH could restore inhibin α-subunit mRNA levels in the testes of hypophysectomized animals. There is also evidence that the effect of Gn's and/or sex steroids on inhibin secretion might require more sophisticated models than those which we have previously used, including experimental manipulations of sex steroid levels (Drummond *et al.*, 1989; Sharpe *et al.*, 1988).

While, as just discussed, FSH is consistently reported to stimulate inhibin secretion by Sertoli cells, it appears that inhibin release and expression are controlled by LH (Risbridger *et al.*, 1989a; Roberts *et al.*, 1989). This led to speculations as to a possible role of, or interaction with, testosterone release on inhibin production. In the human testis measurement of hormone levels in the spermatic vein indicated well-defined and coincidental pulses of both inhibin and testosterone, suggesting that the mechanisms responsible for the secretion of both hormones might be similar (Winters, 1990). In the rat, however, testosterone does not appear to exert direct gonadal effects on inhibin secretion, but might inhibit it via an FSH-dependent mechanism (Handelsman *et al.*, 1989; Sun *et al.*, 1989).

In the rat we could demonstrate an inverse relationship between FSH and irIα levels between 15 and 26 days after birth (Rivier *et al.*, 1988a). This stage of

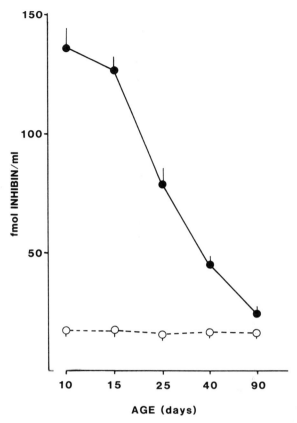

FIG. 5. Measurement of plasma irIα in intact (●) or castrated (○) male rats. Blood samples were obtained 48 hours after surgery. Each point represents the mean ± SEM of six animals.

sexual development also corresponded to the time when immunoneutralization of endogenous inhibin was capable of increasing plasma FSH levels. After day 26 plasma irIα values markedly decreased (Maddocks and Sharpe, 1990; Rivier *et al.*, 1988a), and testicular inhibin expression as well as inhibin immunohisto-chemical staining also showed a marked decline. Furthermore, we found that the amount of irIα present in testicular extracts, while *increasing* when expressed on an absolute basis (picomoles of inhibin per whole testis), *decreased* when expressed on the basis of concentration (femtomoles of inhibin per milligram of testis weight). Other investigators have reported similar findings (Feng *et al.*, 1989; Keinan *et al.*, 1989). In the ram plasma inhibin values change in parallel with developing and regressing stages of the testicular cycle (Lincoln and McNeilly, 1989), and in the rat the expression of the α and β subunits also appears to depend on the stage of spermatogenesis (Bhasin *et al.,* 1989). Interestingly, both a positive and a negative correlation between inhibin and FSH secretion could be demonstrated, which depended on the stage of testicular activity. Thus, it is possible that in species (e.g., the rat) in which the various stages of testicular activity cannot be easily distinguished, a functional relationship between the secretion of both hormones cannot be demonstrated.

III.   Role of Endogenous Inhibin

The classical approach to investigations regarding the physiological role played by a secretagogue is to inject animals with antibodies or antagonists to these secretagogues and to measure the biological consequences of this manipulation. In the field of GnRH, in particular, this approach has significantly helped our understanding of the role and the importance of the decapeptide in modulating reproductive functions (reviewed by Karten and Rivier, 1986). With regard to inhibin, the availability of antibodies to the 32-kDa protein has also started to yield valuable information concerning the possible physiological role of this secretagogue.

A.   FEMALE

1.   *Basal and GnRH-Induced Secretion*

The injection of antibodies raised against the amino-terminal portion of the α chain of inhibin has indicated that removal of endogenous inhibin in female rats younger than 18 days of age did not measurably alter FSH (or LH) secretion (Culler and Negro-Vilar, 1988; Rivier and Vale, 1987). These results suggested that endogenous inhibin did not play a physiological role in modulating Gn release in the young animal. After day 18 administration of the antibodies always caused marked and sustained elevations of plasma FSH (but not LH) levels in the immature (Saito *et al.,* 1989; Culler and Negro-Vilar, 1988) and mature (Rivier *et al.,* 1988b) rat at all stages of the estrous cycle (Rivier *et al.,* 1986; Culler and Negro-Vilar, 1988) (Fig. 6). In the sheep, however, the role of inhibin as a modulator of FSH secretion seems to be restricted to the breeding season (Findlay *et al.,*1988).

Two essential questions asked by investigators in the field of inhibin were, first, whether, in addition to elevating baseline plasma FSH levels, inhibin also modified the pattern of secretion of this particular Gn; and second, whether inhibin altered the pattern of LH release. Using follicular fluid (FF) as a source of inhibin, Lumpkin *et al.,* (1984) reported that the peripheral injection of this material into ovariectomized rats reduced FSH, but not LH, peak frequency and amplitude, and inhibited the FSH, but not LH, response to GnRH. DeGreef *et*

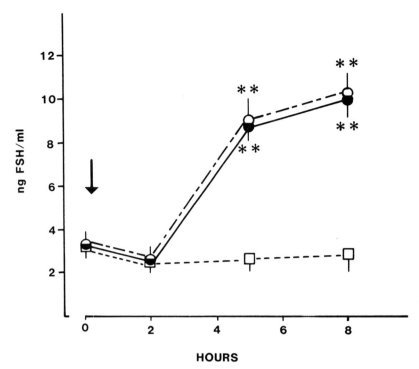

FIG. 6. Effect of the intravenous administration of normal sheep serum (control, □) or anti-inhibin serum to diestrus-1 (●) or -2 (○) female rats. Control animals were in diestrus-1. Each point represents the mean ± SEM of six animals. **, $p \leq 0.01$.

al., (1987) also observed an inhibitory action of FF on FSH, but not LH, pulses in the gonadectomized female rats, and further reported that infusion of FF into the brain did not measurably alter FSH release. In the intact ewe FF suppressed plasma FSH concentrations and increased LH pulse amplitude, a phenomenon which was explained by the reduced negative feedback effects of estradiol occurring as a result of the FF-induced reduction in FSH release (Wallace and McNeilly, 1986). Finally, Mercer et al. (1987) reported that the administration of purified FF to hypothalamic-pituitary-disconnected sheep reduced FSH, but not LH, mRNA levels. However, in this preparation FF reduced LH pulse amplitude, a result which the authors attributed to an interaction between inhibin and GnRH at the level of the pituitary.

It should be noted at this point that there is no consensus as to whether inhibin alters the GnRH-induced release of FSH alone (Lumpkin et al., 1984) or of both Gn's (Campen, 1988; Farnworth et al., 1988; Fukuda et al., 1987; Kotsuji et al., 1988; Martin et al., 1986; Simpson et al., 1987). Together, these results suggest that inhibin (as it is present in purified FF) acts within the periphery, but not the brain, to interfere with the pulsatile secretion of FSH normally observed after the removal of sex steroid feedback. Furthermore, because measurement of portal blood GnRH levels in ewes injected subcutaneously with FF did not show any changes in GnRH secretion, it appears that inhibin (FF) suppresses FSH (and possibly LH) release by a direct action at the pituitary level, and not on GnRH-secreting neurons (Li *et al.*, 1989).

Experiments designed to further investigate a possible pituitary site of interaction between GnRH and inhibin have shown that in acutely castrated (Rush and Lipner, 1979) or long-term ovariectomized (Charlesworth *et al.*, 1984; Koiter *et al.*, 1983; Lumpkin *et al.*, 1984) rats, porcine FF inhibited the response of FSH, but not LH, to GnRH. In *in vitro* studies exposure of cultured pituitary cells to purified inhibin or the 32-kDa protein is reported to inhibit GnRH-induced LH as well as FSH secretion (Farnworth *et al.*, 1988; Simpson *et al.*, 1987; Kotsuji *et al.*, 1988; Campen, 1988), a phenomenon possibly mediated by the ability of inhibin to decrease the number of GnRH receptors in pituitary cells (Wang *et al.*, 1988).

Both LH and FSH are secreted in a pulsatile manner. Simultaneous measurement of portal blood levels of GnRH and peripheral blood values of the Gn's in the intact and the gonadectomized rat have indicated a strong correlation between the pulse pattern of the decapeptide and that of LH, even though the occurrence of "silent" GnRH pulses (i.e., occurring in the absence of LH pulses) is higher in the presence than in the absence of the gonads (Levine and Duffy, 1988; Urbanski *et al.*, 1988). FSH secretion of the intact rat, on the other hand, does not appear to be associated with GnRH release in any consistent manner (Levine and Duffy, 1988), while the castrated animal shows a much higher correlation between GnRH and FSH pulses (Urbanski *et al.*, 1988). This discrepancy between the apparent presence (in the gonadectomized rat) or absence (in the intact rat) of dependency of FSH release on endogenous GnRH could be interpreted as supporting the existence of a gonadal factor specifically regulating FSH secretion.

The respective role of GnRH, sex steroids, and inhibin in modulating pulses parameters (i.e., frequency and amplitude) as well as mean basal Gn secretion has been addressed by the use of GnRH antisera or antagonists, porcine FF, and antiinhibin sera. The administration of a GnRH antiserum (Culler and Negro-Vilar, 1986, 1987) or antagonist (Fig. 7) to castrated male rats immediately lowers plasma LH levels as well as abolishes LH pulses. In contrast, these treatments only reduce mean plasma FSH values and might (Fig. 8) or might not (Culler and Negro-Vilar, 1986) alter pulse amplitude. Thus, it is presently believed that all aspects of LH secretion are dependent on endogenous GnRH, while only basal FSH release depends on the decapeptide. With regard to the role of inhibin, we have already discussed studies done in ovariectomized rats showing that the injection of FF reduced FSH peak frequency and amplitude, while

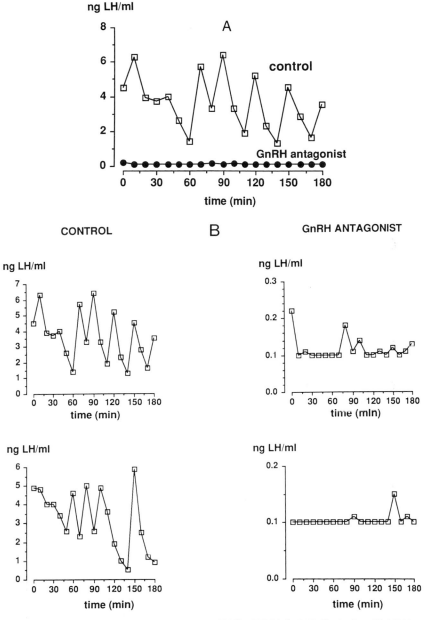

FIG. 7. Effect of the GnRH antagonist [AcD2Nal[1], 4ClDPhe[2], D3Pal[3], Arg[5], DGlu[6](AA), DAla[10]]-GnRH (50 μg intravenously, −8 hours) on LH secretion in diestrus female rats. Each line represents one animal. (A) Mean plasma LH values of one control and one antagonist-treated rat when the results are expressed on the same scale. (B) The scales are different for control and treated rats, to better illustrate the difference in the pattern of LH secretion in both groups of animals.

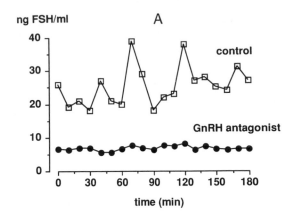

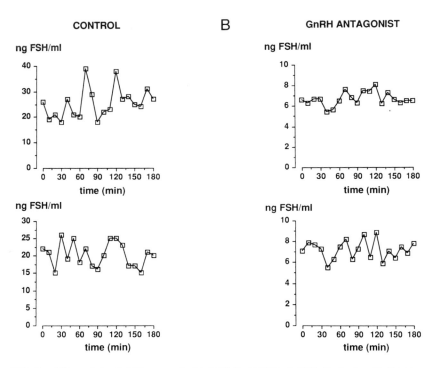

FIG. 8. Effect of the GnRH antagonist [AcD2Nal[1], 4ClDPhe[2], D3Pal[3], Arg[5], DGlu[6](AA), DAla[10]]-GnRH (50 µg intravenously, −8 hours) on FSH secretion in diestrus female rats. Each line represents one animal. (A) Mean plasma FSH values of one control and one antagonist-treated rat when the results are expressed on the same scale. (B) The scales are different for control and treated rats, to better illustrate the difference in the pattern of FSH secretion in diestrus female rats.

none of these parameters appeared altered in the case of LH (Lumpkin *et al.*, 1984). Numerous other studies in the rat have confirmed the selective effect of FF on FSH secretion (reviewed by Channing *et al.*, 1985; Grady *et al.*, 1985).

The role of endogenous inhibin has also been addressed in experiments using passive immunoneutralization. Because the antiinhibin serum does not alter Gn secretion in the absence of the gonads (C. Rivier, unpublished observations), these experiments were carried out in intact female rats in the diestrus-1 or -2 stage of the cycle. According to Culler and Negro-Vilar (1989), the intravenous injection of an antiinhibin serum, administered 1 or 18 hours before blood sampling, elevated baseline levels of both LH and FSH and, while not altering FSH pulsatile secretion, significantly increased LH pulse amplitude and frequency. In addition, pituitary sensitivity to GnRH was markedly augmented in terms of LH, but not FSH, secretion. [It should be noted here that opposite results were obtained in the ewe, in which removal of endogenous inhibin increased FSH, but not LH, release in response to GnRH (Findlay *et al.*, 1988).] The explanation proposed to account for the discrepancy between these results and earlier studies showing that FF suppressed all parameters of pulsatile FSH secretion was the difference between long-term ovariectomized and intact female rats, and the resulting differences in the sensitivity of the brain–pituitary axis to secretagogues (Culler and Negro-Vilar, 1989).

In contrast to Culler and Negro-Vilar's report, we observed that the injection of an antiinhibin serum to diestrus-1 female rats, while markedly increasing baseline FSH release, did not change baseline LH levels measured 15 hours later (Figs. 9 and 10). This observation agrees with our previously published results (Rivier *et al.*, 1986, 1987; and Vale, 1987b) regarding the secretory pattern of the two Gn's in female rats injected with an antiinhibin serum. In two other separate experiments we found no evidence that removal of endogenous inhibin for 6 hours consistently altered the ability of GnRH to stimulate LH secretion (Fig. 11). It is, however, possible that the antiinhibin serum might have induced some increased pituitary responsiveness to GnRH in terms of FSH secretion.

At present, there is no easy way to reconcile this series of contrasting results. As discussed earlier, the frequency of LH and FSH pulses measured in intact or gonadectomized rats is believed to depend primarily on the pulsatile release of GnRH (Levine and Duffy, 1988; Urbanski *et al.*, 1988). It is therefore improbable that changes in pituitary sensitivity, caused by the removal of endogenous inhibin, could account for changes in the frequency of Gn pulses. They could, on the other hand, at least partially explain an increase in pulse amplitude. It should be remembered that GnRH antagonists or antisera completely abolish LH pulses, while their effect on FSH pulses are still controversial. This suggests that pulsatile FSH secretion might be regulated by a factor distinct from the decapeptide GnRH. Because of the hypothesis proposed by Culler and Negro-Vilar (1989) that endogenous inhibin cannot represent this factor, the possible role of

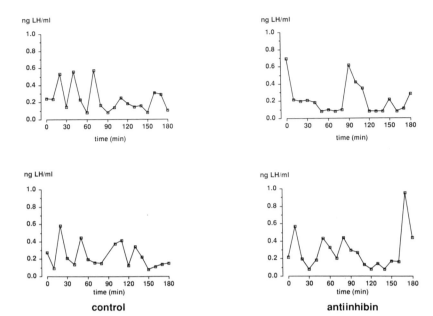

FIG. 9.   Pattern of LH secretion in diestrus-2 female rats injected with normal sheep serum (control) or an antiinhibin serum. Treatments were administered intravenously 6 hours before beginning blood sampling. Each panel represents results from one animal.

an FSH-releasing factor distinct from the decapeptide GnRH (Lumpkin *et al.*, 1987; Mizunuma *et al.*, 1983) might need to be more closely investigated.

2.   *Fertility*

Because removal of endogenous inhibin is accompanied by a marked increase in the plasma FSH levels of female rats and ewes [a condition known to cause superovulation (Fowler and Edwards, 1957; Geiger *et al.*, 1980; Mizumachi *et al.*, 1990)], we reasoned that this treatment might affect folliculogenesis. Indeed, as illustrated in Fig. 12 the administration of an antiinhibin serum (raised against the amino-terminal portion of the α subunit) to diestrus-1 or -2 female rats caused a marked increase in the number of tubal ova shed during the subsequent estrus (Rivier and Vale, 1989a) [an observation previously reported with the use of antisera raised against purified FF (Cummins *et al.*, 1986; Henderson *et al.*, 1984)]. Because infusion of exogenous FSH over a similar time course also increased the number of maturing follicles (Rivier and Vale, 1989a), we suggested that the effect of removal of endogenous inhibin was primarily mediated through elevated circulating FSH levels. Immunization of ewes against a pure recombinant preparation of the α subunit of bovine inhibin also increased the ovulation rate (Forage *et al.*, 1987). Interestingly, immunization of female sheep

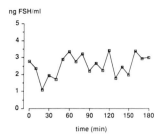

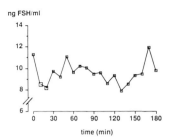

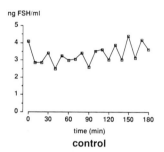

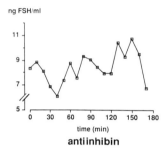

control   **antiinhibin**

FIG. 10.   Pattern of FSH secretion in diestrus-2 female rats injected with normal sheep serum (control) or an antiinhibin serum. Treatments were administered intravenously 6 hours before beginning blood sampling. Each panel represents results from one animal.

against the amino-terminal peptide (αN) of the α subunit of inhibin significantly impaired fertility in the sheep (Findlay *et al.,* 1989). This raised the novel hypothesis that the αN peptide, through as yet unidentified mechanisms, might play a facilitating role, while inhibin plays an inhibitory action, on fertility (Findlay *et al.,* 1989).

B.   MALE

In agreement with results discussed earlier suggesting that the role of endogenous inhibin in modulating FSH secretion in the male rat might be restricted to the early part of sexual development (Hermans *et al.,* 1980), we (Rivier *et al.,* 1988a) and others (Culler and Negro-Vilar, 1988) observed that immunoneutralization of endogenous inhibin only increased plasma FSH levels of young (i.e., <26 days of age) male rats. This observation suggests a functional relationship between inhibin and FSH secretion (illustrated in Fig. 13), which takes place until the relatively high plasma FSH levels characteristic of the adult male rat are established. Before a major role of inhibin in the adult male rat is ruled out, however, at least two possibilities must be considered. First, it is

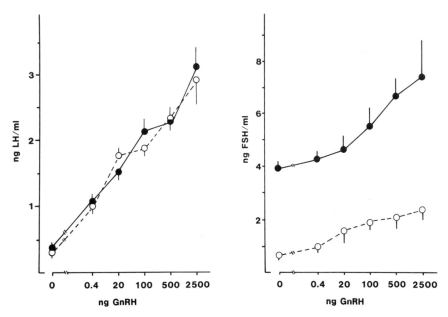

FIG. 11. Effect of the administration of an antiinhibin serum (●) (raised against the amino-terminal portion of the α subunit) 6 hours before the intravenous injection of the vehicle or several doses of GnRH. Blood samples were obtained 10 minutes after treatment. Each point represents the mean ± SEM of six diestrus-1 female rats. ○, Normal rat serum.

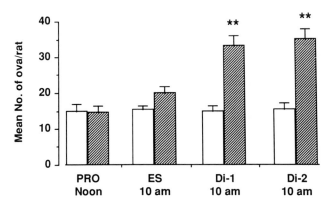

FIG. 12. Effect of the intravenous administration of normal sheep serum (□) or antiinhibin serum (▨) to female rats at the time of the cycle indicated on the abcissa. The oviducts were flushed on the subsequent estrus, and the tubal ova were counted under a microscope. **, $p \leq 0.01$ from control animals at the corresponding time of treatment; PRO, proestrus; ES, estrus; Di-1, Di-2, diestrus-1 and -2.

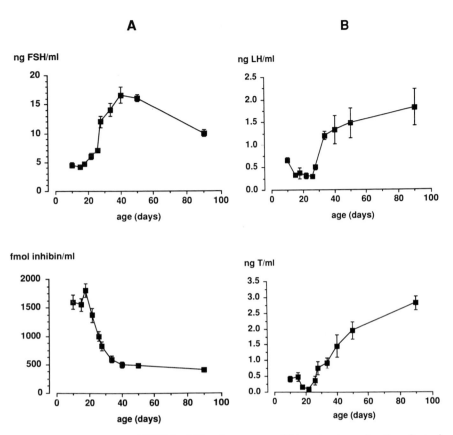

FIG. 13. Plasma levels of FSH irIα, LH, and testosterone (T) in male rats as a function of sexual development. Values are expressed as LH- and FSH-RP-2 (with materials provided by the National Pituitary and Hormone Distribution Program of the National Institute of Diabetes, Digestive and Kidney Diseases) or as a function of highly purified 32-kDa ovine inhibin, respectively. Blood samples were obtained by decapitation. Each point represents the mean ± SEM of five animals.

possible that some inhibin antisera might be more effective in neutralizing inhibin activity from ovarian than from testicular sources (vanDijk *et al.*, 1986). Consequently, the antibodies used might not have been capable of completely neutralizing endogenous inhibin in the male rat. Second, there is some recent evidence that testosterone might mask the role of inhibin in the adult male rat (Culler and Negro-Vilar, 1989).

There is, on the other hand, increasing evidence that, at least in the adult male, the paracrine role of inhibin might be more important than its endocrine (i.e., peripheral) role, particularly as it interacts with activin at the level of the gonads (LaPolt *et al.*, 1989; Lin *et al.*, 1989; Ying and Becker, 1989). In particular, inhibin can enhance LH-stimulated Leydig cell androgen biosynthesis (Hsueh *et al.*, 1987), and, conversely, Leydig cell activity modulates inhibin secretion by Sertoli cells in seemingly complex ways, which do not necessarily depend on testosterone (Drummond *et al.*, 1989). Additional evidence for a paracrine role of inhibin comes from experiments showing that inhibin might regulate spermatogenesis (Bhasin *et al.*, 1989; Voglmayr *et al.*, 1990). These results suggest the existence of important local (i.e., intratesticular) interactions between Leydig and Sertoli cells in the regulation of inhibin production in particular, and gonadal function in general.

IV. Conclusion

Inhibin, a molecule whose role was originally restricted to the specific inhibition of FSH secretion, is now recognized as an essential regulator of pituitary and gonadal function through complex effects of its own, as well as interactions with other secretagogues (e.g., activin, follistatin, Gn's, sex steroids, and GnRH). In the female endogenous inhibin appears to regulate both pituitary and gonadal activity, while in the adult male (rat), the role of the protein might be mostly restricted to testicular function. Finally, the observation that the inhibin subunits are expressed in various tissues throughout the body (Meunier *et al.*, 1988c; Roberts *et al.*, 1989) suggests that inhibin might additionally play a number of as yet unrecognized functions.

ACKNOWLEDGMENTS

This work was supported by National Institutes of Health Grants HD-13527 and DK-26741 and Award B86.29A/ICCR from the Population Council, and was conducted in part by The Clayton Foundation for Research, California Division. C.R. and W.V. are Clayton Foundation Investigators. The authors thank Leatrice Gandara, Rosalia Chavarin, David Hutchinson, Diane Jolley, and Joan Vaughan for expert technical assistance and Bethany Coyne for secretarial assistance.

REFERENCES

Au, C. L., Robertson, D. M., and DeKretser, D. M. (1985). *J. Endocrinol.* **105**, 1–6.
Au, C. L., Robertson, D. M., and DeKretser, D. M. (1986). *Biol. Reprod.* **35**, 37–43.
Bardin, C. W., Morris, P. L., Chen, C. L., Shaha, C., Voglmayr, J., Rivier, J., Speiss, J., and Vale, W. W. (1987). *Proc. Serono Symp.* **42**, 179–190.
Bardin, C. W., Morris, P. L., Shaha, C., Feng, Z. M., Rossi, V., Vaughan, J., Vale, W. W., Voglmayr, J., and Chen, C.-L. C. (1989). *Ann. NY. Acad. Sci.* **564**, 10–23.
Basseti, S. G., Winters, S. J., Keeping, H. S., and Zeleznik, A. J. (1990). *J. Clin. Endocrinol. Metab.* **70**, 590–594.
Bhasin, S., Krummen, L. A., Swerdloff, R. S., Morelos, B. S., Kim, W. H., DiZerega, G. S., Ling, N., Esch, F., Shimasaki, S., and Toppari, J. (1989). *Endocrinology (Baltimore)* **124**, 987–991.

Bicsak, T. A., Tucker, E. M., Cappel, S., Vaughan, J. M., Rivier, J., Vale, W., and Hsueh, A. J. W. (1986). *Endocrinology (Baltimore)* **119**, 2711–2719.

Bicsak, T. A., Vale, W., Vaughan, J., Tucker, E. M., Cappel, S., and Hsueh, A. J. W. (1987). *Mol. Cell. Endocrinol.* **49**, 211–217.

Bicsak, T. A., Cajander, S. B., Vale, W., and Hsueh, A. J. W. (1988). *Endocrinology (Baltimore)* **122**, 741–748.

Blake, C. A., and Kelch, R. P. (1981). *Endocrinology (Baltimore)* **109**, 2175–2179.

Buckler, H. M., McLachlan, R. I., McLachlan, V. B., Healy, D. L., and Burger, H. G. (1988). *J. Clin. Endocrinol. Metab.* **66**, 798–803.

Buckler, H. M., Healy, D. L., and Burger, H. G. (1989). *J. Endocrinol.* **122**, 279–285.

Campen, C. A., and Vale, W. (1988). *Biochem. Biophys. Res. Commun.* **157**, 844–849.

Channing, C. P., Gordon, W. L., Liu, W. K., and Ward, D. N. (1985). *Proc. Soc. Exp. Biol. Med.* **178**, 339–361.

Charlesworth, M. C., Grady, R. R., Shin, L., Vale, W. W., Rivier, C., Rivier, J., and Schwartz, N. B. (1984). *Neuroendocrinology* **38**, 199–205.

Condon, T. P., Heber, D., Stewart, J. M., Sawyer, C. H., and Whitmoyer, D. I. (1984). *Neuroendocrinology* **38**, 357–361.

Culler, M. D., and Negro-Vilar, A. (1986). *Endocrinology (Baltimore)* **118**, 609–612.

Culler, M. D., and Negro-Vilar, A. (1987). *Endocrinology (Baltimore)* **120**, 2011–2021.

Culler, M. D., and Negro-Vilar, A. (1988). *Mol. Cell. Endocrinol.* **58**, 263–273.

Culler, M. D., and Negro-Vilar, A. (1989). *Endocrinology (Baltimore)* **124**, 2944–2953.

Cummins, L. J., O'Shea, T., Al-Obaidi, S. A. R., Bindon, B. M., and Findlay, J. K. (1986). *J. Reprod. Fertil.* **77**, 365–372.

Davis, S. R., Dench, F., Nikolaidis, I., Clements, J. A., Forage, R. G., Krozowski, Z., and Burger, H. G. (1986). *Biochem. Biophys. Res. Commun.* **138**, 1191–1195.

Davis, S. R., Carson, R. S., Krozowski, Z., and Burger, H. G. (1988). *Gynecol. Endocrinol.* **2**, 223–232.

Davis, S. R., Matheson, B., Burger, H., and Krozowski, Z. (1989). *Mol. Cell. Endocrinol.* **61**, 123–128.

DeGreef, W. J., Eilers, G. A. M., DeKonnig, J., Karels, B., and DeJong, F. H. (1987). *J. Endocrinol.* **113**, 449–455.

DeJong, F. H. (1988). *Physiol. Rev.* **68**, 555–607.

DePaolo, L. V., Shander, D., Wise, P. M., Barraclough, C. A., and Channing, C. P. (1979a). *Endocrinology (Baltimore)* **105**, 647–654.

DePaolo, L. V., Wise, P. M., Anderson, L. D., Barraclough, C. A., and Channing, C. P. (1979b). *Endocrinology (Baltimore)* **104**, 402–408.

Drummond, A. E., Risbridger, G. P., and DeKretser, D. M. (1989). *Endocrinology (Baltimore)* **125**, 510–515.

Farnworth, P. G., Robertson, D. M., DeKretser, D. M., and Burger, H. G. (1988). *J. Endocrinol.* **119**, 233–241.

Feng, Z.-M., Bardin, C. W., and Chen, C.-L. C. (1989). *Mol. Endocrinol.* **3**, 939–948.

Findlay, J. K., Doughton, B., Robertson, D. M., and Forage, R. G. (1988). *J. Endocrinol.* **120**, 59–65.

Findlay, J. K., Tsonis, C. F., Doughton, B., Brown, R. W., Bertram, K. C., Braid, F. H., Hudson, F. C., Tierney, M. L., Goss, N. H., and Forage, R. G. (1989). *Endocrinology (Baltimore)* **124**, 3122–3124.

Findlay, J. K., Clarke, I. J., and Robertson, D. M. (1990). *Endocrinology (Baltimore)* **126**, 528–535.

Forage, R. G., Brown, R. W., Oliver, K. J., Atrache, B. T., Devine, P. L., Hudson, G. C., Goss, N. H., Bertram, K. C., Tolstoshev, P., Robertson, D. M., DeKretser, D. M., Doughton, B., Burger, H. G., and Findlay, J. K. (1987). *J. Endocrinol.* **114**, R1–R4.

Fowler, R. E., and Edwards, R. G. (1957). *J. Endocrinol.* **15**, 374–384.

Fraser, H. M., Robertson, D. M., and DeKretser, D. M. (1989). *J. Endocrinol.* **121**, R9–R12.

Fujii, T., Hoover, D. J., and Channing, C. P. (1983). *J. Reprod. Fertil.* **69**, 307–314.

Fukuda, M., Miyamoto, K., Hasegawa, Y., Ibuki, Y., and Igarashi, M. (1987). *Mol. Cell. Endocrinol.* **51**, 41–50.

Geiger, J. M., Plas-Roser, L., and Aron, C. (1980). *Biol. Reprod.* **22**, 837–845.

Gonzales, G. F., Risbridger, G. P., and DeKretser, D. M. (1989). *Endocrinology (Baltimore)* **124**, 1661–1668.

Grady, R. R., Shin, L., Charlesworth, M. C., Cohen-Becker, I. R., Smith, M., Rivier, C., Rivier, J., Vale, W., and Schwartz, N. B. (1985). *Neuroendocrinology* **40**, 246–252.

Grootenhuis, A. J., Steenbergen, J., Timmerman, M. A., Dorsman, A. M. R. D., Schaaper, W. M. M., Meloen, R. H., and DeJong, F. H. (1989). *J. Endocrinol.* **122**, 293–301.

Handelsman, D. J., Spaliviero, J. A., Kidston, E., and Robertson, D. M. (1989). *Endocrinology (Baltimore)* **125**, 721–729.

Hasegawa, Y., Miyamoto, K., Yazaki, C., and Igarashi, M. (1981). *Endocrinology (Baltimore)* **109**, 130–135.

Hasegawa, Y., Miyamoto, K., Iwamura, S., and Igarashi, M. (1988). *J. Endocrinol.* **118**, 211–219.

Hasegawa, Y., Miyamoto, K., and Igarashi, M. (1989). *J. Endocrinol.* **121**, 91–100.

Healy, D. L., McLachlan, R. I., Robertson, D. M., DeKretser, D. M., and Burger, H. G. (1988). *Ann. N.Y. Acad. Sci.* **541**, 162–178.

Henderson, K. M., Franchimont, P., Lecomte-Yerna, M. J., Hudson, N., and Ball, K. (1984). *J. Endocrinol.* **102**, 305–309.

Hermans, W. P., vanLeeuwen, E. C. M., Debets, M. H. M., and DeJong, F. H. (1980). *J. Endocrinol.* **86**, 79–92.

Hillier, S. G., Wickings, E. J., Saunders, P. T. K., Dixson, A. F., Shimasaki, S., Swanston, I. A., Reichert, L. E., Jr., and McNeilly, A. S. (1989). *J. Endocrinol.* **123**, 65–73.

Hsueh, A. J. W., and Jones, P. B. C. (1981). *Endocr. Rev.* **2**, 437.

Hsueh, A. J. W., Bicsak, T. A., Vaughan, J., Tucker, E., Rivier, J., and Vale, W. (1987). *Proc. Natl. Acad. Sci. U.S.A.* **84**, 5082–5086.

Kaneko, H., Taya, K., and Sasamoto, S. (1987). *Life Sci.* **41**, 1823–1830.

Karten, M. J., and Rivier, J. E. (1986). *Endocr. Rev.* **7**, 44–66.

Keinan, D., Madigan, M. B., Bardin, C. W., and Chen, C. L. C. (1989). *Mol. Endocrinol.* **3**, 29–35.

Kimura, J., Katoh, M., Taya, K., and Sasamoto, S. (1983). *J. Endocrinol.* **97**, 313–318.

Klaij, I. A., Toebosch, A. M. W., Themmen, A. P. N., Shimasaki, S., DeJong, F. H., and Grootegoed, J. A. (1990). *Mol. Cell. Endocrinol.* **68**, 45–52.

Knight, P. G., Beard, A. J., Wrathall, J. H. M., and Castillo, R. J. (1989). *J. Mol. Endocrinol.* **2**, 189–200.

Koiter, T. R., VanDerSchaaf-Verdonk, G. C. J., Kuiper, H., Pols-Valkhof, N., and Schuiling, G. A. (1983). *J. Endocrinol.* **99**, 1–8.

Kotsuji, F., Winters, S. J., Keeping, H. S., Attardi, B., Oshima, H., and Troen, P. (1988). *Endocrinology (Baltimore)* **122**, 2796–2802.

LaPolt, P. S., Soto, D., Su, J.-G., Campen, C. A., Vaughan, J., Vale, W., and Hsueh, A. J. W. (1989). *Mol. Endocrinol.* **3**, 1666–1673.

Lee, V. W. K., McMaster, J., Quigg, H., Findlay, J., and Leversha, L. (1981). *Endocrinology (Baltimore)* **108**, 2403–2405.

Lee, V. W. K., McMaster, J., Quigg, H., and Leversha, L. (1982). *Endocrinology (Baltimore)* **111**, 1849–1854.

Levine, J. E., and Duffy, M. T. (1988). *Endocrinology (Baltimore)* **122**, 2211–2221.

Li, J. Y., Francis, H., and Clarke, I. J. (1989). *J. Neuroendocrinol.* **1**, 61–64.

Lin, T., Calkins, J. H., Morris, P. L., Vale, W., and Bardin, C. W. (1989). *Endocrinology* **125,** 2134–2140.

Lincoln, G. A., and McNeilly, A. S. (1989). *J. Endocrinol.* **120,** R9–R13.

Lumpkin, M. D., DePaolo, L. V., and Negro-Vilar, A. (1984). *Endocrinology (Baltimore)* **114,** 201–206.

Lumpkin, M. D., Moltz, J. H., Yu, W. H., Samson, W. K., and McCann, S. M. (1987). *Brain Res. Bull.* **18,** 175–178.

Maddocks, S., and Sharpe, R. M. (1990). *Endocrinology (Baltimore)* **126,** 1541–1550.

Main, S. J., Davies, R. V., and Setchell, B. P. (1978). *J. Endocrinol.* **79,** 255–270.

Mann, G. E., McNeilly, A. S., and Baird, D. T. (1989). *J. Endocrinol.* **123,** 181–188.

Martin, G. B., Wallace, J. M., Taylor, P. L., Fraser, H. M., Tsonis, C. G., and McNeilly, A. S. (1986). *J. Endocrinol.* **111,** 287–296.

McCullagh, D. R. (1932). *Science* **76,** 19–20.

McLachlan, R. I., Healy, D. L., Robertson, D. M., DeKretser, D. M., and Burger, H. G. (1986a). *Lancet* **2,** 1233–1234.

McLachlan, R. I., Robertson, D. M., Burger, H. G., and DeKretser, D. M. (1986b). *Mol. Cell. Endocrinol.* **46,** 175–185.

McLachlan, R. I., Healy, D. L., Robertson, D. M., Burger, H. G., and DeKretser, D. M. (1987a). *Fertil. Steril.* **48,** 1001–1005.

McLachlan, R. I., Robertson, D. M., Healy, D. L., Burger, H. G., and DeKretser, D. M. (1987b). *J. Clin. Endocrinol. Metab.* 65, 954–961.

McNeilly, A. S., and Baird, D. T. (1989). *J. Endocrinol.* **122,** 287–292.

Meijs-Roelofs, H. M. A., Kramer, P., and Sander, H. J. (1983). *J. Endocrinol.* **98,** 241–249.

Mercer, J. E., Clements, J. A., Funder, J. W., and Clarke, I. J. (1987). *Mol. Cell. Endocrinol.* **53,** 251–254.

Meunier, H., Cajander, S. B., Roberts, V. J., Rivier, C., Sawchenko, P. E., Hsueh, A. J. W., and Vale, W. (1988a). *Mol. Endocrinol.* **2,** 1352–1363.

Meunier, H., Rivier, C., Evans, R. M., and Vale, W. (1988b). *Proc. Natl. Acad. Sci. U.S.A.* **85,** 247–251.

Meunier, H., Rivier, C., Hsueh, A. J. W., and Vale, W. (1988c). "Conrad International Workshop on Nonsteroidal Gonadal Factors, January 6–8, 1988, Norfolk, VA" (G. D. Hodgen, Z. Rosenwaks, and J. M. Spieler, eds.), pp. 47–53. Jones Inst. Press, Norfolk, Virginia.

Meunier, H., Roberts, V. J., Sawchenko, P. E., Cajander, S. B., Hsueh, A. J. W., and Vale, W. (1989). *Mol. Endocrinol.* **3,** 2062–2069.

Mizumachi, M., Voglmayr, J. K., Washington, D. W., Chen, C.-L. C., and Bardin, C. W. (1990). *Endocrinology (Baltimore)* **126,** 1058–1063.

Mizunuma, H., Samson, W. K., Lumpkin, M. D., Moltz, J. H., Fawcett, C. P., and McCann, S. M. (1983). *Brain Res. Bull.* **10,** 623–629.

Morris, P. L., Vale, W. W., Cappel, S., and Bardin, C. W. (1988). *Endocrinology (Baltimore)* **122,** 717–725.

Negro-Vilar, A., Ojeda, S. R., and McCann, S. M. (1973). *Endocrinology (Baltimore)* **93,** 729–735.

Odell, W. D., and Swerdloff, R. S. (1976). *Recent Prog. Horm. Res.* **32,** 245–275.

Ojeda, S. R., Andrews, W. W., Advis, J. P., and White, S. S. (1980). *Endocr. Rev.* **1,** 228–257.

Risbridger, G. P., Clements, J., Robertson, D. M., Drummond, A. E., Muir, J., Burger, H. G., and DeKretser, D. M. (1989a). *Mol. Cell. Endocrinol.* **66,** 119–122.

Risbridger, G. P., Hancock, A., Robertson, D. M., Hodgson, Y., and DeKretser, D. M. (1989b). *Mol. Cell. Endocrinol.* **67,** 1–9.

Rivier, C., and Vale, W. (1987). *Endocrinology (Baltimore)* **120,** 1688–1690.

Rivier, C., and Vale, W. (1989a). *Endocrinology (Baltimore)* **125,** 152–157.

Rivier, C., and Vale, W. (1989b). *Endocrinology (Baltimore)* **124**, 195–198.

Rivier, C., Rivier, J., and Vale, W. (1986). *Science* **234**, 205–208.

Rivier, C., Meunier, H., Vaughan, J., and Vale, W. (1987). *Exerpta Med. Int. Congr. Ser. Proc. Reinier De Graff Symp., 6th* pp. 3–7.

Rivier, C., Cajander, S., Vaughan, J., Hsueh, A. J. W., and Vale, W. (1988a). *Endocrinology (Baltimore)* **123**, 120–126.

Rivier, C., Vale, W., and Rivier, J. (1988b). *Proc. J. Int. Henri-Pierre Klotz Endocrinol. Clin.* **28**, 104–118.

Rivier, C., Roberts, V., and Vale, W. (1989). *Endocrinology (Baltimore)* **125**, 876–882.

Roberts, V., Meunier, H., Vaughan, J., Rivier, J., Rivier, C., Vale, W., and Sawchenko, P. (1989). *Endocrinology (Baltimore)* **124**, 552–554.

Robertson, D. M., Giacometti, M., Foulds, L. M., Lahnstein, J., Goss, N. H., Hearn, M. T. W., and DeKretser, D. M. (1989). *Endocrinology (Baltimore)* **125**, 2141–2149.

Rodgers, R. J., Stuchbery, S. J., and Findlay, J. K. (1989). *Mol. Cell. Endocrinol.* **62**, 95–101.

Roseff, S. J., Bangah, M., Kettel, L. M., Vale, W., Rivier, J., Burger, H. G., and Yen, S. S. C. (1989). *J. Clin. Endocrinol. Metab.* **69**, 1033–1039.

Rush, M. E., and Lipner, H. (1979). *Endocrinology (Baltimore)* **105**, 187–194.

Rush, M. E., Ashiru, O. A., Lipner, H., Williams, A. T., McRae, C., and Blake, C. A., (1981). *Endocrinology (Baltimore)* **108**, 2316–1223.

Saito, S., Roche, P. C., McCormick, D. J., and Ryan, R. J. (1989). *Endocrinology (Baltimore)* **125**, 898–905.

Sander, H. J., vanLeeuwen, E. C. M., and DeJong, F. H. (1984). *J. Endocrinol.* **103**, 77–84.

Sander, H. J., Meijs-Roelofs, H. M. A., Kramer, P., and vanLeeuwen, E. C. M., (1985). *J. Endocrinol.* **107**, 251–257.

Sander, H. J., Meijs-Roelofs, H. M. A., vanLeeuwen, E. C. M., Kramer, P., and vanCappellen, W. A. (1986). *J. Endocrinol.* **111**, 159–166.

Schwartz, N. B. (1969). *Recent Prog. Horm. Res.* **25**, 1–55.

Schwartz, N. B., and Talley, W. L. (1978). *Biol. Reprod.* **17**, 820–828.

Shaha, C., Morris, P. L., Chen, C.-L. C., Vale, W., and Bardin, C. W. (1989). *Endocrinology (Baltimore)* **125**, 1941–1950.

Shander, D., Anderson, L. D., and Barraclough, C. A. (1980). *Endocrinology (Baltimore)* **106**, 1047–1053.

Sharpe, R. M., Kerr, J. B., and Maddocks, S. (1988). *Mol. Cell. Endocrinol.* **60**, 243–247.

Simpson, W. G., Vernon, M. W., Maley, B. E., and Rush, M. E. (1987). *Gynecol. Obstet. Invest.* **24**, 232–240.

Sugino, K., Nakamura, T., Takio, K., Titani, K., Miyamoto, K., Hasegawa, Y., Igarashi, M., and Sugino, H. (1989). *Biochem. Biophys. Res. Commun.* **159**, 1323–1329.

Sun, Y. T., Robertson, D. M., Gonzalez, G., Risbridger, G. P., and DeKretser, D. M. (1989). *J. Reprod. Fertil.* **87**, 795–801.

Suzuki, T., Miyamoto, K., Hasegawa, Y., Abe, Y., Ui, M., Ibuki, Y., and Igarashi, M. (1987). *Mol. Cell. Endocrinol.* **54**, 185–195.

Swerdloff, R. S., Walsh, P. C., Jacobs, H. S., and Odell, W. D. (1971). *Endocrinology (Baltimore)* **88**, 120–128.

Toebosch, A. M. W., Robertson, D. M., Trapman, J., Klaassen, P., dePaus, R. A., DeJong, F. H., and Grootegoed, J. A. (1988). *Mol. Cell. Endocrinol.* **55**, 101–105.

Toebosch, A. M. W., Robertson, D. M., Klaij, A., DeJong, F. H. and Grookegoed, J. A. (1989) *J. Endocrinol.* **122**, 757–762.

Torney, A. H., Hodgson, Y. M., Forage, R., and DeKretser, D. M. (1989). *J. Reprod. Fertil.* **86**, 391–399.

Tsafriri, A., Vale, W., and Hsueh, A. J. W. (1989). *Endocrinology (Baltimore)* **125**, 1857–1862.

Tsatsoulis, A., Shalet, S. M., Robertson, W. R., Morris, I. D., Burger, H. G., and DeKretser, D. M. (1988). *Clin. Endocrinol.* **29**, 659–665.

Tsonis, C. G., Baird, D. T., Campbell, B. K., Leask, R., and Scaramuzzi, R. J. (1988). *J. Endocrinol.* **116**, R3–R5.

Tsukamoto, I., Taya, K., Watanabe, G., and Sasamoto, S. (1986). *Life Sci.* **39**, 119–125.

Turner, I. M., Saunders, P. T. K., Shimasaki, S., and Hillier, S. G. (1989). *Endocrinology (Baltimore)* **125**, 2790–2792.

Uilenbroek, J. T. J., DeWolff-Exalto, E. A., and Welschen, R. (1976). *Ann. Biol. Anim., Biochim., Biophys.* **16**, 297–305.

Ultee-VanGessel, A. M., and DeJong, F. H. (1987). *J. Endocrinol.* **113**, 103–110.

Urbanski, H. F., Pickle, R. L., and Ramirez, V. D. (1988). *Endocrinology (Baltimore)* **123**, 413–419.

Vale, W., Rivier, C., Hsueh, A., Campen, C., Meunier, H., Bicsak, T., Vaughan, J., Corrigan, A., Bardin, W., Sawchenko, P., Petraglia, F., Yu, J., Plotsky, P., Spiess, J., and Rivier, J. (1988). *Recent Prog. Horm. Res.* **44**, 1–34.

Vale, W., Hsueh, A., Rivier, C., and Yu, J. (1989). *In* "Peptide Growth Factors and Their Receptors: Handbook of Experimental Pharmacology" (M. A. Sporn and A. B. Roberts, eds.). Springer-Verlag, Berlin, in press.

vanDijk, S., Steenbergen, J., Gielen, J. T., and DeJong, F. H. (1986). *J. Endocrinol.* **111**, 255–261.

Vaughan, J. M., Rivier, J., Corrigan, A. Z., McClintock, R., Campen, C. A., Jolley, D., Voglmayr, J. K., Bardin, C. W., Rivier, C., and Vale, W. (1988). *In* "Methods in Enzymology" (P. M. Conn, ed.), Vol. 168, pp. 588–617. Academic Press, San Diego, California.

Veeramachaneni, D. N. R., Schanbacher, B. D., and Amann, R. P. (1989). *Biol. Reprod.* **41**, 499–503.

Voglmayr, J. K., Mizumachi, M., Washington, D. W., Chen, C.-L. C., Bardin, C. W. (1990). *Biol. Reprod.* **42**, 81–86.

Wallace, J. M., and McNeilly, A. S. (1986). *J. Endocrinol.* **111**, 317–327.

Wang, Q. F., Farnworth, P. G., Findlay, J. K., and Burger, H. G. (1988). *Endocrinology (Baltimore)* **123**, 2161–2166.

Wang, Q. F., Farnworth, P. B., Findlay, J. K., and Burger, H. G. (1989). *Endocrinology (Baltimore)* **124**, 363–368.

Weinbauer, G. F., Bartlett, J. M. S., Fingscheidt, U., Tsonis, C. G., DeKretser, D. M., and Nieschlag, E. (1989). *J. Reprod. Fertil.* **85**, 355–362.

Winters, S. J. (1990). *J. Clin. Endocrinol. Metab.* **70**, 548–550.

Woodruff, T. K., Meunier, H., Jones, P. B. C., Hsueh, A. J. W., and Mayo, K. E. (1987). *Mol. Endocrinol.* **1**, 561–568.

Woodruff, T. K., D'Agostino, J., Schwartz, N. B., and Mayo, K. E. (1988). *Science* **239**, 1296–1299.

Woodruff, T. K., D'Agostino, J., Schwartz, N. B., and Mayo, K. E. (1989). *Endocrinology (Baltimore)* **124**, 2193–2199.

Ying, S.-Y., and Becker, A. (1989). *Proc. Annu. Meet. Endocr. Soc. 71st (Abst)*.

Zhang, Z., Lee, V. W. K., Carson, R. S., and Burger, H. G. (1988). *Mol. Cell. Endocrinol.* **56**, 35–40.

Zhiwen, Z., Carson, R. S., Herington, A. C., Lee, V. W. K., and Burger, H. G. (1987a). *Endocrinology (Baltimore)* **120**, 1633–1638.

Zhiwen, Z., Herington, A. C., Carson, R. S., Findlay, J. K., and Burger, H. G. (1987b). *Mol. Cell. Endocrinol.* **54**, 213–220.

DISCUSSION

J. L. Vaitukaitis.   Have you ascertained whether that antiserum has any effect on FSH action at the cellular level?

C. Rivier.   No.

J. L. Vaitukaitis.   Have you infused synthetic inhibin at levels that mimic those present in normal physiological concentrations to ascertain the effect on circulating FSH levels?

C. Rivier.   No, we do not have enough inhibin to do such studies. The inhibin which is available has been used only in *in vitro* studies. We have not been able to do *in vivo* studies.

J. L. Vaitukaitis.   The reason I ask these questions is because one could easily rationalize that if the antiinhibin serum had a negative effect on FSH action at the cellular level, then one would expect a reciprocal rise of pituitary FSH secretion. Then everything could be accounted for in the paracrine or autocrine.

C. Rivier.   Yes, that is correct.

C. W. Bardin.   We have immunized some rams with recombinant inhibin α, and have found that during the nonbreeding season there is no change in basal gonadotropin secretion, but in the breeding season one gets a marked rise in FSH and LH, but yet a blunting of testosterone secretion. At least this is one species that appears to be different from the rat. What do you know about other species differences?

C. Rivier.   We do not know all that much about possible species differences because, as I have already noted, there is not enough inhibin to do the *in vivo* studies. However, if we compare, for example, the concomitant secretion rates of inhibin and FSH under a number of physiological conditions to determine whether they are parallel or dissociated, we see marked species differences. In the female species differences can be seen during follicular maturation. For example, during proestrus and estrus in the female rat, we see opposite secretory rates of inhibin and FSH. However, this is not true in all stages of the human menstrual cycle, particularly in some stages, when it appears that inhibin loses its ability to inhibit FSH secretion (i.e., when there is a parallel rise in the levels of FSH and inhibin). To my knowledge, possible species differences have not really been studied much in the male for the simple reason that demonstrating a functional role of inhibin in modulating FSH secretion in the male has been a problem.

W. F. Crowley.   In regard to the relationship of inhibin levels and FSH in the human male, we have obtained the Australian inhibin radioimmunoassay that is basically the assay used to describe all of the inhibin physiology in the human to date. Using recombinant α inhibin, Drs. Alan Schneyer and Tony Mason and I found that it is completely cross-reactive. In other words, we were able to displace all of the 32-kDa inhibin tracer from the Australian antibody with this recombinant α inhibin only. Second, to compound the problem of trying to go from one species to another, we used Western blotting to determine that there is a free α inhibin in the circulation of the human. Taken together, these findings make this assay quite suspect, and this is particularly true in the human male. One of the areas in which this problem is evident is the failure of the Australian group to find any correlation, negative or positive, between FSH and inhibin levels, particularly in the human male. In fact, Klinefelter's patients have the highest inhibin levels known without FSH administration, which is very counterintuitive. These previous assertions from this group about the α cross-activity to that antibody are based on its non-cross-reactivity with reduced and carboxymethylated α subunit. In the gonadotropin area this would not be a very meaningful statement, and I think the confirmational aspects of inhibin are going to be quite similar to gonadotropin where all epitopes have been quite conformational. Thus, I think it is even harder to compare one species to another for inhibin on the basis of the immunoassay data available right now, particularly with free α existing in the circulation.

C. Rivier.   I think that this may be particularly true under conditions of elevated FSH secretion (such as in Klinefelter's syndrome) because of the data showing that FSH will specifically increase the α message.

W. F. Crowley. I would like to ask Drs. Rivier and Schwartz to comment on the discrepancies in the results of the *in situ* hybridization studies of their groups, which are confusing, for example, the absence of α-mRNA levels in the corpus luteum in some studies and the presence in others. In addition, precise follicular distribution of this message needs clarification.

C. Rivier. In the corpus luteum of the rat, we see low levels of α message.

N. B. Schwartz. It is not the immunocytochemistry, but the message we have measured. We see no α or β inhibin in the corpus luteum. We have not seen the increase in the α message on the afternoon of proestrus that Dr. Rivier found, but essentially our data are very similar.

J. Kirkland. Have you had the opportunity to utilize bioassays for LH and FSH in the anti-inhibin serum and in the GnRH antagonist experiments?

C. Rivier. No, we have not, but I would like Dr. Crowley to comment on the comparison between the bioassay and the radioimmunoassays for LH and FSH for that before we go too far into that type of discussion.

W. F. Crowley. Our group is "struck" by the differences which exist between the two major FSH bioassay systems which have been described in terms of bio (B) and immuno (I) ratios, for example, across the menstrual cycle: the Hsueh group finds absolutely no changes in the B/I ratios and the Beitins group finds very dramatic changes. Second, we are very concerned about the first step of the Hsueh assay, which uses polyethylene glycol to strip the circulating of "interfering substances" since Dr. Schaeyer of our group has demonstrated that there are both small and large circulating inhibitors to the FSH receptor assay. Third, when we study the FSH radio receptor assays (i.e., merely the binding of the FSH to its receptor), we find that these substances may play a very important role in the action of FSH in certain biological conditions. Consequently, we view the bioassay of FSH as an area of active controversy, rather than established fact.

S. M. Rosenthal. Have you done similar studies on male gonadectomized rats in terms of the pituitary *in situ* hybridization and immunocytochemistry which showed the colocalization of inhibin and FSH in ovariectomized rats?

C. Rivier. We have just started doing such studies but we do not have any results yet.

S. M. Rosenthal. Can you comment on the possible physiological significance of this colocalization in pituitary cells?

C. Rivier. The only suggestion we have comes from studies done by Dr. Burger's group in Australia, which show that inhibin may enhance or stimulate the degradation of LH and FSH in the gonadotrophs. Whether inhibin has any such effect in the whole animal is at present unclear, but this might be one of the autocrine effects of inhibin in the pituitary. We do not believe that the pituitary secretes measurable amounts of inhibin into the circulation. When we gonadectomize an animal, we see a 95% decrease in the levels of circulating inhibin, so whatever amount the pituitary contributes in terms of circulating inhibin cannot amount to much. When Wylie Vale and colleagues measured inhibin in the culture medium of pituitary cells, they saw some low levels of at least the α chain, so I think that if there is really an effect on the pituitary, this effect is going to be found within the pituitary itself.

Structure of the Lutropin/Choriogonadotropin Receptor

Deborah L. Segaloff,*,[1] Rolf Sprengel,† Karoly Nikolics,‡
and Mario Ascoli*[2]

*The Population Council, New York, New York 10021, †Zentrum für Molekulare Biologie
Heidelberg, University of Heidelberg, Federal Republic of Germany, and ‡Department of
Developmental Biology, Genentech, Inc., South San Francisco, California 94080

I. Introduction

The lutropin/choriogonadotropin (LH/CG) receptor plays a pivotal role in reproductive physiology. This cell surface receptor is present on testicular Leydig cells and on ovarian theca, interstitial, and luteal cells, as well as mature granulosa cells. In both males and females the LH/CG receptor recognizes the pituitary hormone LH. In the pregnant female, however, this same receptor also recognizes the placental hormone human choriogonadotropin (hCG). LH and hCG are each composed of two dissimilar subunits, α and β, which are joined by noncovalent interactions (Pierce, 1988; Strickland et al., 1985). They are members of a family of glycoprotein hormones which also includes the pituitary hormones follitropin (FSH) and thyrotropin (TSH) (Pierce, 1988; Pierce and Parsons, 1981). The glycoprotein hormones of a given species are all composed of an identical α subunit, and different (but homologous) β subunits. It has been shown that although both subunits of the glycoprotein hormones are necessary for binding, it is the β subunit which dictates the binding specificity of the hormone (Pierce et al., 1971; Reichert, 1972; Williams et al., 1980). As the amino acid sequences of the β subunits of LH and hCG are highly conserved, it is not surprising that either LH or hCG can bind to the LH/CG receptor, and they each elicit almost identical biological responses (Ascoli and Puett, 1978; Buettner and Ascoli, 1984; Huhtaniemi and Catt, 1981; Lee and Ryan, 1972; Reichert et al., 1973; Strickland and Puett, 1981).

On binding LH or hCG, the LH/CG receptor activates a G_s protein which

---

[1] Present address: Department of Physiology and Biophysics, University of Iowa College of Medicine, Iowa City, Iowa 52242.

[2] Present address: Department of Pharmacology, University of Iowa College of Medicine, Iowa City, Iowa 52242.

261

stimulates adenylyl cyclase (Hunzicker-Dunn and Birnbaumer, 1985). The resulting increase in cAMP in turn stimulates the cAMP-dependent protein kinase (Hunzicker-Dunn and Birnbaumer, 1985). The primary result of this response in LH/CG receptor-bearing gonadal cells is an increase in the synthesis and secretion of steroids (Gore-Langton and Armstron, 1988; Hall, 1988). Studies to date indicate that the cAMP second messenger system is the predominant, if not the sole, second messenger pathway stimulated by either LH or hCG (Ascoli *et al.*, 1989; Hunzicker-Dunn and Birnbaumer, 1985; Pereira *et al.*, 1987). It should also be pointed out that although differences in the duration of the response of a target cell to ovine, bovine, or porcine LH versus hCG have been observed (Segaloff *et al.*, 1981; Strickland and Puett, 1981), these differences can be attributed to the higher affinity (and slower rate of hormone–receptor dissociation) of hCG for the LH/CG receptor as compared to LH from these species (Strickland and Puett, 1981). Therefore, it is generally believed that both LH and hCG bind to and activate the LH/CG receptor similarly. However, because of the greater availability of hCG and because of its slower dissociation rate from the LH/CG receptor (which makes radioligand assays easier), hCG is the hormone usually used experimentally to study the LH/CG receptor.

The responsiveness of a given target cell to LH or hCG can be modulated by one or both of two general kinds of mechanisms. One of these is an alteration in the number of cell surface LH/CG receptors. This can be an increase in the numbers of receptors, one example of which occurs during the FSH-dependent differentiation of granulosa cells (Erickson *et al.*, 1979; Richards *et al.*, 1979; Segaloff and Limbird, 1983). LH/CG receptors can also be down-regulated. Examples of the down-regulation of the LH/CG receptor include the homologous down-regulation of the receptor after exposure to LH or hCG (Ascoli, 1982, 1984, 1985b; Catt *et al.*, 1980; Freeman and Ascoli, 1981; Lloyd and Ascoli, 1983), which results from an increase in the internalization and degradation of the hormone–receptor complex (Ascoli, 1982, 1984; Ascoli and Segaloff, 1987; Lloyd and Ascoli, 1983), and also the heterologous down-regulation of the receptor by certain other hormones, growth factors, and second messenger analogs (Ascoli, 1981; Lloyd and Ascoli, 1983; Mondschein and Schomberg, 1981; Rebois and Patel, 1985).

The responsiveness of the target cell to LH or hCG might also be modulated by alterations in the "functional" activity of the receptor which can occur independently of (or in addition to) changes in receptor numbers. A classical example of this phenomenon is that of desensitization, in which the ability of the receptor to activate adenylyl cyclase is attenuated. Again, this might occur in a homologous manner, after exposure of the cells to LH or hCG (Ekstrom and Hunzicker-Dunn, 1989; Ezra and Salomon, 1981; Rebois and Fishman, 1986), or it might occur in a heterologous manner after exposure of the cells to certain other hormones, growth factors, or second messenger analogs (Inoue and Rebois, 1989; Pereira *et al.,* 1988a; Pereira *et al.,* 1988b; Rebois and Patel, 1985). By analogy with the β-adrenergic receptor (Sibley *et al.,* 1987), it has been hypothesized that the desensitization of the LH/CG receptor occurs as a result of receptor phosphorylation. However, this remains to be demonstrated.

Indeed, for the regulation of both LH/CG receptor levels and the LH/CG receptor functional activity, it has been difficult to study the molecular mechanisms underlying these phenomena. This has been due arily to our lack of knowledge about the structure of the receptor. Structural studies have been hampered by the low abundancy of this receptor. Nonetheless, we have recently made sufficient progress in this area, which is the subject of the present review. Focusing on data from our laboratories, we first consider how chemical cross-linking of [^{125}I]hCG to the LH/CG receptor, immunoprecipitation of a biosynthetically labeled LH/CG receptor, and purification of the rat luteal LH/CG receptor have led to the estimation of the overall size and structure of this receptor. We then discuss how studies on the cloning of the rat luteal receptor have yielded more detailed information on the structure and function of the LH/CG receptor. Last, we discuss how antibodies developed to the receptor have confirmed the topology of this receptor and are being used to address structure–function relationships of this receptor. Other issues concerning the LH/CG receptor (i.e., the mechanism of action and regulation) must be covered in a more extensive review.

II. Structure of the LH/CG Receptor as Determined by Biochemical Approaches

A.   CHEMICAL CROSS-LINKING OF [^{125}I]hCG TO THE LH/CG RECEPTOR

One approach to elucidate the size and organization of the LH/CG receptor used by our own (Ascoli and Segaloff, 1986) and other laboratories (for a review see Ascoli and Segaloff, 1989) was the analysis of products resulting from the chemical cross-linking of [^{125}I]hCG to target cells. These experiments were complicated by the possibility that either or both of the hormone subunits become cross-linked to a receptor protein. To aid in the interpretation of our results, therefore, MA-10 cells (a clonal line of murine Leydig tumor cells that have functional LH/CG receptors; for a review see Ascoli, 1985a) were allowed to bind hCG that was specifically labeled in either the α or the β subunit. After washing to remove the unbound hormone, the cells were exposed to bifunctional succinimidyl esters, and then the iodinated cross-linked products were resolved by sodium dodecyl sulfate (SDS) polyacrylamide gel electrophoresis.

Figure 1 shows the results of a typical experiment in which hCG was cross-linked to MA-10 cells and then analyzed in the presence of reducing agents. It

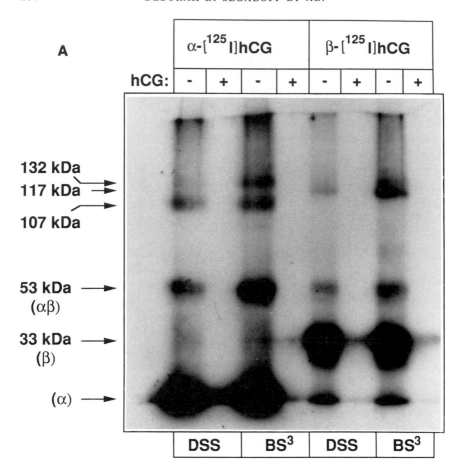

A

α-[^{125}I]hCG   β-[^{125}I]hCG

hCG: - + - + - + - +

132 kDa
117 kDa
107 kDa

53 kDa
(αβ)

33 kDa
(β)

(α)

DSS   BS^3 DSS   BS^3

FIG. 1.   Cross-linking of α- and β-labeled hCG to MA-10 cells. MA-10 cells were incubated (at 4°C) with hCG iodinated in either the α or the β subunit. Incubations were done with the labeled hormone alone or together with an excess of hCG (to prevent binding of the labeled hormone), as indicated. After washing the cells to remove the free hormone, the cells bearing the receptor-bound hormone were incubated with the indicated cross-linker [disuccinimidyl suberate (DSS) or bis(sulfosuccinimidyl)suberate (BS^3)] and subsequently analyzed on SDS gels in the presence of disulfide reducing agents. (A) Autoradiogram of the gel. (B) Densitometric scan of a selected area of the gels shown in (A). (From Ascoli and Segaloff, 1986.)

was determined (by cross-linking free iodinated hormone) that the 53-kDa band, the 33-kDa band, and the radioactivity at the tracking dye correspond to the two hCG subunits cross-linked to each other, the free β subunit, and the free α subunit, respectively. When the cells were allowed to bind α-labeled hCG, hormone–receptor complexes corresponding to 107 and 132 kDa were observed.

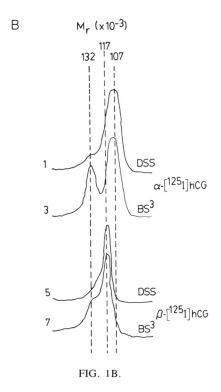

FIG. 1B.

In contrast, when hCG iodinated in the β subunit was used, cross-linked complexes of 117 and 132 kDa were identified.

In most experiments the 132-kDa band is typically faint, and sometimes it is not apparent. It is more readily discerned by examining the densitometric scans of the gel (see Fig. 1). Inasmuch as the 132-kDa band was observed when either α- or β-labeled hCG was used, we concluded that this represents a receptor protein cross-linked to both subunits of hCG. Since the 107-kDa band is observed only when using α-labeled hCG and the 117-kDa band is seen only when using β-labeled hCG, it was concluded that they represent the α or β subunit of hCG, respectively, cross-linked to a receptor component. An approximation of the molecular masses of the receptor component(s) that have been cross-linked to hCG can be determined by subtracting the molecular masses (as observed on SDS gels) of the intact hormone (53 kDa), the β subunit (33 kDa), and the α subunit (22 kDa) from the 132-, 117-, and 107-kDa complexes, respectively. The results of these calculations are shown in Table I. It can be seen that the molecular masses of the receptor protein(s) in the three cross-linked complexes are 79, 84, and 85 kDa. Because the sizes of the receptor protein(s) thus deduced are so similar, these data suggest that the 132-, 117-, and 107-kDa cross-linked

TABLE I
Identification of the Cross-linked Products Detected in MA-10 Cells[a]

Cross-linked product		Cross-linked ligand		Receptor
Identity	kDa[b]	Identity	kDa[b]	(kDa[b])
(α–β)-R	132 ± 3	α–β	53 ± 5	79
(α)-R	107 ± 7	α	22 ± 1	85
(β)-R	117 ± 1	β	33 ± 3	84
			$\bar{X}$ ± SEM =	83 ± 2

[a]From Ascoli and Segaloff (1986).

[b]These molecular masses are higher than the real molecular masses of hCG or its subunits because of the anomalous migration of these highly glycosylated molecules on SDS gels.

products correspond to a single LH/CG receptor protein (with an average molecular mass of 83 kDa) cross-linked to different forms of the hormone.

These data also show that when the LH/CG receptor is occupied by hCG, both the α and the β subunits are in close enough proximity to the receptor to become chemically cross-linked to it (by cross-linking reagents of 7–13 Å). Although the efficiency of cross-linking of the β-labeled hormone to the receptor is typically lower than that observed with the α-labeled hormone, this should not necessarily be interpreted as an indication that the α subunit is in closer physical proximity to the receptor, as there are other alternative explanations for these results. For example, one would predict more difficulties in detecting cross-linked products with the β-labeled hCG simply because the specific radioactivity of this derivative is 25–50% lower than that of α-labeled hCG (Ascoli, 1980). Furthermore, the preferential cross-linking of the α subunit might simply reflect the distribution and/or availability of reactive groups. Thus, while the α subunit contains six lysyl residues, the β subunit contains only four (Strickland *et al.*, 1985).

As would be predicted, the cross-linking of [^{125}I]hCG to the LH/CG receptor on MA-10 cells could be prevented by the inclusion of an excess of either unlabeled hCG or unlabeled LH (Ascoli and Segaloff, 1986). Furthermore, as shown in Fig. 2, the cross-linking of either α-labeled hCG or α-labeled ovine LH to MA-10 cells resulted in the appearance of a 107-kDa cross-linked complex. These data are consistent with previous studies showing that hCG and LH bind to the same cell surface receptor (Ascoli and Puett, 1978; Buettner and Ascoli, 1984; Huhtaniemi and Catt, 1981; Lee and Ryan, 1972; Reichert *et al.*, 1973; Strickland and Puett, 1981).

In other cross-linking experiments we compared the results of cross-linking α-labeled hCG to MA-10 murine Leydig tumor cells versus porcine granulosa cells. The results are shown in Fig. 3 and show that similar cross-linked products were

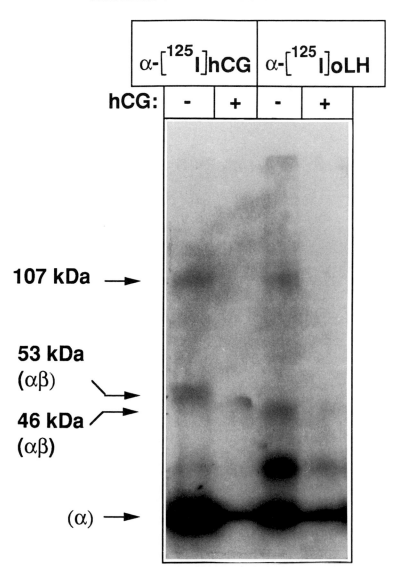

FIG. 2. Cross-linking of α-labeled hCG or ovine LH (oLH) to MA-10 cells. MA-10 cells were incubated (at 4°C) with either hCG or oLH iodinated in the α subunit. Incubations were done with the labeled hormone alone or together with an excess of hCG, as indicated. After washing the cells to remove the free hormone, the cells bearing the receptor-bound hormone were incubated with disuccinimidyl suberate and subsequently analyzed on SDS gels in the presence of disulfide reducing agents. (From Ascoli and Segaloff, 1986.)

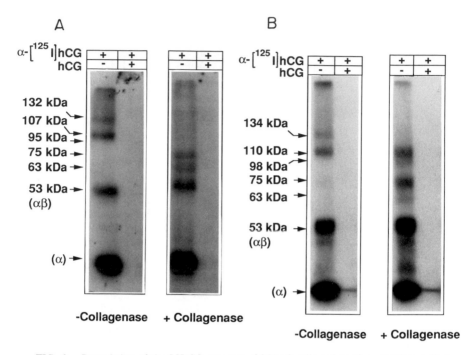

FIG. 3.   Degradation of the LH/CG receptor of MA-10 cells and porcine granulosa cells by collagenase type I. (A) MA-10 cells or (B) primary cultures of porcine granulosa cells (cultured in the presence of cholera toxin to induce LH/CG receptors) were preincubated with or without collagenase type I, as indicated. After washing, the cells were incubated with α-labeled hCG alone or together with an excess of unlabeled hCG. After cross-linking with disuccinimidyl suberate, the cross-linked products were analyzed on SDS gels in the presence of disulfide reducing agents. (Modified from Ascoli and Segaloff, 1986.)

observed, suggesting that the overall size and structure of the LH/CG receptor are similar in these two cell types from different species.

Also shown in Fig. 3 are the results of treatment of either MA-10 cells or cultured granulosa cells with collagenase (the crude preparations typically used to disperse ovarian or testicular tissues) prior to the binding of hCG. The cross-linking of [^{125}I]hCG (labeled in the α subunit) to collagenase-treated cells yields several smaller hormone–receptor complexes (as observed in SDS gels analyzed in the presence of reducing agents) that are not observed in untreated cells. Thus, in collagenase-treated cells there is a decrease in the intensity of the 132-kDa (αβ)–receptor complex and the 107-kDa (α)–receptor complex and a concomitant increase in complexes of 95, 75, and 63 kDa. Similar results are observed with collagenase-treated porcine granulosa cells (see Fig. 3). As the degradation products of the LH/CG receptor from collagenase-treated MA-10 cells and collagenase-treated procine granulosa cells are similar, these data also suggest that the overall structures of the receptor in these two cell types are similar.

The data on collagenase treatment of LH/CG receptor-bearing cells are also important because they show that this receptor is readily susceptible to proteolysis by enzyme(s) present in collagenase preparations typically used to disperse gonadal tissues. This degradation is dependent on the concentration of collagenase used and the time of exposure to collagenase (Ascoli and Segaloff, 1986). With increasing times of incubation with collagenase, there appears to be a precursor–product relationship between the 95-kDa complex and the 75- and 63-kDa complexes (Ascoli and Segaloff, 1986). Although it has not been rigorously shown whether these smaller cross-linked products correspond to a receptor fragment cross-linked to the α subunit only or the α and β subunits of hCG, if one assumes that they are cross-linked only to the α subunit (which is the predominant result when using α-labeled hCG), then the 95-, 75-, and 63-kDa complexes would correspond to the α subunit of hCG cross-linked to receptor degradation products of 63, 52, and 41 kDa.

Interestingly, however, when the cross-linked products from collagenase-treated cells are analyzed on SDS gels in the absence of reducing agents, the receptor appears to be entirely intact (Ascoli and Segaloff, 1986). These results suggest that collagenase [specifically enzymes that contaminate collagenase preparations] "nicks" the LH/CG receptor and that, normally, the nicked receptor is held together by disulfide bonds. As such, when the nicked receptor is exposed to disulfide reducing agents, the smaller receptor fragments are released. This proposal is consistent with the observations that collagenase-treated cells bind hCG with normal affinity and stimulate steroid production with normal efficacy (Ascoli and Segaloff, 1986).

It is important to note that, as documented by Rajaniemi and co-workers, endogenous proteases in gonadal tissues also degrade or nick the LH/CG receptor (Kellokumpu and Rajaniemi, 1985a,b). As with the collagenase-treated receptor, LH/CG receptor exposed to these proteases also binds hCG. Furthermore, the sizes of the receptor fragments generated by endogenous proteases are similar to those generated by collagenase treatment. The proteolytic effects of collagenase can be inhibited by the metal chelating agent ethylenediaminetetraacetic acid (EDTA) (Ascoli and Segaloff, 1986). Inhibition of the proteolysis of the LH/CG receptor by endogenous proteases requires EDTA and also N-ethylmaleimide and phenylmethylsulfonyl fluoride (Kellokumpu and Rajaniemi, 1985a,b).

Thus, when studying the structure of the LH/CG receptor, one must keep in mind that because the receptor binds hormone, it does not necessarily mean that it is structurally intact. Studies with collagenase or endogenous proteases suggest that this receptor might be nicked (and held together by internal disulfide bonds) in spite of having normal hCG-binding activity. Therefore, if appropriate precautions to inhibit proteolysis are not taken, it would be difficult to distinguish a nicked receptor from a receptor composed of multiple subunits. As discussed in a recent review (Ascoli and Segaloff, 1989), we believe that this could account for many of the discrepant reports on the structure of the LH/CG receptor that have been published by different laboratories.

B.   "INDIRECT IMMUNOPRECIPITATION" OF A BIOSYNTHETICALLY LABELED LH/CG RECEPTOR

Another experimental approach that we have used to examine the overall structure of the LH/CG receptor is that which we have termed an "indirect immunoprecipitation" of the receptor (Kim *et al.*, 1987). These experiments were done prior to having antibodies to the LH/CG receptor available. Nonetheless, we were able to immunoprecipitate the hormone–receptor complex from biosynthetically labeled cells with an antibody to the hormone. MA-10 cells were biosynthetically labeled with [^{35}S]cysteine, and then were allowed to bind unlabeled hCG (under conditions in which there was no internalization of the hormone–receptor complex). After washing to remove the unbound hormone, the cells were solubilized with detergent. A critical aspect of this protocol is that, under the conditions used, hCG remains associated with the solubilized receptor. Thus, one solubilizes a hormone–receptor complex, which is held together by noncovalent interactions, in which the receptor (not the hormone) is radiolabeled. After partially purifying the hormone–receptor complex on a wheat germ agglutinin (WGA) agarose column, the complex was immunoprecipitated using an antibody to hCG and protein A–Sepharose. The radiolabeled receptor could then be specifically eluted from the immunoprecipitate using an isotonic pH 3 glycine solution and resolved by SDS polyacrylamide gel electrophoresis. Therefore, in this experimental design we were able to visualize the free (not hormone-occupied) receptor. To verify that a given radiolabeled band on the gel was, in fact, the LH/CG receptor, three independent negative controls were performed. In one, the LH/CG receptor was down-regulated (to 5% of control) prior to and during the biosynthetic labeling. In the second, hCG was not incubated with the labeled cells. In the third, preimmune antisera was substituted for the immune anti-hCG.

The results of a typical indirect immunoprecipitation are shown in Fig. 4. It is readily apparent that a number of radiolabeled bands are immunoprecipitated. However, if one compares the results from the positive control cells with those from the three negative controls discussed above, there is only one band (at 93 kDa) that is present in the control, but not in the negative controls. In the experiment shown the gel was analyzed in the absence of disulfide reducing

$$\left[{}^{35}S\right]\text{Cysteine}$$

93 kDa→

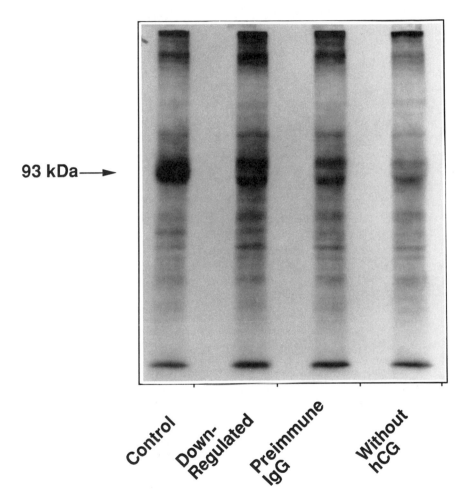

Control   Down-Regulated   Preimmune IgG   Without hCG

FIG. 4. Immunoprecipitation of the LH/CG receptor from MA-10 cells metabolically labeled with [^{35}S]cysteine. The LH/CG receptor of [^{35}S]cysteine-labeled cells was immunoprecipitated as described in the text and by Kim *et al.* (1987) and analyzed on an SDS gels run in the presence of disulfide reducing agents. (From Kim *et al.*, 1987.)

agents. The same results were also obtained when the experiment was performed in the presence of reducing agents (Kim *et al.,* 1987). Thus, data from the indirect immunoprecipitation of the biosynthetically labeled LH/CG receptor also suggest that this receptor is a single polypeptide. The size of the LH/CG receptor observed in these experiments (i.e., 93 kDa) differs from that observed by chemical cross-linking of the hormone to the receptor (83 kDa). However, it should be pointed out that in the cross-linking approach one is visualizing the hormone–receptor complex on the SDS gel and must estimate the size of the receptor alone by subtracting the contribution of the hormone to the molecular mass of the complex. In contrast, the indirect immunoprecipitation method allowed us to visualize the free receptor on the SDS gel. Given the different ways in which the size of the receptor is determined by these two methods, we believe that there is, in fact, relatively good agreement on the estimated size of the receptor. Of the two estimates, however, clearly that determined by the indirect immunoprecipitation (i.e., 93 kDa) must be more accurate.

Therefore, using two independent experimental approaches (and two different target cells) to evaluate the overall size and structure of the LH/CG receptor, we found this receptor to be composed of a single polypeptide whose size (on SDS gels) appeared to be 93 kDa.

C.   PURIFICATION OF THE LH/CG RECEPTOR

There are three characteristics of the LH/CG receptor that have traditionally made it difficult to purify. These are (1) its low abundance in the ovaries and the testes of most species, (2) the rapid loss of hCG binding on solubilization of the receptor, and (3) the susceptibility of this receptor to proteolysis. Advances in recent years, however, have contributed to solving these problems.

Thus, with regard to an appropriate source of starting material for LH/CG receptor purifications, it has been found that the ovaries of pseudopregnant rats appear to be a uniquely rich source of LH/CG receptor. Crude homogenates prepared from this tissue have a specific hCG-binding capacity of 0.4–1.3 pmol/mg of protein (Bruch *et al.,* 1986; Keinanen *et al.,* 1987; Kusuda and Dufau, 1986; Roche and Ryan, 1989), which is approximately 10- to 50-fold higher than that of homogenates prepared from porcine luteal tissue, rat testis, or mouse Leydig cell tumors (D. L. Segaloff and M. Ascoli, unpublished observations; Minegishi *et al.,* 1987; Wimalasena *et al.,* 1985). The theoretical binding capacity for a homogeneous preparation of rat luteal LH/CG receptor (assuming a 1:1 binding stoichiometry to a 93-kDa monomer) would be about 11,000 pmol/mg. Thus, one would need a 8500- to 27,500-fold purification from a rat luteal homogenate to obtain pure LH/CG receptor. This degree of purification has been done successfully for other cell surface receptors (Benovic *et al.,* 1984).

As related to the loss of hCG-binding activity on solubilization of the LH/CG

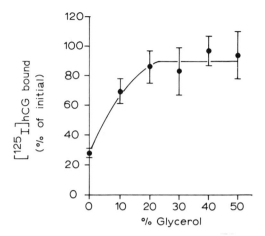

FIG. 5. Effects of glycerol on the stability of detergent-solubilized LH/CG receptor. MA-10 cells were extracted with 1% Triton X-100 containing the indicated concentrations of glycerol. Half of the soluble extracts was used immediately to determine hCG-binding activity; the other half was stored in the indicated concentration of glycerol at 4°C for 24 hours before measuring binding activity. The data show the binding activity of the extracts that had been stored for 24 hours, expressed as a percentage of the binding activity of the extracts that had not been stored. (From Ascoli, 1983.)

receptor, we found that the inclusion of glycerol in the buffers used to solubilize and store the receptor prevents this loss of binding activity (Ascoli, 1983). The binding activity of the solubilized receptor is maximal when concentrations of glycerol of 20% or greater are utilized. Once solubilized, the receptor must be maintained in glycerol (of at least 20%) to preserve its binding activity. As shown in Fig. 5, in the absence of glycerol during storage of the receptor at 4°C, there is a 70% loss in binding activity within 24 hours. In contrast, if glycerol (20% or greater) is included in the same incubation, there is only a 5–10% loss in binding activity. Though not shown, it is possible to store the LH/CG receptor for at least 3 days in 20% glycerol at 4°C without any further loss in binding activity. Thus, most investigators now include glycerol in all buffer used to solubilize and store LH/CG receptor preparations.

Last, as discussed in Section II,A, the LH/CG receptor is readily susceptible to proteolysis both by endogenous proteases (Kellokumpu and Rajaniemi, 1985a,b) and by those that contaminate crude preparations of collagenase (Ascoli and Segaloff, 1986). This proteolysis can result in nicking of the receptor protein, such that the nicked receptor can bind hCG normally and thus can be purified by hCG affinity chromatography. It has been well documented by Rajaniemi and co-workers that the proteolysis (and/or nicking) of the LH/CG receptor by endogenous proteases can be inhibited by the inclusion of an inhibitor cocktail containing phenylmethylsulfonyl fluoride, N-ethylmaleimide, and EDTA in all buffers (Kellokumpu and Rajaniemi, 1985a,b).

Given the above information, we devised a purification scheme for the LH/CG receptor using ovaries from pseudopregnant rats as the starting material (Rosemblit *et al.*, 1988). To prevent receptor proteolysis, all manipulations were done at 4°C or on ice and all buffers contained *N*-ethylmaleimide, phenylmethylsulfonyl fluoride, and EDTA as protease inhibitors. A crude membrane fraction was prepared, and the LH/CG receptor was then solubilized in Nonidet P-40 containing glycerol to maintain hCG-binding activity. The solubilized LH/CG receptor was purified sequentially by WGA and hCG affinity chromatography. Given the low dissociation rate of hCG from the LH/CG receptor (Ascoli and Segaloff, 1987; Roche and Ryan, 1985), it is possible to wash to affinity resin quite extensively prior to elution of the bound receptor (Rosemblit *et al.*, 1988).

Another critical aspect to the purification of the LH/CG receptor is the method used to elute the receptor from the affinity resin. It is desirable that the elution be done quantitatively, specifically, and in such a way that the hormone-binding activity of the eluted receptor is preserved. Since we had previously shown that isotonic pH 3 glycine buffer is capable of quantitatively dissociating the cell surface LH/CG receptor–hormone complex without destroying the biological activity of the receptor (Ascoli, 1982; Segaloff and Ascoli, 1981), this buffer was used for the elution of the receptor from the affinity resin. The resulting (neutralized) purified receptor showed high-affinity binding for hCG (120 ± 29 pM), similar to that observed in the initial detergent extracts (128 ± 29 pM).

Figure 6 shows a silver-stained SDS gel of the material obtained after the WGA chromatography only, and after sequential WGA and hCG affinity chromatography. It is readily apparent that although the WGA-purified material is still quite impure, the WGA- and affinity-purified material appears to consist primarily of a 93-kDa protein, which we presume is the LH/CG receptor. Although the WGA chromatography achieves only a 10% enrichment of the receptor, it serves to remove some proteins which otherwise would copurify with the receptor through the affinity resin and appear in close proximity to the 93-kDa region of the SDS gels. It should also be pointed out that we typically observe some minor lower-molecular-mass contaminants in the WGA- and affinity-purified preparation, which are not apparent on the gel shown. Although we have not done a rigorous determination of the specific hCG-binding capacity of the WGA- and affinity-purified material, we estimate that the 93-kDa protein represents approximately 80% of the total protein purified.

The assumption that the 93-kDa protein purified by WGA and hCG affinity chromatography is the LH/CG receptor is consistent with previous estimations of the size and structure of the LH/CG receptor made by chemical cross-linking (Ascoli and Segaloff, 1986) and by indirect immunoprecipitation studies (Kim *et al.*, 1987) (see Sections II,A and II,B). To substantiate our identification further, however, we performed two additional experiments (Rosemblit *et al.*, 1988). In one, we performed parallel purifications from the ovaries of control pseudopreg-

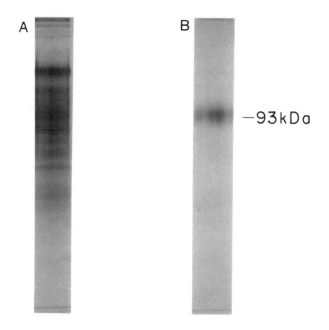

FIG. 6. Purified rat luteal LH/CG receptor. LH/CG receptor was purified from rat luteal tissue as described by Rosemblit *et al.* (1988), except that the chromatography on wheat germ agglutinin (WGA) preceded the chromatography on the hCG affinity resin. Material purified by WGA only (A) or WGA and affinity chromatography (B) was resolved on an SDS gel run in the absence of disulfide reducing agents, and the gels were silver stained.

nant rats and from the ovaries of pseudopregnant rats which had been treated with hCG 24 hours prior to sacrificing to down-regulate the hCG-binding activity in their ovaries (Conti *et al.*, 1977). The result of this down-regulation is a decrease in the hCG-binding activity of the tissue. Although this has been assumed to be a true loss of receptor protein, this has not been directly demonstrated. However, even if the receptor protein is present, it should not be capable of binding to the hCG affinity resin (due to its decreased binding activity). Therefore, by this criterion alone, the LH/CG receptor protein should not be present in the hCG affinity-purified material from down-regulated extracts. As shown in Fig. 7, silver-stained SDS gels of the material purified from the down-regulated ovaries did not reveal a 93-kDa protein, in spite of deliberate overstaining of the gel. Note that when overstained, the lower-molecular-mass proteins copurified with the receptor are readily observed.

In another experiment [^{125}I]hCG was used to probe blots prepared from SDS gels of the crude luteal detergent extract and the WGA- and affinity-purified material (Rosemblit *et al.*, 1988). As shown in Fig. 8, specific [^{125}I]hCG binding

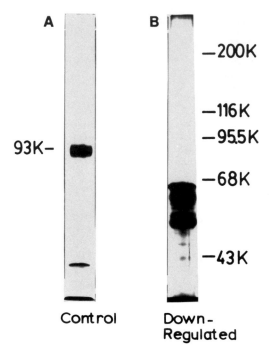

FIG. 7. Purification of the LH/CG receptor from control or down-regulated rat luteal tissue. Luteal membranes from control rats (A) or rats treated with hCG to down-regulate the hCG-binding activity (B) were solubilized and chromatographed on hCG affinity and wheat germ agglutinin–agarose columns, as described by Rosemblit et al. (1988). The resulting materials were analyzed on SDS gels in the presence of disulfide reducing agents, and the gels were silver stained. The gel containing the material purified from down-regulated ovaries (B) was deliberately overdeveloped to ensure the absence of the 93-kDa band, leading to an exaggeration of the contaminants present. (From Rosemblit et al., 1988.)

was observed to the 93-kDa protein in both samples, confirming the identity of this protein as the LH/CG receptor.

As shown in Fig. 9, when the purified rat luteal LH/CG receptor is analyzed on SDS gels in the presence or absence of reducing agents, only a single band of 93 kDa is observed. Thus, these results are again consistent with the LH/CG receptor's being composed of a single polypeptide.

Therefore, by chemical cross-linking of hCG to the LH/CG receptor (in MA-10 murine Leydig tumor cells and in porcine granulosa cells), by indirect immunoprecipitation of the biosynthetically labeled LH/CG receptor (in MA-10 cells), and by LH/CG receptor purification (from rat luteal tissue), we have consistently observed that the LH/CG receptor is composed of a single polypeptide with an estimated molecular mass of 93 kDa.

A Initial Extract **B** Purified Receptor

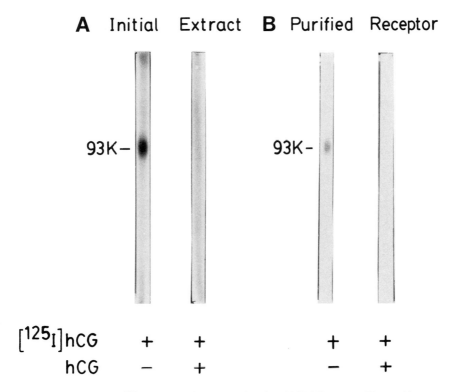

93K—   93K—

$[^{125}I]$hCG   +   +   +   +

hCG   −   +   −   +

FIG. 8. Binding of $[^{125}I]$hCG to Western blots of rat luteal LH/CG receptor. Western blots were prepared from SDS gels of a crude detergent extract of rat luteal membranes (A) or from purified LH/CG receptor (B) run in the absence of reducing agents. The blots were then incubated with $[^{125}I]$hCG alone or together with an excess of unlabeled hCG, as indicated. (From Rosemblit *et al.*, 1988.)

These results are in general agreement with those reported by Keinanen *et al.* (1987), Roche and Ryan (1989), Sojar and Bahl (1989), Kusuda and Dufau (1986), Minegishi *et al.* (1987), Rapoport *et al.* (1985), Rebois *et al.* (1981), and Rebois (1982). However, alternate structures invoking multiple subunits (joined covalently or noncovalently) have been proposed by a number of investigators (for a review see Ascoli and Segaloff, 1989). As discussed in Section II,A and in a recent review (Ascoli and Segaloff, 1989), we have argued that much of the data indicating multiple subunits for the LH/CG receptor can be explained by proteolysis (and/or nicking) of the receptor during the experimental procedures used.

It should be pointed out that although the apparent molecular mass of the denatured LH/CG receptor is 93 kDa, the apparent molecular mass of the non-denatured receptor has been reported to be 190–220 kDa (Dufau *et al.*, 1973;

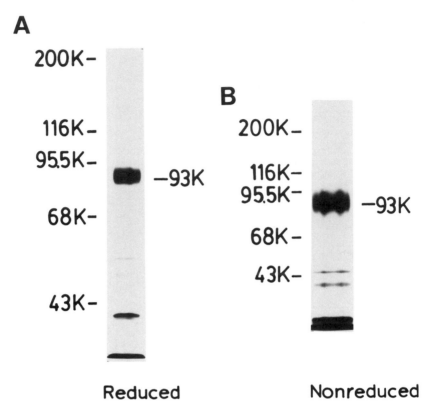

FIG. 9. Purified rat luteal LH/CG receptor analyzed in the absence or presence of disulfide reducing agents. Rat luteal LH/CG receptor, purified as described (Rosemblit *et al.*, 1988), was analyzed on SDS gels in the presence (A) or absence (B) of disulfide reducing agents, and the gels were then silver stained. (From Rosemblit *et al.*, 1988.)

Rebois *et al.*, 1987). Whether these data reflect a different tertiary structure of the receptor under denaturing versus nondenaturing conditions, or whether the receptor exits in the plasma membrane as a noncovalently associated oligomer of the 93-kDa polypeptide remains to be determined.

Prior to the cloning and expression of the LH/CG receptor cDNA (see below), all of the methods we and other investigators have used to study the structure of this receptor have, at one point or another in the experimental design, relied on the binding of hCG to the receptor. Thus, one caveat to bear in mind is that the 93-kDa LH/CG "receptor" identified and purified by these methods could represent an hCG-binding component of the receptor and that an additional protein(s) not identified (or copurified) by hCG binding might be required for coupling to the G_s protein.

III. Structure of the LH/CG Receptor as Determined by Cloning and Expression of a cDNA for the Rat Luteal LH/CG Receptor

A. ISOLATION OF A cDNA FOR THE RAT LUTEAL RECEPTOR

Rat luteal LH/CG receptor that was purified by WGA and hCG affinity chromatography was further purified by SDS gel electrophoresis. The 93-kDa receptor protein was electroblotted from the gel and was used directly for determining the amino-terminal amino acid sequence. In other experiments the 93-kDa receptor protein was electroeluted from the gel and was subjected to cleavage with lysyl C endopeptidase or with CNBr (McFarland *et al.*, 1989). The resulting fragments were purified and then were subjected to amino-terminal amino acid sequence analysis. The amino acid sequences thus obtained are shown in Table II.

Oligonucleotides based on the amino-terminal amino acid sequence of the intact receptor (underlined residues of lhrk in Table II) and on one of the internal amino acid sequences (underlined residues of lhrr in Table II) were used to prime a preparation of rat luteal cDNA. The polymerase chain reaction (PCR) was then used (Tung *et al.*, 1989), generating a 622-nucleotide cDNA. As predicted, the 5' end of this cDNA encoded for the amino-terminal sequence of the intact receptor, and the 3' end encoded for the internal amino acid sequence on which one of the oligonucleotide primers was based. Fortuitously, this cDNA also encoded for other amino acid sequences derived from receptor peptides. Thus,

TABLE II
Amino Acid Sequences Determined from Purified LH/CG Receptor Peptides[a]

Peptide	Amino acid sequence[b]
CNBr-derived peptides	
lhrk	KELSGSRKEPEPNDFAPDGAL̲XXPGP
lhrr	MXXESVTLKLYGNCFEEVQ
lhrf	MX(S)G̲AFOGATGPSILD̲(P)V
	(E) (I)
lhrc	M(D)YA(G)LXVLI(G)LINILDXF
	(G) (F) (F)
	(A)
	(N)
Lysyl C-endopeptidase peptides	
lhr26	KXYGNXFEVVQ
lhr28	KNLLYIEPGSF

[a]From McFarland *et al.* (1989). Copyright © 1989 by the American Association for the Advancement of Science.

[b]The underlined sequences were used to design the oligonucleotides used in the polymerase chain reaction (see text).

this PCR fragment appeared to be a partial cDNA for the LH/CG receptor. The PCR fragment was then used to screen a rat luteal λgt10 cDNA library, ultimately yielding a cDNA that has 43 nucleotides of a 5'-flanking region, 2100 nucleotides that represent the entire coding region, and 759 nucleotides of a 3'-flanking region (Fig. 10).

B.   CHARACTERISTICS OF THE cDNA FOR THE RAT LUTEAL LH/CG RECEPTOR

The nucleotide sequence of the rat LH/CG receptor cDNA and the deduced amino acid sequence are shown in Fig. 10. The open reading frame is 2100 nucleotides, encoding for a protein of 700 amino acids. The first 26 amino acids appear to be a signal sequence, as the subsequent 25 amino acids correspond to the amino acid sequence determined from the purified LH/CG receptor (lhrk in Table II). All of the amino acid sequences determined from LH/CG receptor peptides can be found within the open reading frame of this cDNA (see solid boxes atop amino acid sequences in Fig. 10). The mature receptor protein (minus the signal peptide) would be 674 amino acids and would be predicted to have a molecular mass of 75 kDa. The difference between this size and that observed for the purified receptor (i.e., 93 kDa) is presumably due to the glycoprotein nature of the receptor. As shown in Fig. 10, the primary sequence of the receptor reveals six potential sites for N-linked glycosylation, and preliminary evidence suggests that most of these sites are glycosylated (McFarland et al., 1989).

Of critical interest was whether the LH/CG receptor would be related to the family of G protein-coupled receptors that have been characterized to date. These receptors include rhodopsin (Findlay and Pappin, 1986; Nathans and Hogness, 1983), and the adrenergic (Dixon et al., 1986; Kobilka et al., 1987; Schofield et al., 1987), muscarinic acetylcholine (Kubo et al., 1986; Liao et al., 1989; Peralta et al., 1987), dopamine (Bunzow et al., 1988), serotonin (Julius et al., 1988; Pritchett et al., 1988), angiotensin (Jackson et al., 1988), and substance K receptors (Masu et al., 1987). All of these receptors appear to be related to each other by significant amino acid homology. Furthermore, they all contain seven regions of hydrophobic amino acids of sufficient length to span the plasma

---

FIG. 10.   The cDNA sequence and the deduced amino acid sequence of the rat luteal LH/CG receptor. Amino acids are numbered beginning with the amino-terminal sequence for the mature intact receptor, with negative numbers encoding the signal sequence. Solid bars above the sequence denote amino acid sequences determined from the purified receptor and receptor peptides (see Table II), with residues differing from those predicted by the open bars. Potential sites for N-linked glycosylation are noted by the inverted solid triangles, and the proposed membrane-spanning regions are enclosed in boxes. Lines above residues (e.g., amino acids 254–255) denote amino acids that are identical to a region of the soybean lectin (Schnell and Etzler, 1987). [From McFarland et al. (1989). Copyright © 1989 by the American Association for the Advancement of Science.]

```
-43 ATACTGGCTCAACCTCGGGAGCTCACACTCAGGCTGGCGGGCC

-26 Met Gly Arg Arg Val Pro Ala Leu Arg Gln Leu Leu Val Leu Ala Val Leu Leu Leu Lys Pro Ser Gln Leu Gln
  1 ATG GGG CGG CGA GTC CCA GCT CTG AGA CAG CTG CTG GTG CTG GCA GTG CTG CTG CTG AAG CCT TCA CAG CTG CAG

 -1 Ser Arg Glu Leu Ser Gly Ser Arg Cys Pro Glu Pro Cys Asp Cys Ala Pro Asp Gly Ala Leu Arg Cys Pro Gly
 76 TCC CGA GAG CTG TCA GGG TCG CGC TGC CCC GAG CCC TGC GAC TGC GCA CCG GAT GGC GCC CTG CGC TGT CCT GGC

 25 Pro Arg Ala Gly Leu Ala Arg Leu Ser Leu Thr Tyr Leu Pro Val Lys Val Ile Pro Ser Gln Ala Phe Arg Gly
151 CCT CGA GCC GGC CTC GCC AGA CTA TCT CTC ACC TAT CTC CCT GTC AAA GTA ATT CCA TCA CAA GCT TTC AGG GGA

 50 Leu Asn Glu Val Val Lys Ile Glu Ile Ser Gln Ser Asp Ser Leu Glu Arg Ile Glu Ala Asn Ala Phe Asp Asn
226 CTT AAT GAG GTC GTA AAA ATT GAA ATC TCT CAG AGT GAT TCC CTG GAA AGG ATA GAA GCT AAT GCC TTT GAC AAC

 75 Leu Leu Asn Leu Ser Glu Leu Leu Ile Gln Asn Thr Lys Asn Leu Leu Tyr Ile Glu Pro Gly Ala Phe Thr Asn
301 CTC CTC AAT TTG TCT GAA CTA CTG ATC CAG AAC ACC AAA AAC CTG CTA TAC ATT GAA CCT GGT GCT TTT ACA AAC

100 Leu Pro Arg Leu Lys Tyr Leu Ser Ile Cys Asn Thr Gly Ile Arg Thr Leu Pro Asp Val Thr Lys Ile Ser Ser
376 CTC CCT CGG TTA AAA TAC CTG AGC ATC TGT AAC ACA GGC ATC CGA ACC TTT CCA GAT GTT ACG AAG ATC TCC TCC

125 Ser Glu Phe Asn Phe Ile Leu Glu Ile Cys Asp Asn Leu His Ile Thr Thr Ile Pro Gly Asn Ala Phe Gln Gly
451 TCT GAA TTT AAT TTC ATT CTG GAA ATC TGT GAT AAT CTA CAC ATA ACC ACC ATA CCC GGG AAT GCT TTC CAA GGG

150 Met Asn Asn Glu Ser Val Thr Leu Lys Leu Tyr Gly Asn Gly Phe Glu Glu Val Gln Ser His Ala Phe Asn Gly
526 ATG AAT AAC GAG TCT GTC ACA CTA AAA CTG TAT GGA AAT GGA TTT GAA GAA GTA CAA AGC CAT GCA TTC AAT GGG

175 Thr Thr Leu Ile Ser Leu Glu Leu Lys Glu Asn Ile Tyr Leu Glu Lys Met His Ser Gly Ala Phe Gln Gly Ala
601 ACG ACT CTA ATC TCG CTG GAG CTA AAA GAA AAC ATC TAC CTG GAG AAG ATG CAC AGT GGA GCC TTC CAG GGG GCC

200 Thr Gly Pro Ser Ile Leu Asp Ile Ser Ser Thr Lys Leu Gln Ala Leu Pro Ser His Gly Leu Glu Ser Ile Gln
676 ACG GGG CCC AGC ATC CTG GAT ATT TCT TCC ACC AAA TTG CAG GCC CTG CCG AGC CAC GGG CTG GAG TCC ATT CAG

225 Thr Leu Ile Ala Leu Ser Ser Tyr Ser Leu Lys Thr Leu Pro Ser Lys Glu Lys Phe Thr Ser Leu Leu Val Ala
751 ACG CTC ATC GCC CTG TCT TCC TAC TCA CTG AAA ACA CTG CCC TCA AAG GAA AAA TTC ACG AGC CTC CTG GTC GCC

250 Thr Leu Thr Tyr Pro Ser His Cys Cys Ala Phe Arg Asn Leu Pro Lys Lys Glu Gln Asn Phe Ser Phe Ser Ile
826 ACG CTG ACC TAC CCC AGC CAC TGC TGC GCC TTC AGG AAT TTG CCG AAG AAA GAA CAG AAT TTT TCA TTT TCC ATT

275 Phe Glu Asn Phe Ser Lys Gln Cys Glu Ser Thr Val Arg Lys Ala Asp Asn Glu Thr Leu Tyr Ser Ala Ile Phe
901 TTT GAA AAC TTC TCC AAA CAA TGC GAA AGC ACA GTT AGA AAA GCA GAT AAT GAG ACG CTT TAT TCC GCA ATC TTT

300 Glu Glu Asn Glu Leu Ser Gly Trp Asp Tyr Asp Tyr Gly Phe Cys Ser Pro Lys Thr Leu Gln Cys Ala Pro Glu
976 GAG GAG AAT GAA CTC AGT GGC TGG GAT TAT GAT TAT GGC TTC TGT TCA CCC AAG ACA CTC CAA TGT GCT CCA GAA

325 Pro Asp Ala Phe Asn Pro Cys Glu Asp Ile Met Gly Tyr Ala Phe Leu Arg Val Leu Ile Trp Leu Ile Asn Ile
1051 CCA GAT GCT TTC AAC CCC TGT GAA GAT ATT ATG GGC TAT GCC TTC CTT AGG GTC CTG ATT TGG CTG ATT AAT ATA

350 Leu Ala Ile Phe Gly Asn Leu Thr Val Leu Phe Val Leu Leu Thr Ser Arg Tyr Lys Leu Thr Val Pro Arg Phe
1126 CTA GCC ATC TTT GGC AAC CTG ACA GTC CTC TTT GTT CTC CTG ACC AGT CGT TAT AAA CTG ACA GTG CCC CGC TTC

375 Leu Met Cys Asn Leu Ser Phe Ala Asp Phe Cys Met Gly Leu Tyr Leu Leu Leu Ile Ala Ser Val Asp Ser Gln
1201 CTC ATG TGT AAT CTC TCC TTT GCA GAC TTT TGC ATG GGG CTC TAC CTG CTG CTC ATT GCC TCC GTC GAC TCC CAA

400 Thr Lys Gly Gln Tyr Tyr Asn His Ala Ile Asp Trp Gln Thr Gly Ser Gly Cys Gly Ala Ala Gly Phe Phe Thr
1276 ACA AAA GGC CAG TAC TAT AAC CAC GCA ATA GAC TGG CAG ACA GGG AGT GGC TGC GGT GCA GCT GGC TTC TTT ACT

425 Val Phe Ala Ser Glu Leu Ser Val Tyr Thr Leu Thr Val Ile Thr Leu Glu Arg Trp His Thr Ile Thr Tyr Ala
1351 GTG TTT GCC AGT GAA CTC TCT GTC TAC ACC CTG ACG GTT ATC ACC CTG GAA AGG TGG CAC ACC ATC ACC TAT GCT

450 Val Gln Leu Asp Gln Lys Leu Arg Leu Arg His Ala Ile Pro Ile Met Leu Gly Gly Trp Leu Phe Ser Thr Leu
1426 GTA CAG CTA GAC CAA AAG CTA AGA CTG AGG CAT GCC ATC CCA ATT ATG CTC GGA GGA TGG CTC TTT TCT ACG CTG

475 Ile Ala Thr Met Pro Leu Val Gly Ile Ser Asn Tyr Met Lys Val Ser Ile Cys Leu Pro Met Asp Val Glu Ser
1501 ATC GCC ACG ATG CCC CTT GTG GGT ATC AGC AAT TAC ATG AAG GTC AGC ATC TGC CTC CCC ATG GAT GTG GAA TCC

500 Thr Leu Ser Gln Val Tyr Ile Leu Ser Ile Leu Ile Leu Asn Val Val Ala Phe Val Val Ile Cys Ala Cys Tyr
1576 ACT CTG TCC CAA GTC TAC ATA TTA TCC ATC TTA ATC CTC AAC GTG GTG GCC TTC GTC GTC ATC TGT GCT TGC TAC

525 Ile Arg Ile Tyr Phe Ala Val Gln Asn Pro Glu Leu Thr Ala Pro Asn Lys Asp Thr Lys Ile Ala Lys Lys Met
1651 ATT AGG ATC TAC TTT GCA GTT CAA AAT CCA GAG CTG ACA GCT CCT AAC AAG GAC ACA AAA ATT GCT AAG AAG ATG

550 Ala Ile Leu Ile Phe Thr Asp Phe Thr Cys Met Ala Pro Ile Ser Phe Phe Ala Ile Ser Ala Ala Phe Lys Val
1726 GCC ATC CTC ATC TTC ACA GAC TTC ACG TGC ATG GCG CCC ATC TCT TTC TTT GCC ATC TCG GCT GCC TTC AAA GTG

575 Pro Leu Ile Thr Val Thr Asn Ser Lys Ile Leu Leu Val Leu Phe Tyr Pro Val Asn Ser Cys Ala Asn Pro Phe
1801 CCC CTT ATC ACT GTC ACC AAC TCG AAA ATC TTA CTG GTC CTT TTT TAT CCT GTC AAT TCT TGT GCC AAT CCA TTT

600 Leu Tyr Ala Ile Phe Thr Lys Thr Phe Gln Arg Asp Phe Leu Leu Leu Leu Ser Arg Phe Gly Cys Cys Lys Arg
1876 CTG TAT GCG ATC TTC ACG AAG ACG TTT CAG AGA GAT TTC CTT CTG CTG AGC CGA TTC GGC TGC TGT AAA CGC

625 Arg Ala Glu Leu Tyr Arg Arg Lys Glu Phe Ser Ala Tyr Thr Ser Asn Cys Lys Asn Gly Phe Pro Gly Ala Ser
1951 CGG GCG GAC CTT TAC AGA AGG AAG GAA TTT TCT GCA TAT ACT TCC AAC TGC AAA AAT GGC TTC CCA GGA GCA AGT

650 Lys Pro Ser Gln Ala Thr Leu Lys Leu Ser Thr Val His Cys Gln Gln Pro Ile Pro Pro Arg Ala Leu Thr His
2026 AAG CCG TCC CAG GCT ACC CTG AAG TTG TCC ACA GTG CAC TGT CAA CAG CCC ATA CCA CCG AGA GCG TTA ACT CAC

2101 TAGCATTACAAAATTGTGCCTAAATATGTTTTTTAAAAAGTGTTTTAGAAAAATATTTATCCTTAGGCACTTCAGGAGAATTGTACCTGCTTCAGAGGAC
2201 GGCCTATAACACTTGGTCACATAAGTTTCAGGAAGGTTTAGAAATTTTTATAGTAATTTAGGCATAATAATTTTTTGTTGAATCTAATACTAAGGAAATC
2301 TAAGTTGTCATTTTTCACGTCTCTGACATTTTTCATTTCAATCTTGTGATTTACATTGTAATCTCCAAATATATTACTTCATAGCAGATTGAAAATTTAA
2401 ACTGGTCTTTGTCCTCAGATAGTTTGATAAATATATTCAAGAGATGCACTGTGCAGTGTGACTGCTAGCCTTGCATGGTAAATAGAAGTTTCTTTAGCCAT
2501 ATTCCAAGTGCTTCACATGTCACACTAGGAGGCACAGATGCAAACTGTTTACATCAGTGAATTCTATTAGCCAGCTCTATTCTTAGAGACTTCTATTTCCC
2601 ATTGACACTCTGCTTAACTTTCCATCTGAAGGCACATGCTGCATATTTGTTTGGCTTACAGATCATGAGTACCTCATGGCCAGGAGCCCATCTCAGCCCA
2701 TCTTGTTCCTCGTCTATCTCAGGATCTTGGAAATGCTACACAGCAAGCATGCCTAGCCAGTTAAACTCCCTAAATCTACACAGGAAAATATTTCTACCAC
2801 CTTAGCATATTGTTTTCGATGATTACATGCTTTCTGTATTTTGCCCTCCTCCTAGTATC
```

FIG. 10.

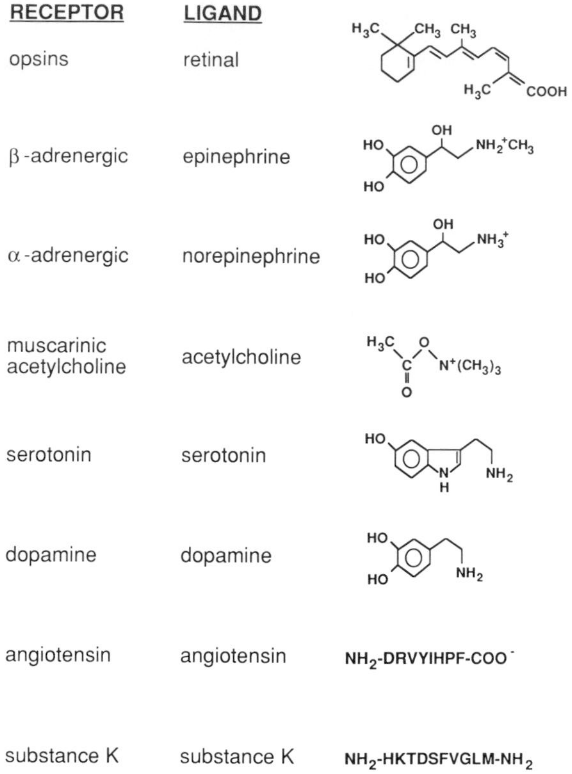

RECEPTOR   **LIGAND**

opsins   retinal

β-adrenergic   epinephrine

α-adrenergic   norepinephrine

muscarinic acetylcholine   acetylcholine

serotonin   serotonin

dopamine   dopamine

angiotensin   angiotensin NH_2-DRVYIHPF-COO$^-$

substance K   substance K NH_2-HKTDSFVGLM-NH_2

FIG. 11. G protein-coupled receptors and their ligands. Shown are the G protein-coupled receptors that had been characterized prior to the cloning of the LH/CG receptor. Also shown are the structures of their respective ligands.

membrane seven times. It has been demonstrated for both rhodopsin and the β-adrenergic receptor that the amino-terminal regions of these receptors are extracellular, the carboxy-terminal regions are intracellular, and they traverse the plasma membrane seven times (Findlay and Pappin, 1986; Wang *et al.*, 1989). By analogy, it is assumed that the other receptors in this family share these features.

Another common feature of the G protein-coupled receptors published to date is that they also bind small ligands. As shown in Fig. 11, the angiotensin and substance K receptors bind small peptides of 10–12 amino acids in length, and the other receptors mentioned bind even smaller relatively hydrophobic molecules. Since it has been shown for rhodopsin and for the β-adrenergic receptor that their respective ligands interact directly with amino acids within their plasma membrane-spanning regions (Dixon *et al.*, 1987; Dohlman *et al.*, 1988; Wang *et al.*, 1989; Wong *et al.*, 1988), one could question whether the particular feature of seven membrane-spanning regions present in these receptors is necessary for the coupling of the receptor to the G protein or if it is required for the binding of these small ligands. In contrast to these G protein-coupled receptors, the LH/CG receptor binds large (i.e., 28–38 kDa) glycoproteins and has been shown to have a large extracellular domain (Ascoli and Segaloff, 1986; Keinanen and Rajaniemi, 1986). Thus, it was of immediate interest to determine which structural features, if any, the LH/CG receptor would share with the other G protein-coupled receptors mentioned above.

To address this question, a comparison was made between the hydropathy plot for the rat luteal LH/CG receptor and those of the rhodopsinlike G protein-coupled receptors. It is readily apparent, as shown in Fig. 12, that the

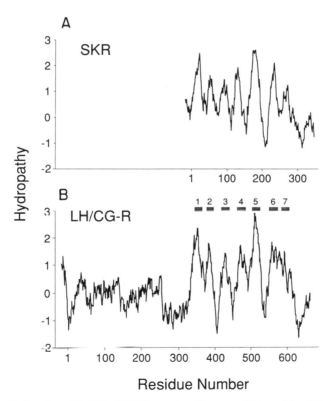

FIG. 12.   Hydropathy plot of the LH/CG receptor. Shown are Kyte and Doolittle hydropathy plots (window of 20 residues) for (A) the substance K receptor (SKR) and (B) the LH/CG receptor (LH/CG-R). The seven putative transmembrane regions of the LH/CG receptor are noted by the solid bars atop them. [From McFarland *et al.* (1989). Copyright © 1989 by the American Association for the Advancement of Science.]

carboxy-terminal half of the LH/CG receptor indeed displays a strikingly similar hydropathy plot to that of the substance K receptor, suggesting that this half of the LH/CG receptor possesses seven membrane-spanning regions. It should be pointed out that of the rhodopsinlike G protein coupled-receptors the substance K receptor gives the best alignment of hydropathy patterns to the LH/CG receptor, due to its relatively short third intracellular cytoplasmic loop (between trans-membrane regions V and VI).

In addition to the similarity of hydropathy plots, the carboxy-terminal half of the LH/CG receptor shows significant amino acid homology with all members of the G protein-coupled receptor family. An alignment of the amino acids within the carboxy-terminal half of the LH/CG receptor with selected members of the G protein-coupled receptor family is shown in Fig. 13. Amino acid identity is highest when the regions of the LH/CG receptor shown in Fig. 13 are compared with the β-adrenergic receptor (26%) and lower when compared with other receptors in this family (18–24%). However, when the full-length sequences are compared, the LH/CG receptor shows greater overall identity with rhodopsin and the substance K receptor (22%, due to the shorter length of their regions between the membrane-spanning domains V and VI) than with the β-adrenergic receptor or the other neurotransmitter receptors (18–21%).

Studies with the β-adrenergic receptor have suggested that the amino acids preceding the fifth and following the seventh membrane-spanning regions might be important for receptor–G_s coupling (O'Dowd et al., 1988; Strader et al., 1987). Interestingly, however, the LH/CG receptor does not appear to share a greater percentage of amino acid identity with the β-adrenergic receptor in these (or any) regions than with those receptors that couple to other G proteins, such as the muscarinic acetylcholine or serotonin receptors (see Fig. 13).

Thus, it appears that the carboxy-terminal half of the LH/CG receptor shares both amino acid and structural homologies with the rhodopsinlike G protein-coupled receptors. In marked contrast, however, the LH/CG receptor also contains a large (i.e., 341 amino acids in length) amino-terminal hydrophilic domain (see Fig. 12). By analogy with rhodopsin and the β-adrenergic receptor, this amino-terminal region would be predicted to be extracellular (see below). An obvious question is whether this large hydrophilic domain of the LH/CG receptor is related to any other cell surface receptors. At the moment, no such similarities have been published. When amino acid sequences are compared, the protein most similar to the extracellular domain of the LH/CG receptor is PG40, a collagen-binding proteoglycan found in the extracellular matrices of connective tissues (Krusius and Ruoslahti, 1986).

Analysis of the amino acids in the extracellular domain, however, does reveal a noteworthy feature. Thus, as shown in Fig. 14, this region contains a 14-fold imperfectly repeated sequence of approximately 25 residues. The amino acids which are aligned and the spacing between them are similar to a repeat motif,

TM-1   TM-2

```
LH/CGR 339 F L R V L I  W L I  N I  L A I  F G N L T V L F V L L T S - - R Y K L - T V P R F L M C N L S F A D F  384
RHO     36 Q F S M L A A Y M F L L I  M L G F P I  N F L T L Y V T V Q H K K L R T P L N Y I  L L N L A V A D L   84
SKR     35 L W T A A Y L A L V L V A V M G N A T V I  W I  I  L A - - - H Q R M R T V T N Y F I  V N L A L A D L  80
ß-2AR   35 G M G I  V M S L I  V L A I  V F G N V L V I  T A I  A K - - - F E R L Q T V T N Y F I  T S L A C A D L  80
5HT-2R  53 W S A L L T T V V I  I  L T I  A G N I  L V I  M A V S L - - - E K K L Q N A T N Y F L M S L A I  A D M  99
```

TM-3

```
LH/CGR  C M G L Y L L L I  A S V D S Q T K G Q Y Y N H A I  D W Q T G - S G C G A A G F F T V F A S E L S V Y  433
RHO     F M V F G G F T T T L Y T S L - - - - - - - - H G Y F V F G P T G C N L E G F F A T L G G E I  A L W   126
SKR     C M A A F N A A F N F V Y A S - - - - - - - - H N I  W Y F G R A F C Y F Q N L F P I  T A M F V S I  Y  122
ß-2AR   V M G L A V V P F G A A H I  L - - - - - - - - M K M W T F G N F W C E F W T S I  D V L C V T A S I  E  122
5HT-2R  L L G F L V M P V S M L T I  L - - - - - - - Y G Y R W P L P S K L C A I  W I  Y L D V L F S T A S I  M  142
```

TM-4

```
LH/CGR  T L T V I  T L E R W H T I  T Y A V Q L D Q K L R L R H A I  P I  M L G G W L F S T L I  A T M P L V G I  483
RHO     S L V V L A I  E R Y V V V C K P M S N F R F - G E N H A I  M G V A F T W V M A L A C A A P P L V G W   175
SKR     S M T A I  A A D R Y M A I  V H P F Q P R L S A P G T R A - - V I  A G I  W L V A L A L A F - P Q C F Y  169
ß-2AR   T L C V I  A V D R Y F A I  T S P F K Y Q S L L T K N K A R V I  I  L M V W I  V S G L T S F L P I  Q M H  172
5HT-2R  H L C A I  S L D R Y V A I  Q N P I  H H S R F N S R T K A F L K I  I  A V W T I  S V G I  S M - P I  P V F  191
```

TM-5

```
LH/CGR  S N Y - - - M K V S I  C L P M D V E S T L - - - S Q V Y I  L S I  L I  L N V V A F - V V I  C A C Y I  R  526
RHO     S R Y I  P E G M Q C S C G I  D Y Y T P H E E T N N E S F V I  Y M F V V H F I  I  P L I  V I  F F C Y G Q  225
SKR     S T I  T T D E G A T K C V V A W P E D S G G K M L L L Y H L I  V I  A L I  Y F L P L V V M F V A Y S V   219
ß-2AR   W Y R A T H Q E A I  N C Y A N E T C C D F - F T N Q A Y A I  A S S I  V S F Y V P L V I  M V F V Y S R   221
5HT-2R  G L Q D D S K V F K E G S C L L A D - - - - - - - D N F V L I  G S F V A F F I  P L T I  M V I  T Y F L   234
```

TM-6

```
LH/CGR  I  Y F A V Q N P E L T A P N K D T K I  A K K M A I  L I  F T D F T - C M A P I  S F F A I  S A A F K V P  575
RHO     L V F T V K E A A A     (8)  Q K A E K E V T R M V I  I  M V I  A F L I  C W L P Y A G V A F Y I  F T H Q G  280
SKR     I  G L T L W R R S V     (12) L Q A K K K F V K T M V L V V V T F A I  C W L P Y H L Y F I  L G T F Q E D  278
ß-2AR   V F Q E A K R Q L Q     (33) C L K E H K A L K T L G I  I  M G T F T L C W L P F F I  V N I  V H V I  Q D N  301
5HT-2R  T I  K S L Q K E A T     (48) I  S N E Q K A C K V L G I  V F F L F V V M W C P F F I  T N I  M A V I  C K E  329
```

TM-7

```
LH/CGR  L I  T V T N S - - - K I  L L V L F Y P V N S C A N P F L Y A I  F T K A F Q R D F L L L L S R F G C  621/674
RHO     S D F G P I  F - - - M T I  P A F F A K T S A V Y N P V I  Y I  M M N K Q F R N C M V T T L C C G K N  326/348
SKR     I  Y C H K F I  Q Q - Y L A L F W L A M S S T M Y N P I  I  Y C C L N H R F R S G F R L A F R C C P W  327/384
ß-2AR   L I  R K E V - - - - Y I  L L N W I  G Y V N S G F N P L I  Y - C R S P D F R I  A F Q E L L C L R R S  345/413
5HT-2R  S C N E N V I  G A L L N V F V W I  G Y L S S A V N P L V Y T L F N K T Y R S A F S R Y I  Q C Q Y K  378/449
```

FIG. 13. Alignment of the carboxy-terminal half of the LH/CG receptor with other receptors that couple to G proteins. The transmembrane regions of the rat LH/CG receptor (LH/CGR) were aligned (see McFarland *et al.*, 1989) with those of bovine rhodopsin (RHO) (Nathans and Hogness, 1983), the bovine substance K receptor (SKR) (Masu *et al.*, 1987), the human β₂-adrenergic receptor (β-2AR) (Schofield *et al.*, 1987), and the rat 5HT-2 serotonin receptor (5HT-2R) (Pritchett *et al.*, 1988). Amino acids that are identical at a given position in three or more of the proteins are enclosed by boxes. Solid bars atop the sequences denote the seven putative transmembrane numbers in parentheses between transmembrane regions V and VI (TM-5 and -6) correspond to the number of residues deleted to maximize the alignment. [From McFarland *et al.* (1989). Copyright © 1989 by the American Association for the Advancement of Science.]

A

```
          (1-11)   R E L S G S R C P E P
  I      (12-38)   C D C A P D G - - A L R C P G P R A G L A R L S L T Y L P -
 II      (39-63)   V K V I P S Q - - A F R G L N E V V - K I E I S Q S D S - -
III      (64-88)   L E R I E A N - - A F D N L L N L S - E L L I Q N T K N - -
 IV      (89-112)  L L Y I E P G - - A F T N L P R L K - Y L S I C N T G - - -
  V      (113-138) I R T L P D V - - T K I S S S E F N F I L E I C D N L H - -
 VI      (139-164) I T T I P G N - - A F Q G M N N E S V T L K L Y G N G - - -
VII      (165-187) F E E V Q S H - - A F N G T T L I S - - L E L K E N I Y - -
VIII     (188-211) L E K M H S G - - A F Q G A T G P S - I L D I S S T K - - -
 IX      (212-233) L Q A L P S H - - - - - G L E S I Q T L I A L S S Y S - - -
  X      (234-251) L K T L P S K - E K F T S L L V A T L - - - - - - - - - -
 XI      (252-273) - - T Y P S H C C A F R N L P K K E Q N F S F S - - - - - -
XII      (274-290) - - - - - - - - - I F E N F S K Q C E S T V R K A D - - - -
XIII     (291-318) N E T L Y S A - - I F E E N E L S G W D Y D Y G F C S P K T
XIV      (319-341) L Q C A P E P - D A F N P C E D I M G Y A F L R - - - - - -
```

B

```
LRG     L x x L P x x - - L L x x L x x L x - x L D L S x N x
Toll    L x x L P x x - - L F x H x x N L x - x L x L x x N x
GPIB    L T T L P x G - - L L x x L P x L x - x L x L S x N x
ACY     a x x a P x x - - - a x x L x x L x - x L x L x x N x
```

FIG. 14.   The leucine-rich repetitive motif in the amino-terminal half of the LH/CG receptor. (A) Alignment of 14 imperfect repeats (numbered I–IV) observed in the amino-terminal half of the LH/CG receptor. Amino acids that are identical or conserved at a given position among the segments are boxed. Dashes indicate the placement of gaps to optimize the periodicity. (B) Consensus sequences for the leucine-rich repetitive motifs observed in the leucine-rich α_2 glycoprotein of human serum (LRG) (Takahashi *et al.*, 1985), the Toll developmental gene of *Drosophila* (Toll) (Hashimoto *et al.*, 1988), the α chain of human platelet glycoprotein 1b (GB1B) (Lopez *et al.*, 1987), and the yeast adenylyl cyclase (ACY) (Kataoka *et al.*, 1985). a, One of three aliphatic amino acids: valine, leucine, or isoleucine. (From McFarland *et al.*, 1989.)

termed a "leucine-rich repeat," that has been recognized in various proteins composing the family of leucine-rich glycoproteins (see Fig. 14). This family includes such widely divergent proteins as PG40 (see above) (Krusius and Ruoslahti, 1986), the α_2 serum glycoprotein (Takahashi *et al.*, 1985), the Toll developmental gene of *Drosophila* (Hashimoto *et al.*, 1988), the yeast adenylyl cyclase (Hashimoto *et al.*, 1988), and the α chain of the human platelet protein 1b (Lopez *et al.*, 1987).

The functional significance of this repeat motif is not clearly understood, although it has been suggested that this structure might, by forming amphipathic helices, be able to interact with both hydrophobic and hydrophilic surfaces. This raises the interesting possibility that such a repeat structure in the extracellular region of the LH/CG receptor could enable the extracellular domain to interact with both the hormone and the hydrophobic transmembrane regions of the receptor or the cell membrane. This possibility remains to be tested experimentally.

The observations noted above suggest that the LH/CG receptor might have originated by a recombination of genes encoding a hormone-binding glycoprotein (related to the family of leucine-rich glycoproteins) and a seven-transmembrane protoreceptor.

There has also been a report from Loosfelt et al. (1989) on the cloning of the porcine testicular LH/CG receptor. As discussed in Section II,A, our studies on the chemical cross-linking of hCG to the LH/CG receptor had suggested that the overall size and structure of this receptor in these two different species were similar. In comparing the deduced amino acid sequences from the cloned cDNAs, there is, in fact, an 87% identity of amino acids between the rat luteal and the porcine testicular LH/CG receptors. The residues that are identical between these two molecules are noted in Fig. 15.

C. FUNCTIONAL ASPECTS OF THE LH/CG RECEPTOR DEDUCED FROM ITS PRIMARY STRUCTURE

From the amino acid sequence of the rat luteal LH/CG receptor, and by analogy with the topography of other G protein-coupled receptors, we postulated that the LH/CG receptor exists in the plasma membrane, with the amino-terminal hydrophilic half being extracellular and the carboxy-terminal half spanning the plasma membrane seven times, ending with a relatively short cytoplasmic tail (see Fig. 15). As discussed below, immunofluorescence studies in intact cells using site-specific antibodies directed toward the amino- and carboxy-terminal regions of the receptor confirm the postulated orientation.

The structure of the LH/CG receptor based on its amino acid sequence is consistent with previous biochemical data suggesting that the LH/CG receptor has a large (i.e., 65 kDa) extracellular domain (Ascoli and Segaloff, 1986; Keinanen and Rajaniemi, 1986; Kellokumpu and Rajaniemi, 1985a,b). Given that hCG and LH are 38- and 28-kDa glycoproteins, respectively, this is not unexpected. Furthermore, it has been shown that a large extracellular region of the receptor is involved (at least in part) in binding hormone. Rajaniemi and co-workers have shown that a 65-kDa water-soluble fragment proteolytically released from rat luteal membranes, resolved by SDS polyacrylamide gel electrophoresis, and transferred to nitrocellulose specifically binds [^{125}I]hCG (Keinanen and Rajaniemi, 1986). It remains to be determined, however, whether the extracellular domain alone can bind hCG (or LH) with the high affinity characteristic of the intact receptor, or whether a subsequent interaction of the hormone/extracellular domain with the transmembrane region of the receptor is necessary for high-affinity binding.

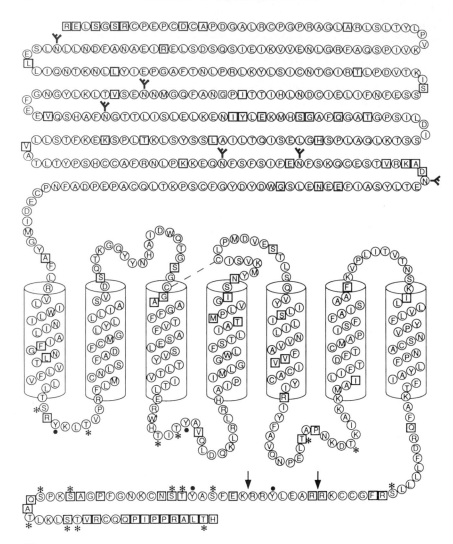

FIG. 15. Postulated topology of the LH/CG receptor in the plasma membrane. Amino acids that are identical between the rat luteal (McFarland *et al.*, 1989) and porcine testicular (Loosfelt *et al.*, 1989) LH/CG receptors are enclosed in circles. Those enclosed in squares are unique to the rat luteal receptor. Amino acids in barrels correspond to the putative transmembrane regions, those amino acids above the barrels being extracellular, those below the barrels being intracellular. Potential sites for N-linked glycosylation in the extracellular region are denoted by (**Y**). A potential disulfide bond between the first and second extracellular loop regions is noted by the dashed line. Potential intracellular sites for phosphorylation are denoted by asterisks (serines and threonines) or solid circles (tyrosines). The two arrows in the cytoplasmic tail point to two clusters of basic amino acids which might represent potential tryptic cleavage sites.

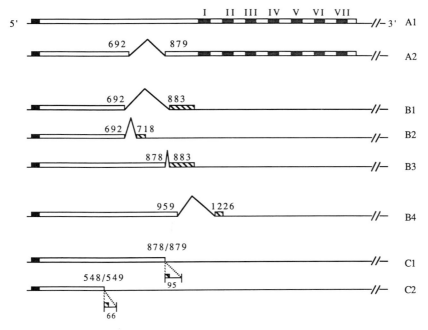

FIG. 16.   Differentially spliced forms of rat ovarian LH/CG receptor cDNA. The top scheme depicts the complete LH/CG receptor cDNA (A1) containing a region encoding the signal sequence (solid bar), a section encoding the extracellular receptor domain (open bar), and the sequence encoding transmembrane regions I–VII. Untranslated regions are represented by thin lines. A2 represents an alternatively spliced version of A1, deleting amino acid residues 206–268. B1–B4 are differentially spliced cDNAs, leading to the translation of a different reading frame (cross-hatched bar) with early termination. C1 and C2 contain 95 and 66 nucleotides, respectively, of presumptive intronic sequences. The positions of the nucleotides (McFarland *et al.*, 1989) which flank all variation points are indicated. In addition to the cDNAs shown, combinations of these variants were also found.

   Interestingly, the sequence analysis of cloned LH/CG receptor cDNAs isolated from the ovarian cDNA library (see Section III,A) revealed an unexpectedly high number of cDNAs encoding truncated forms of the LH/CG receptor (Fig. 16). One such cDNA (A2) is missing 186 nucleotides encoding a variant receptor which lacks 62 residues of the extracellular domain. The deleted region includes residues homologous to a soybean lectin (see below). Other cDNA variants displayed similar deletions and some carried insertions presumably of intronic origin. As seen in Fig. 16, many of these variants lead to frameshifts which introduce premature translational termination. Some of these variants are predicted to generate the extracellular domain of the LH/CG receptor lacking the transmembrane regions. These variants are likely to be created by alternative, incomplete, or incorrect splicing events. Similarly truncated LH/CG receptor cDNAs were isolated from a porcine testicular library by Loosfelt *et al.* (1989).

We are currently investigating the potential biological significance of these findings. It is possible that if extracellular domains of this receptor were expressed, they could act as competitive inhibitors of the receptor or as carriers of LH and hCG.

The overall structure of the LH/CG receptor is unique in that, unlike other G protein-coupled receptors characterized to date, it possesses this large extracellular domain that seems to be involved in ligand binding. As the other rhodopsinlike G protein-coupled receptors all bind small ligands and these ligands are thought to interact directly with amino acids within the plasma membrane-spanning regions (Dixon *et al.*, 1987; Dohlman *et al.*, 1988; Wang *et al.*, 1989; Wong *et al.*, 1988), it appears that the mechanism of the translation of ligand binding to G protein coupling in the LH/CG receptor must be inherently different from that of the rhodopsinlike receptors. Whether such a mechanism involves interaction of the hormone and/or extracellular domain of the LH/CG receptor with the transmembrane regions of this receptor after hormone binding or the information is transferred by more indirect conformational changes remain challenging questions to be addressed.

Another feature contained within the extracellular domain is a site where 10 of 12 amino acids (244–255; Fig. 10) are identical to a region of the soybean lectin. This is of interest because it is well known that although deglycosylated forms of hCG or LH bind to the LH/CG receptor with high affinity, they elicit little, if any, stimulation of cAMP production (Matzuk *et al.*, 1989; Moyle *et al.*, 1975; Sairam and Bhargavi, 1985). Although it is tempting to speculate that this site in the LH/CG receptor might be involved in the signal transduction process elicited by glycosylated hormones, it should be pointed out that in the soybean lectin this sequence is not thought to be involved in carbohydrate binding (Schnell and Etzler, 1987). Analysis of receptors lacking this domain should help to clarify whether it does have any biological role.

In examining the amino acid sequence of the regions of the receptor that are believed to be exposed cytoplasmically, it is apparent that numerous serines, threonines, and tyrosines are present within the intracellular loops and within the cytoplasmic tail (see Fig. 15), raising the possibility that the function and/or levels of this receptor are modulated by phosphorylation. It is also apparent that there are two clusters of basic amino acids (see Fig. 15) which might represent potential tryptic cleavage sites. Although preliminary data (see below) suggest that at least some of the mature receptor is not cleaved at either of these sites, it remains possible that such a cleavage occurs under some conditions and that it, too, might be related to receptor function.

D. FUNCTIONAL EXPRESSION OF THE LH/CG RECEPTOR cDNA

The cloning of the rat luteal LH/CG receptor cDNA was done based on amino acid sequence data derived from receptor that was purified (in part) by hCG affinity chromatography. Therefore, from the outset we had to consider that we might have cloned the cDNA for the hCG-binding subunit of the receptor and that an additional protein(s) might be necessary for the coupling of the receptor to G_s. However, once cloned, the observed homology between the carboxy-terminal half of the LH/CG receptor and other G protein-coupled receptors made it reasonable to predict that this cDNA would, in fact, encode for a receptor that could both bind hormone and activate cAMP formation.

To test the functional activity of the cloned LH/CG receptor cDNA, it was subcloned into an expression vector under the transcriptional control of the cytomegalovirus promoter, and this was used to transiently transfect human kidney 293 cells (McFarland et al., 1989).

When α-labeled hCG was bound and cross-linked to the transfected cells and the cross-linked products were analyzed on SDS gels, a receptor–hormone complex of 107 kDa was observed. These results are identical to those observed when the same experiment is done with MA-10 cells (see Section II,A) and suggest that the same-size LH/CG receptor (i.e., 93 kDa) is present in the transfected cells. Thus, the 293 cells appear to posttranslationally process the 75-kDa receptor protein encoded by the LH/CG receptor cDNA to a 93-kDa mature receptor. Furthermore, this mature expressed receptor specifically binds hCG.

As shown in Fig. 17, transfected cells incubated with increasing concentrations of [^{125}I]hCG bound hCG in a concentration-dependent and saturable manner (whereas mock transfected cells did not bind [^{125}I]hCG at all). In additional experiments the affinities of hCG and ovine LH were determined in transfected cells using a competition assay with trace amounts of [^{125}I]hCG. These experiments show that hCG binds with an affinity of 100 pM, which is comparable to that observed with the purified rat luteal LH/CG receptor (see Section II,C). As would be predicted, ovine LH binds with a lower affinity (7.4 nM). At the concentrations tested (up to 180 ng/ml) neither hFSH nor hTSH displaced bound [^{125}I]hCG.

The results presented in Fig. 17 also show that the addition of increasing concentrations of hCG to 293 cells transfected with the LH/CG receptor expression vector showed a dose-dependent and saturable increase in the production of cAMP. These data confirm that the 93-kDa LH/CG receptor protein we have identified and purified is not simply a hormone-binding subunit of the receptor, but is sufficient for both hormone binding and activation of adenylyl cyclase. More complete dose curves show that the EC_{50}s for hCG- and ovine LH-stimulated cAMP production are 36 pM. Furthermore, the maximal amount of cAMP produced in response to hCG or ovine LH is comparable to that elicited by isoproterenol, which binds to endogenous β-adrenergic receptors on the 293 cells. High concentrations (i.e., 50 ng/ml) of hTSH or hFSH elicited little, if any, increase in cAMP levels in the transfected 293 cells.

These results show that the cloned cDNA for the LH/CG receptor encodes for a 93-kDa receptor that both binds hormones and activates adenylyl cyclase.

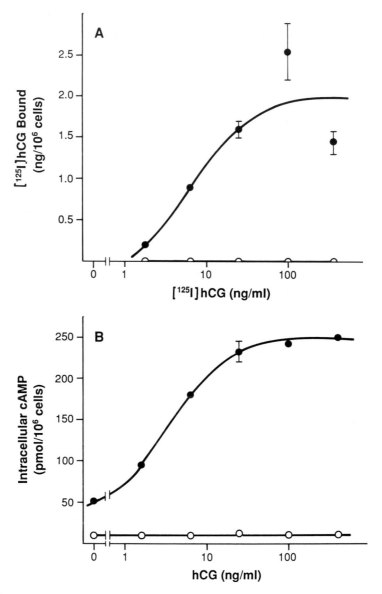

FIG. 17.   Functional expression of the LH/CG receptor cDNA. Kidney 293 cells were transiently transfected with (●) or without (○) an expression vector containing the rat luteal LH/CG receptor cDNA and were assayed for [125I]hCG binding (A) or hCG-stimulated cAMP production (B) 42 hours later. [From McFarland *et al.* (1989). Copyright © 1989 by the American Association for the Advancement of Science.]

Furthermore, the binding specificity of the expressed receptor for the different glycoprotein hormones, the binding affinities for hCG and ovine LH, and the EC_{50}s for hCG and ovine LH-stimulated cAMP production are comparable to the endogenous LH/CG receptors of gonadal tissues (Buettner and Ascoli, 1984; Conti *et al.*, 1977; Payne *et al.*, 1980; Pereira *et al.*, 1987).

A more complete characterization of the properties of the LH/CG receptor expressed from the cloned cDNA is in progress. Preliminary data suggest that, in addition to binding hormone and activating adenylyl cyclase, the expressed receptor is also capable of hormone-dependent desensitization of adenylyl cyclase activation, hormone-dependent internalization, and hormone-dependent down-regulation of receptor levels. Therefore, the data collected thus far suggest that the LH/CG receptor expressed from the cDNA described is fully functional.

E. LH/CG RECEPTOR mRNAs

When the ovary of a rat 9 days pregnant was examined by *in situ* hybridization with the antisense strand of the LH/CG receptor cDNA, intense hybridization to the corpora lutea was observed (McFarland *et al.*, 1989). Much fainter hybridization was also observed to the theca and interstitial cells. Hybridization to granulosa cells of the small immature follicles (which do not yet express hCG-binding activity) was not observed.

A Northern blot analysis of total RNA isolated from different tissues of the rat is shown in Fig. 18. Ovaries from pseudopregnant rats and ovaries and testes from adult cycling rats show hybridization of the LH/CG receptor cDNA to mRNAs of 6.7, 4.3, 2.6, and 1.2 kb. Importantly, no hybridization is observed in rat liver, lung, or kidney. Furthermore, within the gonadal tissues tested, the relative abundance of LH/CG receptor mRNA is comparable to the relative degree of [^{125}I]hCG binding to these tissues (Ascoli and Segaloff, 1989; Roche and Ryan, 1985, 1989). The apparent discrepancy between the sizes of hybridizing mRNA species we previously reported (McFarland *et al.*, 1989) and those reported here is due to the fact that, whereas the previous report used DNA markers for the determination of mRNA sizes, the data in Fig. 17 were calculated using RNA markers.

It should be pointed out that the open reading frame of the complete LH/CG receptor is 2.1 kb. Since one of the different LH/CG receptor mRNA species is only 1.2 kb, it might represent a mRNA that encodes for a truncated form of the receptor. Although there are no direct data yet to show that a truncated form of the LH/CG receptor protein exists physiologically, as discussed in Section III,C, it is an interesting hypothesis that deserves further experimentation.

It is also important to note that it is not known which of the larger mRNAs (6.7, 4.5, or 2.6 kb) that hybridize to the LH/CG receptor cDNA is used for the translation of the LH/CG receptor protein.

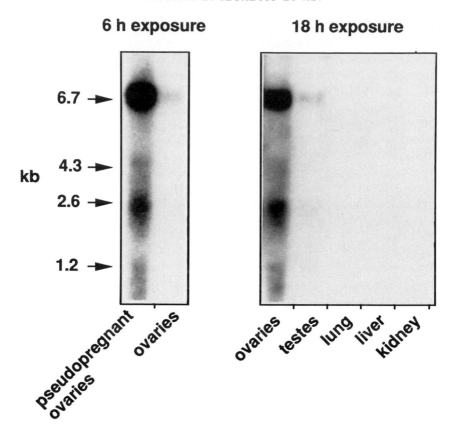

FIG. 18. Northern blot analysis of LH/CG receptor cDNA hybridization to RNA of different tissues. Total RNA from the ovaries of pseudopregnant rats or from the ovaries, testes, lung, liver, or kidney of adult rats (as indicated) were used to prepare a Northern blot which was probed with a polymerase chain reaction-generated LH/CG receptor cDNA fragment corresponding to nucleotides 1–622 (McFarland *et al.*, 1989). Shown are 6-hour and overnight (18-hour) exposures of the same blot. The sizes of the observed bands have been calculated using RNA molecular size markers. [Modified from McFarland *et al.* (1989). Copyright © 1989 by the American Association for the Advancement of Science.]

IV. Topology of the LH/CG Receptor as Determined by Antireceptor Antibodies

We have recently begun using site-specific antibodies toward regions of the rat luteal LH/CG receptor to directly ascertain the topology of this receptor in the plasma membrane. Polyclonal antibodies have been raised toward synthetic peptides corresponding to specific regions of the rat luteal receptor. One of these, anti-LHR02, is directed toward amino acids 194–206 (see Fig. 10), which are in the amino-terminal half of the receptor. This antiserum is specific for the LH/CG receptor, as determined by its ability to recognize only the 93-kDa receptor on Western blots prepared from WGA-purified rat luteal extracts. Primary cultures of rat luteal cells were incubated with immunoglobulin Gs (IgGs) prepared from this antiserum and were visualized by indirect immunofluorescence. In contrast to IgGs prepared from the preimmune serum, the immune anti-LHR02 IgGs resulted in fluorescently labeled luteal cells. This immunofluorescence could be diminished if the cells were incubated with anti-LHR02 in the presence of the peptide LHR02. As these cells were intact, these data confirm that the amino-terminal region of the LH/CG receptor is, in fact, extracellular.

An antiserum to the extreme carboxy-terminal region of the LH/CG receptor, designated anti-LHR06, was also prepared. The peptide used as the antigen corresponds to amino acids 661–674 of the receptor (see Fig. 10), which is in the putative cytoplasmic tail of the receptor. When used to probe Western blots prepared from WGA-purified rat luteal extracts, anti-LHR06 bound only to a 93-kDa LH/CG receptor protein. As mentioned in Section III,C, there are two clusters of basic amino acids (at positions 623–625 and 630–632) that raised that possibility that the mature LH/CG receptor terminates at one of these positions (due to tryptic cleavage), rather than at the position suggested by the stop codon found in the cDNA. Thus, the finding that LHR06 (which was raised to a peptide derived from the extreme carboxy terminus predicted by the cDNA) recognizes the 93-kDa LH/CG receptor protein indicates that at least some of the mature receptor is not proteolyzed.

The anti-LHR06 antiserum was also used for immunofluorescent detection of the LH/CG receptor in primary cultures of rat luteal cells. When intact luteal cells were incubated with this antiserum, no immunofluorescence was observed. These data are consistent with the proposed intracellular location of the carboxy-terminal region of the receptor. Moreover, when the cells were permeabilized with detergent first and then incubated with anti-LHR06, an intense immunofluorescence, which could be blocked by coincubation with the peptide LHR06, was observed. These data, again, suggest that the carboxy-terminal region of the LH/CG receptor is not cleaved in all or some receptor molecules and confirm that the carboxy-terminal domain of the receptor is, in fact, cytoplasmic and available for antibody binding.

V. Antibodies to the LH/CG Receptor Which Interfere with hCG Binding

The first anti-LH/CG receptor antiserum which we developed (Rosemblit et al., 1988) was raised against a homogenous preparation of rat luteal receptor purified by WGA chromatography, affinity chromatography, and SDS electrophoresis. The 93-kDa receptor was electroeluted from the gel and used as the antigen. Perhaps not surprisingly, the resulting antiserum, although quite specific for the LH/CG receptor on nitrocellulose, had no effect on [^{125}I]hCG binding.

Since then, we have developed three antisera to the LH/CG receptor which interfere with [^{125}I]hCG binding. One of these is a polyclonal antiserum raised against the WGA- and affinity-purified receptor. By avoiding further purification on an SDS gel, this receptor was not denatured, but it was about 80% pure when used as an antigen. The resulting antiserum, designated #145, is quite specific for the receptor, as assayed by Western blotting. Unlike #145, the other two antireceptor antisera that affect [^{125}I]hCG binding are both site specific. One of these is anti-LHR02, which was described in Section IV, and is directed against amino acids 194–206 in the extracellular domain. The other, designated anti-LHR04, is directed toward the first 14 amino acids in the amino terminus.

Although data thus far show that anti-LHR04 inhibits [^{125}I]hCG binding to the detergent-solubilized rat luteal LH/CG receptor, we have not yet determined whether this inhibition is due to an effect of the antiserum on the affinity of the receptor for the hormone or an effect on the apparent number of binding sites. However, preliminary data on antisera #145 and anti-LHR02 on [^{125}I]hCG binding to the detergent-solubilized receptor show that they inhibit binding by apparently different mechanisms. Thus, antiserum #145 decreases the apparent number of hCG-binding sites, but has no effect on the affinity of the receptor for hCG. In contrast, anti-LHR02 appears to decrease the affinity of the receptor for hCG without having an effect on the apparent number of hCG-binding sites.

In additional experiments we tested the ability of anti-LHR02 and #145 to immunoprecipitate the free and hCG-occupied receptors. Although both antisera were capable of immunoprecipitating the free receptor, only the #145 antireceptor antiserum was capable of immunoprecipitating the hormone–receptor complex. Together, these data suggest that antiserum #145 (which is toward the intact native LH/CG receptor) inhibits hCG binding by interacting with the extracellular domain of the receptor at sites other than those directly involved in hormone binding. In contrast, the data thus far with anti-LHR02 (which is directed toward amino acids 194–206 in the extracellular domain) suggest that it binds to a site which is (or is sterically close to) a domain involved in hormone binding.

Another aspect of the antisera described here is that neither anti-LHR02 (to amino acids 194–206) or anti-LHR04 (to amino acids 1–14) appears to inhibit binding of [^{125}I]hCG to the solubilized porcine luteal LH/CG receptor. Antiserum #145 (to the intact receptor) does so, but only at concentrations about 200-fold higher than that required for a comparable inhibition of binding to the rat luteal receptor. These observations are somewhat surprising, given the high degree of amino acid identity (i.e., 87%) over the entire sequences of the rat and porcine LH/CG receptors. Nonetheless, three of the 13 and six of 14 amino acids of peptides LHR02 and LHR04, respectively, are different between the rat and porcine sequences (see Fig. 15).

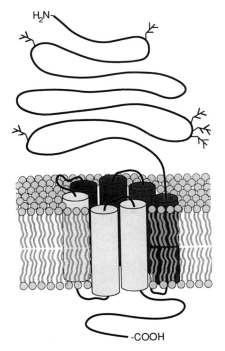

FIG. 19.   A postulated model for the LH/CG receptor in the plasma membrane. Above the membrane bilayer is the extracellular space; below is cytoplasmic. [From McFarland *et al.* (1989). Copyright © 1989 by the American Association for the Advancement of Science.]

Further studies using different site-specific antireceptor antibodies, in addition to mutagenesis studies of the receptor cDNA, should help to elucidate those areas of the LH/CG receptor that are involved in binding hormone.

VI.   Summary

In summary, the LH/CG receptor is a single polypeptide which contains a large hydrophilic domain that is situated extracellularly, attached to a region that spans the plasma membrane seven times, the carboxy-terminal region being intracellular (see Fig. 19). This topology was predicted by the amino acid sequence and has been confirmed by our immunofluorescence studies. The extracellular domain, which is related to a family of leucine-rich glycoproteins, is presumably involved in binding the large glycoprotein hormones hCG and LH. The carboxy-terminal half of the receptor, which is related to the family of rhodopsinlike receptors, is (by analogy with these receptors) presumably involved in the coupling of the receptor to the G protein.

Our transfection studies confirm that this single polypeptide is capable of binding hormone and activating adenylyl cyclase. Therefore, not only is the structure of the LH/CG receptor unique compared to other cell surface receptors characterized to date, but also its structure suggests that the mechanism of the translation of hormone binding to G protein coupling in this receptor is different from other G protein-coupled receptors whose ligands are much smaller and intercalcate among the transmembrane helices.

We predict that, due to the homology among the glycoprotein hormones, the structures of the FSH and TSH receptors share extensive amino acid and structural homology with the LH/CG receptor.

Last, our newly acquired knowledge about the structure of the LH/CG receptor, and the development of a cDNA and antibodies for this receptor, should enable more detailed studies on the function and regulation of the LH/CG receptor, not previously possible.

ACKNOWLEDGMENTS

We would like to acknowledge the invaluable contributions of our collaborator Peter H. Seeburg as well as members of our laboratories and other collaborators who have participated in some of the studies discussed here: M. I. Keller-Sarmiento, I. C. Kim, J. Klein, M. Kohler, K. C. McFarland, D. Phillips, H. Phillips, M. Rodriguez, N. Rosemblit, H. Wang, and Y. Xie. We also thank Wayne Bardin for his support and for his critical review of the manuscript and the National Hormone Pituitary Program for their gifts of purified glycoprotein hormones. The studies from our own laboratories were supported in part by Genentech, Inc., and by National Institute of Child Health and Human Development Grant HD-22196 (to D.L.S.), National Cancer Institute Grant CA-40629 (CA-23603 while at Vanderbilt University) (to M.A.), and DFG and BRFT grants (to P. H. Seeburg).

NOTE ADDED IN PROOF

Since this paper was presented, we have cloned the FSH receptor cDNA (Sprengel *et al.*, 1990), and two other laboratories have reported the cloning of the TSH receptor cDNA (Libert *et al.*, 1989; Nagayama *et al.*, 1989; Parmentier *et al.*, 1989). As we had predicted, the FSH and TSH receptors share both amino acid and structural homology with the LH/CG receptor. Similar to the LH/CG receptor, the FSH and TSH receptors are each composed of a single polypeptide that confers both the ability to bind hormone and the ability to activate G_s when occupied by hormone.

REFERENCES

Ascoli, M. (1980). *Biochim. Biophys. Acta* **629,** 409–417.
Ascoli, M. (1981). *J. Biol. Chem.* **256,** 179–183.
Ascoli, M. (1982). *J. Biol. Chem.* **257,** 13306–13311.
Ascoli, M. (1983). *Endocrinology (Baltimore)* **113,** 2129–2134.
Ascoli, M. (1984). *J. Cell Biol.* **99,** 1242–1250.
Ascoli, M. (1985a). *In* "The Receptors" (P. M. Conn, ed.), Vol. 2, pp. 368–400. Academic Press, Orlando, Florida.

Ascoli, M. (1985b). *In* "Luteinizing Hormone Action and Receptors" (M. Ascoli, ed.), pp. 199–217. CRC Press, Boca Raton, Florida.

Ascoli, M., and Puett, D. (1978). *Proc. Natl. Acad. Sci. U.S.A.* **75**, 99–102.

Ascoli, M., and Segaloff, D. L. (1986). *J. Biol. Chem.* **261**, 3807–3815.

Ascoli, M., and Segaloff, D. L. (1987). *Endocrinology (Baltimore)* **120**, 1161–1172.

Ascoli, M., and Segaloff, D. L. (1989). *Endocr. Rev.* **10**, 27–44.

Ascoli, M., Pignataro, O. P., and Segaloff, D. L. (1989). *J. Biol. Chem.* **264**, 6674–6681.

Benovic, J. L., Shorr, R. G. L., Caron, M. G., and Lefkowitz, R. J. (1984). *Biochemistry* **23**, 4510–4518.

Bruch, R. C., Thotakura, N. R., and Bahl, O. P. (1986). *J. Biol. Chem.* **261**, 9495–9460.

Buettner, K., and Ascoli, M. (1984). *J. Biol. Chem.* **259**, 15078–15084.

Bunzow, J. R., Van Tol, H. H. M., Grandy, D. K., Albert, P., Salon, J., Christie, M., Machida, C. A., Neve, K. A., and Civelli, O. (1988). *Nature (London)* **336**, 783–787.

Catt, K. J., Harwood, J. P., Clayton, R. N., Davies, T. F., Chan, V., Katikineni, M., Nozu, K., and Dufau, M. L. (1980). *Recent Prog. Horm. Res.* **36**, 557–622.

Conti, M., Harwood, J. P., Dufau, M. L., and Catt, K. J. (1977). *J. Biol. Chem.* **252**, 8869–8874.

Dixon, R. A. F., Kobilka, B. K., Strader, D. J., Benovic, J. L., Dohlman, H. G., Frielle, T., Bolanowski, M. A., Bennett, C. D., Rands, E., Diehl, R. E., Mumford, R. A., Slater, E. E., Sigal, I. S., Caron, M. G., Lefkowitz, R. J., and Strader, C. D. (1986). *Nature (London)* **321**, 75–79.

Dixon, R. A. F., Sigal, I. S., Candelore, M. R., Register, R. B., Scattergood, W., Rands, E., and Strader, C. D. (1987). *EMBO J.* **6**, 3269–3275.

Dohlman, H. G., Caron, M. G., Strader, C. D., Amlaiky, N., and Lefkowitz, R. J. (1988). *Biochemistry* **27**, 1813–1817.

Dufau, M., Charreau, E. H., and Catt, K. J. (1973). *J. Biol. Chem.* **248**, 6973–6981.

Ekstrom, R. C., and Hunzicker-Dunn, M. (1989). *Endocrinology (Baltimore)* **124**, 956–963.

Erickson, G. F., Wang, C., and Hsueh, A. J. W. (1979). *Nature (London)* **279**, 336–338.

Ezra, E., and Salomon, Y. (1981). *J. Biol. Chem.* **256**, 5377–5382.

Findlay, J. B. C., and Pappin, D. J. C. (1986). *Biochem. J.* **238**, 625–642.

Freeman, D. A., and Ascoli, M. (1981). *Proc. Natl. Acad. Sci. U.S.A.* **78**, 6309–6313.

Gore-Langton, R. E., and Armstrong, D. T. (1988). *In* "The Physiology of Reproduction" (E. Knobil, J. D. Neill, L. L. Ewing, G. S. Greenwald, C. L. Markert, and D. W. Pfaff, eds.), Vol. 1, pp. 331–385. Raven, New York.

Hall, P. F. (1988). *In* "The Physiology of Reproduction" (E. Knobil, J. D. Neill, L. L. Ewing, G. S. Greenwald, C. L. Markert, and D. W. Pfaff, eds.), Vol. 1, pp. 975–998. Raven, New York.

Hashimoto, C., Hudson, K. L., and Anderson K. V. (1988). *Cell (Cambridge, Mass.)* **52**, 269–279.

Huhtaniemi, I. T., and Catt, K. J. (1981). *Endocrinology (Baltimore)* **108**, 1931–1938.

Hunzicker-Dunn, M., and Birnbaumer, L. (1985). *In* "Luteinizing Hormone Action and Receptors" (M. Ascoli, Ed.), pp. 57–134. CRC Press, Boca Raton, Florida.

Inoue, Y., and Rebois, R. V. (1989). *J. Biol. Chem.* **264**, 8504–8508.

Jackson, T. R., Blair, L. A. C., Marshall, J., Goedert, M., and Hanley, M. R. (1988). *Nature (London)* **335**, 437–440.

Julius, D., MacKermott, A. B., Axel, R., and Jessell, T. M. (1988). *Science* **241**, 558–564.

Kataoka, T., Broek, D., and Wigler, M. (1985). *Cell (Cambridge, Mass.)* **43**, 493–505.

Keinanen, K. P., and Rajaniemi, H. J. (1986). *Biochem. J.* **239**, 83–87.

Keinanen, K. P., Kellokumpu, S., Metsikko, M. K., and Rajaniemi, H. J. (1987). *J. Biol. Chem.* **262**, 7920–7926.

Kellokumpu, S., and Rajaniemi, H. (1985a). *Mol. Cell. Endocrinol.* **42**, 157–162.

Kellokumpu, S., and Rajaniemi, H. (1985b). *Endocrinology (Baltimore)* **116**, 707–714.

Kim, I.-C., Ascoli, M., and Segaloff, D. L. (1987). *J. Biol. Chem.* **262**, 470–477.

Kobilka, B. K., Matsui, H., Kobilka, T. S., Yang-Feng, T. L., Francke, U., Caron, M. G., Lefkowitz, R. J., and Regan, J. W. (1987). *Science* **238,** 659–656.

Krusius, T., and Ruoslahti, E. (1986). *Proc. Natl. Acad. Sci. U.S.A.* **83,** 7683–7687.

Kubo, T., Fukuda, K., Mikami, A., Maeda, A., Takahashi, H., Mishina, M., Haga, T., Haga, K., Ichiyama, A., Kangawa, K., Kojima, M., Matsuo, H., Hirose, T., and Numa, S. (1986). *Nature (London)* **323,** 411–416.

Kusuda, S., and Dufau, M. (1986). *J. Biol. Chem.* **261,** 16161–16168.

Lee, C. Y., and Ryan, R. J. (1972). *Proc. Natl. Acad. Sci. U.S.A.* **69,** 3520–3523.

Liao, C.-F., Themmen, A. P. N., Joho, R., Barberis, C., Birnbaumer, M., and Birnbaumer, L. (1989). *J. Biol. Chem.* **264,** 7328–7337.

Libert, F., Lefort, A., Gerard, C., Parmentier, M., Perret, J., Ludgate, M., Dumont, J. B., and Vassart, G. (1989). *Biochem. Biophys. Res. Commun.* **5,** 1250–1255.

Lloyd, C. E., and Ascoli, M. (1983). *J. Cell Biol.* **96,** 521–526.

Loosfelt, H., Misrahi, M., Atger, M., Salesse, R., Vu Hai-Luu Thi, M. T., Jolivet, A., Guiochon-Mantel, A., Sar, S., Jallal, B., Garnier, J., and Milgrom, E. (1989). *Science* **245,** 525–528.

Lopez, J. A., Chumg, D. W., Fujikawa, K., Hagen, F. S., Papayannopoulou, T., and Roth, G. J. (1987). *Proc. Natl. Acad. Sci. U.S.A.* **84,** 5615–5619.

Masu, Y., Nakayama, K., Tamaki, H., Harada, Y., Kuno, M., and Nakanishi, S. (1987). *Nature (London)* **329,** 836–838.

Matzuk, M. M., Keene, J. L., and Boime, I. (1989). *J. Biol. Chem.* **264,** 2409–2414.

McFarland, K. C., Sprengel, R., Phillips, H. S., Kohler, M., Rosemblit, N., Nikolics, K., Segaloff, D. L., and Seeburg, P. H. (1989). *Science* **245,** 494–499.

Minegishi, T., Kusuda, S., and Dufau, M. L. (1987). *J. Biol. Chem.* **262,** 17138–17143.

Mondschein, J. S., and Schomberg, D. W. (1981). *Science* **211,** 1179–1180.

Moyle, W. R., Bahl, O. P., and Marz, L. (1975). *J. Biol. Chem.* **250,** 9163–9169.

Nagayama, Y., Kaufman, K. D., Seto, P., and Rapoport, B. (1989). *Biochem. Biophys. Res. Commun.* **165,** 1184–1190.

Nathans, J., and Hogness, D. S. (1983). *Cell (Cambridge, Mass.)* **34,** 807–814.

O'Dowd, B. F., Hnatowich, M., Regan, F. W., Leader, W. M., Caron, M. G., and Lefkowitz, R. J. (1988). *J. Biol. Chem.* **263,** 15985–15992.

Parmentier, M., Libert, F., Maenhaut, C., Lefort, A., Gerard, C., Perret, J., Van Sande, J., Dumont, J. E., and Vassart, G. (1989). *Science* **246,** 1620–1622.

Payne, A. H., Downing, J. R., and Wong, K.-L. (1980). *Endocrinology (Baltimore)* **106,** 1424–1429.

Peralta, E. G., Winslow, J. W., Peterson, G. L., Smith, D. H., Ashkenazi, A., Ramachandran, J., Schimerlik, M. I., and Capon, D. J. (1987). *EMBO J.* **6,** 3923–3929.

Pereira, M. E., Segaloff, D. L., Ascoli, M., and Eckstein, F. (1987). *J. Biol. Chem.* **262,** 6093–6100.

Pereira, M. E., Segaloff, D. L., and Ascoli, M. (1988a). *Endocrinology (Baltimore)* **122,** 2232–2239.

Pereira, M. E., Segaloff, D. L., and Ascoli, M. (1988b). *J. Biol. Chem.* **263,** 9761–9766.

Pierce, J. G. (1988). *In* "The Physiology of Reproduction" (E. Knobil, J. D. Neill, L. L. Ewing, G. S. Greenwald, C. L. Markert, and D. W. Pfaff, eds.), Vol. 1, pp. 1335–1348. Raven, New York.

Pierce, J. G., and Parsons, T. F. (1981). *Annu. Rev. Biochem.* **50,** 465–495.

Pierce, J. G., Bahl, O. P., Cornell, J. S., and Swaminathan, N. (1971). *J. Biol. Chem.* **246,** 2321–2324.

Pritchett, D. B., Bach, A. W. J., Wozny, M., Taleb, O., Dal Toso, R., Shih, J. C., and Seeburg, P. H. (1988). *EMBO J.* **7,** 4135–4140.

Rapoport, B., Hazum, E., and Zor, U. (1985). *J. Biol. Chem.* **259,** 4267–4271.

Rebois, R. V. (1982). *J. Cell Biol.* **94,** 70–76.

Rebois, R. V., and Fishman, P. H. (1986). *Endocrinology (Baltimore)* **118,** 2340–2348.

Rebois, R. V., and Patel, J. (1985). *J. Biol. Chem.* **260,** 8026–8031.

Rebois, R. V., Omedeo-Sale, F., Brady, R. O., and Fishman, P. H. (1981). *Proc. Natl. Acad. Sci. U.S.A.* **78,** 2086–2089.

Rebois, R. V., Bradley, R. M., and Titlow, C. C. (1987). *Biochemistry* **26,** 6422–6428.

Reichert, L. E. (1972). *Endocrinology (Baltimore)* **90,** 1119–1122.

Reichert, L. E., Lawson, G. M., Leidenberger, F. L., and Trowbridge, C. G. (1973). *Endocrinology (Baltimore)* **93,** 938–946.

Richards, J. S., Uilenbroek, T. J., and Jonassen, J. A. (1979). *Adv. Exp. Med. Biol.* **112,** 11–26.

Roche, P. C., and Ryan, R. J. (1985). *In* "Luteinizing Hormone Action and Receptors" (M. Ascoli, ed.), pp. 17–56. CRC Press, Boca Raton, Florida.

Roche, P. C., and Ryan, R. J. (1989). *J. Biol. Chem.* **264,** 4636–4641.

Rosemblit, N., Ascoli, M., and Segaloff, D. L. (1988). *Endocrinology (Baltimore)* **123,** 2284–2290.

Sairam, M. R., and Bhargavi, G. N. (1985). *Science* **229,** 65–67.

Schnell, D. J., and Etzler, M. E. (1987). *J. Biol. Chem.* **262,** 7220–7225.

Schofield, P. R., Rhee, L. M., and Peralta, E. G. (1987). *Nucleic Acids Res.* **15,** 3636.

Segaloff, D. L., and Ascoli, M. (1981). *J. Biol. Chem.* **256,** 11420–11423.

Segaloff, D. L., and Limbird, L. E. (1983). *Proc. Natl. Acad. Sci. U.S.A.* **80,** 5631–5635.

Segaloff, D. L., Puett, D., and Ascoli, M. (1981). *Endocrinology (Baltimore)* **108,** 632–637.

Sibley, D. R., Benovic, J. L., Caron, M. G., and Lefkowitz, R. J. (1987). *Cell (Cambridge, Mass.)* **48,** 913–922.

Sojar, H. T., and Bahl, O. P. (1989). *J. Biol. Chem.* **264,** 2552–2559.

Sprengel, R., Braun, T., Nikolics, K., Segaloff, D. L., and Seeburg, P. H. (1990). *Mol. Endocrinol.* **4,** 525–530.

Strader, C. D., Dixon, R. A. F., Cheung, A. H., Candelore, M. R., Blake, A. D., and Sigal, I. S. (1987). *J. Biol. Chem.* **262,** 16439–16443.

Strickland, T. W., and Puett, D. (1981). *Endocrinology (Baltimore)* **109,** 1933–1942.

Strickland, T. W., Parsons, T. F., and Pierce, J. G. (1985). *In* "Luteinizing Hormone Action and Receptors" (M. Ascoli, ed.), pp. 1–16. CRC Press, Boca Raton, Florida.

Takahashi, N., Takahashi, Y., and Putman, F. W. (1985). *Proc. Natl. Acad. Sci. U.S.A.* **82,** 1906–1910.

Tung, J.-S., Daugherty, B. L., O'Neill, S. W., Han, J., and Mark, G. E. (1989). *In* "PCR Technology" (H. A. Erlich, ed.), pp. 99–104. Stockton, New York.

Wang, H., Lipfert, L., Malbon, C. C., and Bahouth, S. (1989). *J. Biol. Chem.* **264,** 14424–14431.

Williams, J. F., Davies, T. F., Catt, K. J., and Pierce, J. G. (1980). *Endocrinology (Baltimore)* **106,** 1353–1359.

Wimalasena, J., Moore, P., Wiebe, J. P., Abel, A., Jr., and Chen, T. T. (1985). *J. Biol. Chem.* **260,** 10689–10697.

Wong, S. K.-F., Slaughter, C., Ruoho, A. E., and Ross, E. M. (1988). *J. Biol. Chem.* **263,** 7925–7928.

DISCUSSION

N. B. Schwartz. What can you tell us about the internalization of these receptors when they are occupied?

D. L. Segaloff. Are you referring to the LH receptor expressed from the cloned cDNA?

N. B. Schwartz. LH plus the receptor. I am referring to the data of Gordon Niswender, which showed a difference between the time of recycling of an hCG-occupied receptor and an LH-occupied receptor.

D. L. Segaloff. I believe what Dr. Niswender was interpreting as differences in the rates of internalization of hCG-versus oLH-occupied receptors could be readily explained by the different rates of dissociation of hCG and oLH from the LH receptor. In fact, in a study done by me and Mario Ascoli, we demonstrated that when the experiments are done such that the rate of hormone–receptor dissociation is taken into account, hCG and oLH are internalized at identical rates. These data have been published in *Endocrinology* [**120**, 1161–1172 (1987)]. With regard to the LH receptor expressed in transfected 293 cells, this receptor does mediate the internalization of hCG, but we have not yet done a detailed characterization of the properties of this phenomenon in the transfected cells to determine if they are indeed identical to those observed in luteal or Leydig cells.

N. B. Schwartz. Have you done this with labeled receptors? Dr. Niswender was doing it with a labeled hormone.

D. L. Segaloff. The way we, Dr. Niswender, and others have examined the internalization of the hormone–receptor complex has always entailed following the fate of the labeled hormone. Theoretically, we would like to be able to biosynthetically label the receptor and study the increased disappearance of the pool of labeled receptors as the hormone–receptor complexes are internalized and degraded. This is difficult to do, however, due to the low concentration of the LH receptor. We are currently in the process of making stable cell lines expressing the cloned cDNA in the hope that we might get one with a higher than normal level of receptor, which would enable us to do these as well as many other experiments which are now technically very difficult to do because of the low levels of receptor in gonadal cells.

J. H. Clark. The fact that the membrane-spanning regions look so much like the other smaller G_s-coupled receptors implies that there might be a small ligand in addition to LH. Is there any evidence for such a ligand?

D. L. Segaloff. There are no data to suggest that such is the case. It should be borne in mind, however, that once the hormone is bound, a portion of the receptor and/or hormone may intercalate within the transmembrane helices.

W. F. Crowley. There have been a number of rather odd effects of LH which have been reported over the years, such as immediate vasodilation of ovarian arterial supply to the corpus luteum, renotropic effects, and rapid direct feedback effects on FSH, suggesting that perhaps LH has extra-gonadal effects. Of course, you also are aware of the clinical syndrome of hyperthyroidism during pregnancy. Have your *in situ* hybridization studies revealed LH receptors in any unusual circumstances which might account for some of these effects?

D. L. Segaloff. We have only done *in situ* hybridizations on the ovary so far. What you are suggesting certainly should be done. We have been collaborating with Roger Cone of Tufts University, who has been screening a library from a patient with Graves' disease with the LH receptor cDNA in the hope of cloning a TSH receptor cDNA. What was originally cloned and sequenced appears to be a human LH receptor cDNA. Whether the LH receptor mRNA in the thyroid is expressed as a functional receptor, we do not yet know. But this raises the interesting question of whether there might also be other tissues that express the LH receptor mRNA and/or protein.

S. P. Bottari. I am aware that there is a lot of pharmacological evidence which tends to indicate that the hCG and LH bind to the same receptor. Nevertheless, I would like to know whether you really have conclusive evidence that there is only one single receptor for these two peptides. I cannot think of any other two peptide hormones or glycoprotein hormones (except for metabolic products such as angiotensin I, II, and II) which, although they can bind to more than one receptor, do not have a specific receptor. For example, for oxytocin and vasopressin, which were also thought to bind a single receptor, I think it has been quite conclusively shown, although they have not yet been cloned, that they have different specific receptors. LH and hCG sharing a single common receptor would be in contradiction to the concept of specificity and selectivity of hormone action. In testes, a target organ for LH, the levels of message are extremely low.

D. L. Segaloff. In answer to your question about both glycoprotein hormones hCG and LH binding to the same receptor, it has been well documented by hormone-binding studies prior to the receptor cloning that both hormones can bind to the same receptor. I am not aware of any data to support your suggestion that there may be different receptors for these two hormones. The data I have discussed demonstrate that the LH receptor expressed from the cloned cDNA can bind either hCG or oLH. Furthermore, the calculated affinities of hCG and oLH for the expressed receptor are comparable to those observed in rat luteal extracts.

S. P. Bottari. I understand that. But, as I said, for example, concerning oxytocin and vasopressin receptors, you could show exactly the same thing; if you look at myometrial membranes, you would find both receptors. However, the difference in binding capacity for both peptides as well as the differences in kinetics clearly indicate two different receptors.

D. L. Segaloff. I do not understand the point of your question.

S. P. Bottari. Very simply, if, for example, you take the uterus from nonpregnant animals, there are basically almost no oxytocin receptors. There are, however, vasopressin receptors which enables one to show that there is high-affinity oxytocin binding to apparently one single population of receptors. So, if you only express, because of certain circumstances, one type of receptor, you may erroneously think that only one receptor exists when you see binding of both peptides to it.

D. L. Segaloff. You cannot rule out the possibility that there may be subtypes of the LH receptor. Nonetheless, the LH receptor we have cloned and expressed can bind either hCG or LH. I would also like to point out that it is not as redundant as it may sound that this receptor binds two polypeptides, if you remember that hCG is only produced by the female during pregnancy and serves the specific function of maintaining the corpus luteum.

G. C. Chamness. Binding affinities for hCG and LH were 30-fold different, but the EC_{50}s were the same. I know that this is not a new observation for peptide hormones. In terms of molecular biology, do we now have a better explanation for this finding?

D. L. Segaloff. One possible explanation is that the conditions for measuring hormone binding and for measuring hormone-stimulated cAMP production are very different. The binding assays are done under equilibrium conditions, e.g., overnight at 4°C. In contrast, cAMP stimulation is assayed during a 30-minute incubation at 37°C, most definitely not equilibrium conditions. In such a short incubation, the similar EC_{50}s for hCG and oLH may, in fact, be more a reflection of the rates of association of the two hormones rather than of their binding affinities. In fact, if I remember correctly, the rates of association of these hormones are very similar. The rate of dissociation of hCG, however, is much slower than that of oLH, and I believe this difference is what is responsible for the vastly different affinities of these two hormones. An interesting point that I would like to make along these lines is that the hCG and oLH have the same affinity for the LH receptor if sodium is removed from the binding media. This was published by Buettner and Ascoli in *J. Biol. Chem.* [**259**, 15078–15084 (1984)]. The molecular basis for the differing affinities of these two hormones in the presence of sodium remains to be determined.

Search for the Gene for Multiple Endocrine Neoplasia Type 2A

Kenneth K. Kidd* and Nancy E. Simpson†

*Departments of Human Genetics, Psychiatry, and Biology, Yale University School of Medicine, New Haven, Connecticut 06510, and the †Departments of Pediatrics and Biology, Queen's University, Kingston, Ontario, Canada K7L 3N6

I. Introduction

Multiple endocrine neoplasia type 2A (MEN 2A) is a hereditary cancer syndrome with a unique tissue distribution. As the name conveys, tumors occur in multiple endocrine glands: the thyroid (specifically the C cells), the adrenals (chromaffin cells in the adrenal medulla), and occasionally the parathyroids. The medullary carcinomas of the thyroid (MTC), while generally slow growing, can metastasize and be life threatening, especially if a vital organ becomes involved. When they become hyperplastic and then neoplastic, the proliferating C cells, which produce calcitonin, cause hypercalcitonemia, but few serious symptoms are associated with the elevated hormone levels. The tumors of the adrenal [pheochromocytomas (PHEOs)] and parathyroid glands are not malignant and are generally slow growing. These tumors are not usually themselves, as tissue masses, the cause of the associated mortality; however, the elevated production of catecholamines by the PHEOs results in hypertension which is a major problem.

Having been briefly mentioned, the hormones themselves are subsequently ignored in this review. We concentrate instead on the genetic mapping and progress toward cloning of the gene causing this disorder. We believe that the normal function of this gene is involved in the differentiation of these endocrine tissues, and thus understanding this gene will be relevant not only to oncology but also to endocrinology.

All MEN 2A families reported to date have been found, if informative, to have the disease locus linked to genetic markers in a small region of chromosome 10 immediately surrounding the centromere. Thus, it seems safe to conclude that over 90%, and possibly all of the families with MEN 2A have an abnormal allele

305

at the same *MEN2A* locus, a locus close to the centromere on chromosome 10. The major groups working on the genetics of MEN 2A are all now engaged in "reverse" genetics—trying to go from knowing the general location of this gene to having actual clones of both the normal and abnormal forms of the gene. Some approaches being used are reviewed here.

The power of genetic linkage to map genes for inherited diseases has increased dramatically in the last decade. MEN 2A is one of many successes. While the step from mapping to cloning is still recognized as difficult, many think the mapping has become easy. Conceptually, it is, but the mapping is also tedious and involves much labor. Because it can serve as a model system, illustrating both the methods and progress in the field over the last few years, the history of what was done to map MEN 2A and the "candidate genes" excluded in the process are reviewed in some detail.

II. Clinical Aspects of the MEN Syndromes

A. OVERVIEW OF THE RELATED SYNDROMES

Three primary hereditary syndromes have been described that involve tumors of one or more of the endocrine glands. They are referred to here as MEN types 1, 2A, and 2B and their respective gene loci as *MEN1, MEN2A,* and *MEN2B.* Other designations, such as MEN I, II, and III and MEN2a and 2b, are found in the literature. The association of MTC and pheochromocytoma was first described by Sipple (1961). Work by Cushman (1962) strengthened the association, and by the late 1960s the syndrome was well established (e.g., Steiner *et al.,* 1968). This syndrome has since been subdivided into MEN 2A (kindreds without mucosal neuromas), the original Sipple's syndrome, which is believed to be distinct from MEN 2B (kindreds with mucosal neuromas) (for a historical review see Sipple, 1984). A fourth syndrome, MTC without PHEO (MTCWP) is also referred to but it is unlikely that its locus is distinct from that of MEN 2A and in this review it is included in the discussion of MEN 2A. The above designations are used, for consistency with the recommendations made at the Third International MEN 2 Workshop held in Heidelberg in September of 1989 (Simpson and Kidd, 1990) and at the Tenth International Workshop on Human Gene Mapping (HGM10) (Kidd *et al.,* 1989b). A fifth syndrome of apparently inherited early-onset (i.e., generally before adulthood) PHEO has also been described (Glowniak *et al.,* 1985; Irvin *et al.,* 1983), but its relationship to the MENs is not known. Although the individual tumors associated with the endocrine neoplasias occur sporadically, the hereditary syndromes appear to be dominantly inherited and are relatively rare.

B.   MEN 1

MEN 1 is characterized by tumors of the parathyroids, the islet cells of the pancreas, and the pituitary gland. In some families the only manifestation is hyperparathyroidism. The Zollinger–Ellison syndrome of intractable peptic ulcer and pancreatic adenomas is thought to be the same entity (Lulu *et al.*, 1968). These patients usually present with hypercalcemia, peptic ulcer, hypoglycemia, and symptoms relating to a pituitary mass. A host of other symptoms related to malfunctioning of the glands involved in this syndrome have been reviewed by Schimke (1986). The syndrome shows an autosomal dominant inheritance pattern in families; however, at the cellular level the normal allele at the locus for this syndrome appears to act as a dominant antioncogene, similar to the normal allele at the retinoblastoma locus, such that tumor cells result from the loss of the normal allele (Thakker *et al.*, 1989; A. E. Bale *et al.*, 1989). Mapping studies using the linkage method have placed the *MEN1* locus on chromosome 11 (Larsson *et al.*, 1988; Nakamura *et al.*, 1989b; A. E. Bale *et al.*, 1989; S. J. Bale *et al.*, 1989), making it clearly distinct genetically from the other endocrine neoplasias. One complication in distinguishing the syndromes is the rare patient from an MEN 2A kindred who also has developed the endocrinopathy associated with MEN 1 (Maton *et al.*, 1989).

C.   MEN 2A

The syndrome MEN 2A is a dominantly inherited condition of high penetrance exposing bearers of the abnormal gene to the risk of developing one or more of the three tumors, MTC, PHEO, and parathyroid adenomas. The usual presenting clinical symptom is a thyroid mass, and often by the time the tumor is recognized, widespread metastases have occurred. The PHEOs present with hypertension and occur in about half of the patients who have the MTC in these families. Although the MTC usually occurs first, it might not be recognized early, and the hypertension resulting from a PHEO might be the first indication of the disease. When it occurs, parathyroid involvement often occurs later than either of the other tumors (Gagel *et al.*, 1987).

In some families only MTCWP occurs, and the tumors are less aggressive than when PHEOs also occur in the family members. These families also show an autosomal dominant inheritance pattern. Farndon *et al.* (1986) have reviewed data on two large families and consider MTCWP to be a distinct clinical entity. Nelkin *et al.* (1989a) have suggested from unpublished data that this syndrome is genetically distinct and the locus is not on chromosome 10. However, in our linkage studies of a family with MTCWP [family S in Simpson *et al.* (1987), originally described by Jackson *et al.* (1973) as the Sla family with MTC and parathyroid adenomas], there were no recombinants between the centromeric marker *D10Z1*, which is the closest marker yet reported to the *MEN2A* locus (Wu *et al.*, 1990; Nakamura *et al.*, 1989a), and the disease locus. This single family gave a LOD score of 2.86 at a recombination frequency of zero between this marker and the syndrome, making it likely that the locus for MTCWP is on chromosome 10. Furthermore, Sobol *et al.* (1989) found no evidence for heterogeneity between the loci for the two clinical types, MEN 2A and MTCWP, in their French families. The two families studied by Noll *et al.* (1988) had MTCWP and gave LOD scores consistent with its being the same locus as *MEN2A*. It is possible, of course, that the MTCWP syndrome is the result of a different mutation at the locus on chromosome 10 than that for MEN 2A, much as sickle cell anemia and β-thalassemia are clinically distinct diseases caused by different mutations in the β-hemoglobin gene. There might also be some families with a different locus causing MTCWP, much as α- and β-thalassemia are caused by mutations on loci on completely different chromosomes.

D. MEN 2B

The third syndrome, MEN 2B, is clinically distinct from MEN 2A. The individuals with this syndrome can be diagnosed by their physical appearance: a marfanoid habitus, a distinctive dysmorphic facial appearance, abnormal ganglionic plexuses of the intestinal tract, and mucosal neuromas (for details of the clinical type, see Schimke, 1986). Again, linkage studies have shown that the *MEN2B* locus is likely to be on chromosome 10, since a LOD score of >4.0 has been noted with the centromeric locus *D10Z1* (C. E. Jackson, personal communication). Although formal proof of identity is not possible, this suggests that this clinically distinct syndrome could result from yet another mutation at the same locus as that for MEN 2A.

E. SCREENING FOR MEN 2A

Because of its clear pattern of inheritance, MEN 2A occurs only among the members of certain families; the children of an affected parent are at a high risk (50%) relative to the general rarity of MEN 2A in the total population. These characteristics provide optimal conditions for the application of cancer screening and prevention programs.

Screening tests are used for early preclinical detection or the actual detection of tumors of the three syndromes. MTC is a tumor of the calcitonin-secreting C cells of the gland, and the presymptomatic sign of the tumor is thought to be C-cell hyperplasia, which results in an excess of calcitonin being secreted, particularly when stimulated with calcium and/or the hormone pentagastrin. Because MTC is the most aggressive of the tumors and results in metastases if left untreated, standard clinical practice for members of families with MTC is regular (annual or biannual) screening for C-cell hyperplasia by measuring their serum calcitonin after stimulation usually with a combined dose of calcium and pentagastrin (Wells *et al.*, 1978). If total thyroidectomy is performed soon after the first positive test, metastases are prevented in most cases (Gagel *et al.*, 1987, 1988). ["Positive" meaning a serum calcitonin concentration considerably above normal, which varies from laboratory to laboratory and among assays; usually at least two tests are done before a clinical decision of "positive" is made.] The average age at presentation of the MTC and/or PHEOs is about 35 years, but at diagnosis of the preclinical state by the screening tests it is about 15 years (Gagel *et al.*, 1982, 1988; Easton *et al.*, 1989).

The PHEOs are recognized by abnormalities of urinary catecholamine excretion, and their measurement has been used to screen for the tumors before the adrenal mass becomes life threatening and before thyroidectomy or other surgery. However, the catecholamine abnormalities are not a reliable indication of adrenal chromaffin cell hyperplasia, the precursor of the PHEOs, as they are for the actual tumors. Thus, testing needs to be frequent, and compliance is often difficult (Gagel *et al.*, 1988).

F. IMPORTANCE OF MEN 2A IN GENERAL CANCER AND ENDOCRINE BIOLOGY

Current evidence favors the notion that the endocrine tumors in MEN 2A derive from a single cell line (Baylin *et al.*, 1976, 1978), probably of neural ectodermal origin (Pearse, 1976). People inheriting the gene for MEN 2A might develop any or all of the three pathological manifestations of the disease. Indeed, it has been stated (Sizemore *et al.*, 1980) that the hallmark of MEN 2A is tumor multiplicity, with multiple glands and sites within those glands affected. While MTC is the most common and clinically most serious manifestation of MEN 2A, the frequency of associated endocrine organ disease is also high. In one large kindred, the ratio of MTC to PHEO to parathyroid hyperplasia was 25:11:16 (Keiser *et al.*, 1973), while in another the ratio of MTC to PHEO was 40:13 (Graze *et al.*, 1978). All three of the tissues which are pathologically affected in MEN 2A are capable of endocrine function, a capability which provides accessible biochemical markers for the early detection of disease.

Largely because the standardized conventions for recording tumors do not distinguish the syndrome MEN 2A from occurrences of other thyroid or adrenal tumors (Mulvihill, 1984), the frequency of MEN 2A in the population is not known. Mulvihill (1977) has estimated that a sizable percentage of cases of MTC do, in fact, represent the inherited MEN 2A syndrome, whether it was recognized or not. Some clinical surveys suggest that between 20 and 25% of all MTC patients have one of the MEN 2 syndromes (Saad *et al.*, 1984). Others have put the frequency of MEN 2A as high as one in 25,000 (Carter *et al.*, 1987). Certainly, it is frequent enough that several large and apparently unrelated kindreds have been identified. Large families are now known from several different countries. The first large kindreds were those reported by Steiner *et al.* (1968) and by Keiser *et al.* (1973) and from the United Kingdom (Ponder, 1984), The Netherlands (Lips *et al.*, 1984), Denmark (Emmertsen, 1984), Japan (Takai *et al.*, 1984), France (Sobol *et al.*, 1989), and Canada (Birt *et al.*, 1977; Partington *et al.*, 1981; Verdy *et al.*, 1984), as well as several different centers in the United States (Wells *et al.*, 1978; Hamilton *et al.*, 1978; Noll *et al.*, 1984; Babu *et al.*, 1984). The N kindred originating from Sicily was described by Hamilton *et al.* (1978) and updated by Kruger *et al.* (1986). One large genealogical study in Sweden identified a common origin of seven Swedish families and one American family (Telenius-Berg *et al.*, 1984). Presumably, some of the other families of European origin also have a common origin. However, the number of independent mutational events cannot even be guessed at based on current information.

Understanding of the pathophysiology of MEN 2A, as one of a small group of clearly inherited cancer syndromes, might elucidate basic mechanisms in the transformation of cells to a neoplastic state. Cavenee *et al.* (1983) have clearly outlined frequent mechanisms of malignant transformation for retinoblastoma. Although this particular familial tumor is quite rare (even when compared to MEN 2A their studies have had a major scientific impact and far-reaching implications for comprehending oncogenesis. Because MEN 2A has significant differences from retinoblastoma (e.g., involvement of multiple tissues and variable late onset), quite different insights might result from understanding more about MEN 2A. Schimke (1986) states: "The multiple endocrine neoplasia syndromes are not common. Yet, because the basic alteration predisposing to neoplasia is a single-gene phenomenon, they have an importance far beyond their low frequency in the population. In our search for the ultimate oncogenic trigger, the multiple endocrine neoplasia syndromes appear to be ideal models for the application of contemporary molecular technology. Understanding the precise pathogenesis of each syndrome might well provide insight into the cause of hereditary malignant disease in particular and carcinogenesis in general."

III. Power of Linkage Studies and "Reverse" Genetics

A. WHAT IS A LINKAGE STUDY?

From a genetic perspective each chromosome is a single long DNA molecule and its genes are actually segments of that molecule. Genetic linkage is a consequence, since long stretches of that molecule, containing many genes, are transmitted intact from generation to generation. When genes or small DNA segments are close together, they are said to be linked and those alleles at the so-called loci on a given chromosome will be transmitted as a block in families. Thus, the particular alleles on the paternal chromosome (inherited from individual's father) or those on the maternal chromosome (inherited from the person's mother) will tend to be transmitted as a block to his or her children and will not be reassorted. This is in clear violation of Mendel's second law—independent assortment— which does apply to genes on separate chromosomes. This tendency for specific alleles at nearby loci to travel together through families is what is meant by genetic linkage. To observe this inherently statistical phenomenon, at least two distinct identifiable alleles must exist at both loci. Loci that have such alleles with common frequencies are useful as marker loci.

If it were not for the phenomenon of recombination, all alleles on any single chromosome would be inherited as a block. However, under exquisitely fine control the maternal and paternal DNA strands constituting a given chromosome pair undergo cross-overs such that in the resulting DNA strand (i.e., chromatid) that becomes the single chromosome (of that pair) included in a gamete, the alleles on one side of the cross-over are the maternally derived alleles and those on the other side are the paternally derived alleles. Cross-overs occur several times along each homologous pair of chromosomes, and they occur independently in each primary gametocyte undergoing meiosis. The occurrence of a cross-over at any particular point along the DNA molecule is quite infrequent, but the probability that one (or more) might occur within an interval between two genes is larger if the interval is larger. The observed frequency of gametes that are recombinant (i.e., that contain a nonparental combination of alleles at two or more loci) increases from effectively zero if two genes are immediately adjacent to 50% when two genes are sufficiently far apart on a chromosome. This upper limit of 50% is exactly what is expected for alleles at loci on separate chromosomes. Thus, it is possible for genes on the same chromosome not to be linked (i.e., to show no deviation from Mendel's second law of independent assortment). In contrast, genes that are linked (i.e., that show significantly more frequent parental combinations of alleles than recombinant or nonparental combinations of alleles) must be on the same chromosome.

In experimental organisms, such as the mouse, *Drosophila melanogaster,* corn, and others, it is possible to set up controlled matings so that one can tell directly from the appearance of the offspring whether the gamete that produced that individual was recombinant or nonrecombinant. From these simple tallies one could directly estimate the recombination frequency and test for whether or not it was significantly different from what was expected by chance alone. Human linkage studies require far more elaborate statistical procedures to extract the necessary information from the families one samples. The two most commonly used statistical approaches today are embodied in the computer programs LIPED (Ott, 1974; Hodge 1979) and LINKAGE (Lathrop *et al.,* 1984). In the case of linkage studies with a disorder such as MEN 2A, it is necessary to define the probabilities of each of the possible genotypes at the *MEN2A* locus based on the observed phenotype of the individual. That phenotype includes the age of the individual, since it is self-evident that an unaffected individual who is only 10 years old but whose parent had MEN 2A is much more likely to have the allele causing MEN 2A (and consequently to develop the disorder some time in the future) than is, for example, that individual's older sibling who is already 30 years old and still unaffected.

Today two types of linkage analyses are commonly done: pairwise and multipoint. The first involves just two loci, either two different markers or the disease locus and a single marker. The results are reported as a set of recombination frequencies (usually given the symbol θ) ranging from zero to 0.5 and the LOD score (often given the symbol Z) associated with each. The LOD score statistic (Morton, 1955; see also Ott, 1985) is based on the odds ratio of the probability of the data at the specific recombination frequency divided by the probability of the data with the two loci not linked. The LOD score is then the logarithm to the base 10 of that odds ratio and by definition is always zero at $\theta = 0.5$, which corresponds to the null hypothesis of no linkage. Positive LOD scores represent evidence for linkage; negative LOD scores represent evidence against linkage. The best (i.e., maximum likelihood) estimate of the true recombination frequency is the one with the maximum value of the LOD score. By convention a LOD score of $+3$ or greater is significant evidence of linkage. A LOD score of -2 or less is significant evidence against linkage and excludes the loci from being closer than the recombination frequency at which the LOD score drops below -2.

Multipoint analyses also yield a set of LOD scores, but the individual scores correspond to a new marker locus or a disease locus being at different positions along a genetic map. This map is defined by the known positions of the several markers being used in the study. The same rules of significance apply. The point on the map at which the LOD score is a positive maximum is the estimate of the position of the "new" locus. Negative LOD scores below -2 exclude the new locus from that region of the map. Examples of both pairwise and multipoint analyses are presented in Sections IV and V. Genetic maps are measured in centimorgan units, which are defined as 1 cM = 1% recombination when measured over small intervals. Map units are additive across intervals, but direct measurements of recombination between two loci can never exceed 50%.

Our complete ignorance of, and hence inability to detect, the primary genetic defect in MEN 2A motivated a linkage study of this disorder. We gain two major benefits from finding linkage of this cancer syndrome to some marker. The first is a greatly increased ability to provide genetic counseling to unaffected family members and to provide the *de facto* equivalent of a diagnosis prior to either the onset of any symptoms or even a positive preclinical screening test. This is a goal that has just now been achieved for MEN 2A, as explained in Section V. The second motivating factor is the ability to do reverse genetics in order to study the primary etiology and the subsequent pathogenesis of MEN 2A in the hopes of identifying an effective preventive therapy.

B.   WHAT IS REVERSE GENETICS?

The genetic map for humans has become a valuable and powerful research tool within the past 5 years. This map allows the linkage mapping of disease loci without knowledge of the intervening pathophysiology. This is a new route for the discovery of major loci for heritable diseases and the subsequent elucidation of the underlying etiology and pathophysiology. The dramatic identification of the gene for cystic fibrosis is one recent success using this approach (Rommens *et al.*, 1989; Riordan *et al.*, 1989; Kerem *et al.*, 1989). The absence of any hypotheses on etiology and the absence of any presymptomatic biological markers made this strategy an attractive approach for studying MEN 2A, because it bypasses the pathophysiologic mysteries that have confounded researchers since the syndrome was described. However, as we describe, finding the location of the gene by linkage analysis, the first step in a reverse genetics strategy, has had its own difficulties and surprises.

Prior to the advent of techniques that identify common normal genetic variation directly in the DNA, there were only a few polymorphic blood groups and enzymes, some serum protein markers, and the human leukocyte antigen (HLA) system available for linkage studies in humans. Although geneticists recognized the value of finding a linked marker, the limitation to fewer than two dozen useful markers largely precluded meaningful linkage studies. In the traditional approach to the genetics of human diseases, investigators searched for the biochemical defect underlying the phenotype in patients and identified the enzyme or structural protein that was abnormal. Once the protein involved was identified, the gene coding for that protein would be identified and mapped. Today that approach is yielding important new understanding of several inherited diseases and usually involves actually cloning of the relevant gene as a piece of genomic DNA or as cDNA (complementary to the processed mRNA). Figure 1 illustrates the contrast between the traditional and new genetic approaches. The figure illustrates why the new approach has been called "reverse genetics," but it is really a typical genetics research paradigm for experimental and domestic organisms. Only because much of the traditional armamentarium of genetics research has not been possible in humans has this misnomer been applied. This new (for humans) genetics approach starts by locating the chromosomal region of a disease gene using DNA polymorphisms. Knowledge of this location and the ability to genotype individuals at the disease locus—without knowledge of either pathophysiology in general or even diagnosis for some specific individuals—allows clinicians to provide improved services to families and allows researchers to design more powerful research protocols to determine pathophysiology. Even

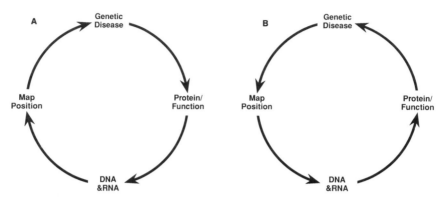

FIG. 1.   (A) The traditional, more biochemical, approach to the genetic investigation of a disease: identify a defective protein involved in the disorder (not possible for disorders such as MEN 2A with no known etiology; see text), purify the protein, clone the gene that makes it, and eventually search for the chromosomal location of the gene (often as an afterthought). (B) The reverse direction of investigation, now possible through application of molecular technology and DNA polymorphisms. This genetic linkage approach has the major advantage of not requiring any knowledge of the etiology or pathophysiology of the disease in question.

more important, mapping the gene is the first step toward cloning the gene itself. Thus, reverse genetics has the potential to locate and clone the disease locus without any knowledge of the process causing the disorder.

In general, for disorders with no clear candidate genes, it has become standard to scan the entire genome with just a few hundred well-placed linkage markers. Botstein *et al.*(1980) advocated this approach and predicted that it would become feasible within a decade. We chose this approach in the early 1980s, when we began our studies of MEN 2A. At the time we started, there were only a few dozen useful markers, but the expectation existed that more would be discovered, sufficient for a complete search of the entire human genome.

C.   DRAMATIC INCREASE IN THE NUMBER OF MARKERS

Extraordinary advances in all aspects of human molecular genetics have occurred over the past decade. One component of those advances is the increase in the number of cloned segments of human DNA. These clones have been classified into two logical types that serve as the resources for a variety of medical applications. First, there are the cloned genes that allow investigations of the normal and abnormal function of genes. For example, studying clinically important abnormal alleles can yield greater understanding of the pathophysiology of the resulting disease. Second, there are the clones that serve as genetic markers, usually because they identify restriction fragment-length polymorphisms (RFLPs). Botstein *et al.* (1980) predicted that about 150–200 evenly spaced RFLPs would allow

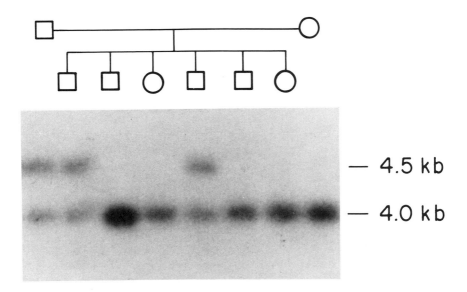

(p9 - 12a, TaqI) Chromosome 10

FIG. 2.   The RFLP at the *D10S5* locus. The electrophoresis of *Taq*I-digested DNA samples was done in lanes corresponding to the family members represented in the pedigree at the top. The probe p9 − 12a was used for hybridizing. The segregation pattern at this locus was the first major hint to the location of *MEN2A* (see Sections IV,E and F).

diseases of unknown etiology to be mapped. They made that prediction when fewer than a dozen RFLPs were known; the roughly 2000 DNA polymorphisms known today (Kidd *et al.*, 1989a; unpublished observations) represent a 200-fold increase over the number of markers known a decade ago.

Figure 2 illustrates an RFLP at the *D10S5* locus. After the DNA samples from all individuals in the family were digested with a restriction enzyme, they were size-fractionated using gel electrophoresis, transferred to a nylon membrane, and then hybridized to a ^{32}P-labeled probe. The probe reconstitutes the DNA double helix only with those fragments bound to the nylon membrane that have the same nucleotide sequence, and their locations are revealed by autoradiography. Here the polymorphism is the occurrence of chromosomes that have the sequence on a 4.5-kb fragment and chromosomes that have it on a 4.0-kb fragment. In this family we can trace the father's two chromosomes. He gave the chromosome with the 4.5-kb fragment (i.e., allele) to his first and third sons; he gave the 4.0-kb allele to his other four children.

Table I is taken from the compilations made as part of the Tenth International

TABLE I

Increase in the Number of Cloned Genes and Polymorphic Markers over the Past Decade[a]

Type of cloned human DNA	Human Gene Mapping Workshop (year)				
	HGM6 (1981)	HGM7 (1983)	HGM8 (1985)	HGM9 (1987)	HGM10 (1989)
Cloned genes					
Total	16	104	249	610	945
Polymorphic	6	35	88	216	391
Anonymous DNA segments					
Total	35	215	559	2057	3417
Polymorphic	18	95	245	977	1495
Cloned DNA					
Total	51	319	808	2667	4362
Polymorphic	24	130	333	1193	1886

[a]The summaries were made at each of the last five Human Gene Mapping Workshops. At each workshop there were a few unassigned RFLPs not tabulated here, but included at the ends of the DNA polymorphism table in the workshop reports (e.g., Kidd *et al.*, 1989a). Data were compiled by Pearson *et al.* (1987) and by Kidd *et al.* (1989a).

HGM Workshop (Kidd *et al.*, 1989a). The top line of Table I gives the total numbers of cloned and mapped human genes known at each of the Workshops held since 1981. This table underestimates the total number of cloned genes, since there is no tabulation available for cloned genes that have not been mapped. However, genes are often mapped soon after they are cloned; so the tabulated numbers might lag behind the total numbers by only a few months. Also in Table I are the numbers of these identified genes known to show at least one DNA polymorphism. While the number known to be polymorphic is a substantial percentage, it is a clear underestimate of the potential, since many of the clones of genes have never been tested to see whether or not they will identify a polymorphism. The total number of DNA polymorphisms, however, has increased even more dramatically than the number of cloned genes, as shown in the bottom line of Table I. This dramatic, virtually exponential, increase in the numbers of mapped RFLPs is attributable mostly to the anonymous segments of human DNA. These segments are anonymous only with respect to function, but are otherwise cloned unique pieces of the human genome that can be precisely mapped and, if polymorphic, can serve as genetic markers for linkage studies.

Figure 3 gives the chromosome-by-chromosome breakdown of polymorphic cloned genes and anonymous DNA segments, showing changes over the last 5 years up to the latest summary at HGM10. There is obviously considerable variation among chromosomes, often correlated with the mapping of clinically relevant genes. For example, chromosomes 4 and 7 have disproportionately more DNA polymorphisms because Huntington's disease (Gusella *et al.*, 1983) and

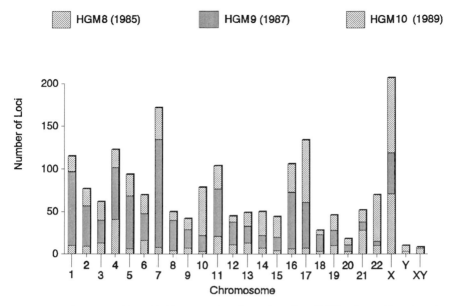

FIG. 3.   Trends in RFLPs. This histogram gives the total number of DNA polymorphisms (mostly RFLPs) mapped to each chromosome at each of the past three HGM workshops. The numbers were compiled from data in the Human Gene Mapping Library database at Yale University.

cystic fibrosis (Tsui *et al.*, 1985) were mapped to these chromosomes, thereby motivating research focused on them. On some chromosomes the numbers of RFLPs were initially disproportionately low; chromosome 10 is the most notable. As an illustration of how rapidly changes can occur, we note that between September 1987 and August 1988 dozens of additional markers were mapped on chromosome 10. Between HGM9 and HGM10 chromosome 10 had the greatest proportional increase in markers for any chromosome, because the gene for MEN 2A had recently been mapped to this chromosome (Mathew *et al.*, 1987; Simpson, *et al.*, 1987). This finding stimulated several groups to develop linkage maps covering chromosome 10 and resulted in chromosome 10's having one of the best linkage maps of any chromosome. This progress is reviewed in detail in Section V,A.

D.   FAMILY MATERIAL AVAILABLE FOR MEN 2A

We do not know the frequency of the abnormal allele at the *MEN2A* gene (more precisely, the *MEN2A* locus). The MEN 2A syndrome is considered to be a rare disorder and yet there are many quite large kindreds that have been identified in the roughly 30 years since Sipple (1961) first published on the association between MTC and PHEO in the early 1960s. The number of families described in the literature is too large to review here. We note some of the largest of the kindreds in Section II,F. Many of these, as well as other large kindreds, are now being used in linkage studies.

IV.   Initial Linkage Studies of MEN 2A

What linkage studies there were through the early 1980s were not very informative, mostly attributable to the paucity of markers available, but they did give exclusions around such classical markers as blood groups and protein polymorphisms (Jackson *et al.*, 1976; Emmertsen *et al.*, 1983; Ferrell *et al.*, 1984). Takai *et al.* (1984) reported evidence against linkage with seven such markers in Japanese families, but only a small region was strictly excluded around each marker. Emmertsen *et al.* (1983) also found cytogenetically visible variants in the centromeric heterochromatin of several chromosomes, but saw several crossovers of *MEN2A*, each arguing strongly against any linkage. Verdy *et al.* (1984) identified a similar centromeric variant on chromosome 16 in the large MEN 2A family they were studying and could exclude *MEN2A* from being within 2% recombination of that location. The suggestion of possible linkage to the P blood group and to HLA was one early hint (Jackson *et al.*, 1976), but it was not supported by subsequent studies (Simpson and Falk, 1982). Similar weak hints of linkage to haptoglobin and group specific component (GC) (Kruger *et al.*, 1986) were resolved by using nearby RFLPs; the *MEN2A* locus was excluded from the entire region between and around those closely linked genes (Kidd *et al.*, 1986b).

A.   1984: EXCLUSION OF THE CANDIDATE GENES
HRAS, CALCA, AND *PTH*

We started our linkage studies of the N kindred in 1982. At that time few RFLPs were known, but several of them seemed to have a special relevance to MEN 2A: *HRAS, CALCA,* and *PTH.* The cellular Harvey-*ras* oncogene homolog (*HRAS*) was the first human oncogene cloned (Shih *et al.*, 1981; Goldfarb *et al.*, 1982) and was thought then to have broad involvement in causing neoplasms; it mapped to the tip of the short arm of chromosome 11 (11p15), close to the locus for insulin and the β-hemoglobin cluster of genes. The structural genes for calcitonin (*CALCA*) and parathyroid hormone (*PTH*) were clearly genes expressed in the tumor cells in MEN 2A, and although no obvious mechanism for causing the tumors could be ascribed to these genes, it seemed reasonable to test their possible involvement; moreover, they mapped into the same chromosome arm (11p) as *HRAS,* raising interesting questions of possible interactions among genes. Needless to say, all of this speculation was clearly rejected by the first linkage study we completed (Kidd *et al.*, 1984); strongly negative LOD scores were obtained for several genes in the region, not only eliminating *HRAS,*

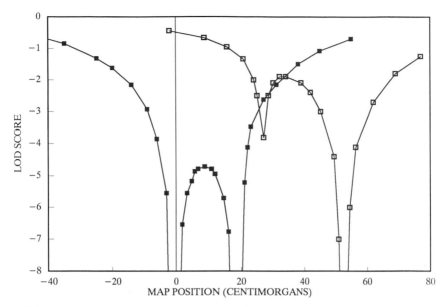

FIG. 4. Two multipoint linkage analyses of *MEN2A*. The curves give the LOD scores for *MEN2A* being at the corresponding positions on the map. The two curves derive from two separate analyses: the first (solid squares) uses *HBBC* (the β-hemoglobin cluster) and *PTH* (parathyroid hormone) (Kidd *et al.*, 1984) and the second (open squares) uses *CALCA* (calcitonin), *D11S16* (an anonymous locus), and *CAT* (catalase) (Pakstis *et al.*, 1987). These markers all map to the distal half of 11p (the short arm of chromosome 11). Based on the best estimate of their relative distances, they have been assigned map positions, from distal to proximal: *HBBC* at 0 cM, *PTH* at 18 cM, *CALCA* at 27 cM, and both *D11S16* and *CAT* at 52 cM. Just these two analyses using five markers exclude *MEN2A* (LOD scores less than 2) from the entire distal half of chromosome 11p.

CALCA, and *PTH* as candidates for the cause of MEN 2A, but also excluding the *MEN2A* locus from being anywhere in this region. Figure 4 shows a multipoint linkage analysis of some of the data used in that study (Kidd *et al.*, 1984), showing how just two of the loci studied excluded the *MEN2A* locus from a region more than 45 cM long. At the time, this was the largest continuous segment of the genome that had been thoroughly screened and rejected. Also in Fig. 4 is a second multipoint analysis of later data (Pakstis *et al.*, 1987) that extended the region of exclusion.

B. 1983–1987: CHROMOSOME 20 DELETION HYPOTHESIS AND ITS REJECTION BY LINKAGE

In the early 1980s the gene for retinoblastoma was mapped as the result of a small cytogenetic deletion being found on chromosome 13 in the cells of many patients (see Sparkes *et al.*, 1980, 1983). Wilms' tumor on the short arm of chromosome 11 showed a similar picture (Koufos *et al.*, 1984; Orkin *et al.*,

1984). These results gave a strong rationale for cytogenetic studies of MEN 2A. Initially in abstracts (Van Dyke *et al.*, 1981) and then in several papers (Van Dyke *et al.*, 1984; Babu *et al.*, 1984, 1987), Jackson and colleagues in Detroit reported finding a small deletion in the middle of the short arm of chromosome 20 (20p−) in the normal somatic tissue of patients with MEN 2A, but the 20p− "deletion" was neither confined to MEN 2A nor found in all patients with MEN 2A. Butler *et al.* (1987a,b) also found the 20p− deletion in 12 of 13 patients, but also in one of seven controls. Others (Hsu *et al.*, 1981; Emmertsen *et al.*, 1983; Gustavson *et al.*, 1983; Zatterale *et al.*, 1984; Wurster-Hill *et al.*, 1986b; Ikeuchi *et al.*, 1987) were not able to find the deletion in the karyotypes of members of their MEN 2A families or found it only in normal control subjects. The significance of this 20p− chromosome has still not been clarified, but was shown not be the cause of the syndrome by linkage studies involving some of the same families in which the 20p− chromosome had been found. Goodfellow *et al.* (1985) first used linkage to test the hypothesis of a gene on 20p by mapping an RFLP, *D20S5*, to exactly the same band, 20p12, that was reported by Van Dyke *et al.* (1984) to be deleted and showing that *MEN2A* was excluded from a region of 13% recombination on either side of this marker. In Japanese families Tateishi *et al.* (1987) also excluded linkage closer than ~12% recombination between *D20S5* and *MEN2A*. The relative positions of two additional markers on chromosome 20 were determined (Goodfellow *et al.*, 1987), and using all three markers, *MEN2A* was excluded from most of chromosome 20 (Farrer *et al.*, 1987a). We concluded that *MEN2A* was not a locus on 20p at the site of the deletion and probably not on 20 at all.

C.   1986: EXCLUSION OF 5% OF THE GENOME

Concomitantly with the above studies, markers scattered throughout the genome were being tested for linkage with *MEN2A*. Choice of markers was motivated primarily by availability as they were being discovered and the probes could be obtained. Kruger *et al.* (1986) and Kidd *et al.* (1986a) summarized data on 43 loci and excluded the *MEN2A* locus from over 5% of the entire genome.

D.   1987: EXCLUSION OF "WHOLE" CHROMOSOMES 13 AND 19

The chromosome 11 and 20 studies were motivated in part by specific hypotheses about the *MEN2A* gene. In contrast, our study of chromosome 13 (Farrer *et al.*, 1987b) and Ponder's study of chromosomes 19 (Carter *et al.*, 1987) were motivated by the availability of sets of markers that allowed each of the chromosomes to be covered nearly completely. In both studies the results excluded the *MEN2A* locus from essentially the entire chromosome. Combined with the scattered exclusions on other chromosomes, nearly 15% of the genome had been excluded by this point.

E.   1987: EXCLUSION OF 32% OF THE GENOME

By the time of the Second International Workshop on MEN 2A in Cambridge, England, in 1986, the combined results from the several published studies, along with results presented at the meeting (Tateishi *et al.*, 1987; Ponder *et al.*, 1987; Pakstis *et al.*, 1987) and unpublished results from our two laboratories, allowed the *MEN2A* locus to be excluded from 32% of the genome (Simpson and Kidd, 1987). At that time only one locus showed a LOD score above 1.0, the RFLP recognized by the probe p9− 12A, now given the locus symbol *D10S5* (see Fig. 2). This locus showed a peak LOD score of 1.7 at 15% recombination (P. J. Goodfellow, cited by Simpson and Kidd, 1987). Such a small value did not even approach statistical significance, and the results were actually moderately negative in the N kindred (Pakstis *et al.*, 1987). Since several dozen RFLP loci had been studied by this time, it was actually likely that a false-positive result with an even higher LOD score would have occurred. Still, it was a clue to be pursued.

F.   1987: DEFINITIVE MAPPING TO CHROMOSOME 10

D10S5, the marker that gave the first clue to the location of *MEN2A*, was the first RFLP marker studied on chromosome 10. This prompted us and others to look at additional families for linkage of a chromosome 10 marker to *MEN2A*. Our initial efforts involved typing two additional families and some additional members in the families already being studied. Table II presents the confusing results we had in early 1987. The first additional marker tested, retinol-binding

TABLE II
Pairwise LOD Scores for MEN2A and D10S5 in Early 1987[a]

Family	Recombination frequency ($\theta_m = \theta_t$)						
	0.00	0.001	0.005	0.10	0.20	0.30	0.40
W	−4.61	−4.16	−1.49	−0.92	−0.32	−0.05	0.04
S	0.42	0.55	1.66	1.84	1.73	1.35	0.73
C	1.31	1.31	1.15	1.00	0.68	0.37	0.11
K	1.35	1.34	1.18	1.00	0.64	0.29	0.06
N	−6.59	−4.48	−1.15	−0.66	−0.29	−0.13	−0.05
Total (all families)	−8.12	−5.44	1.35	2.26	2.44	1.83	0.89
				$\theta = 0.16, \hat{Z} = 2.50$			
Total (S, C, and K only)	3.08	3.20	3.99	3.84	3.05	2.01	0.90
				$\theta = 0.05, \hat{Z} = 3.99$			

[a]The initial results with *D10S5* were confusing: Two families gave negative LOD scores; three gave positive LOD scores. If the differences were just chance (which we now know they were), the results did not quite reach statistical significance, because the LOD score was only 2.50. However, if there really were genetic heterogeneity, the three "linked" families gave a singificant LOD score of 3.99 for close linkage. Heterogeneity tests done on these data gave a borderline result of $p = 0.06$, so we could not conclude that linkage existed between *MEN2A* and *D10S5*. All five families now show linkage of *MEN2A* to *RBP3*.

protein 3, interstitial (the official symbol is now "*RBP3*," but initially it was published as "*IRBP*") resolved the confusion in our families and gave highly significant statistical evidence of linkage. Positive results from two groups were published simultaneously in 1987 (Mathew *et al.*, 1987; Simpson *et al.*, 1987). This confirmation prompted other groups to use RBP3 for linkage studies in their families. Two additional groups have published their findings confirming linkage of *MEN2A* to *RBP3* (Sobol *et al.*, 1988; Narod *et al.*, 1989; Yamamoto *et al.*, 1989). Other groups also have positive results, but have not published them in full (Noll *et al.*, 1988; H. Donis-Keller, personal communication). Ponder's group, in collaboration with several other research groups, have studied additional families (Nakamura *et al.*, 1989a); our laboratories in Kingston and New Haven have also now studied additional families, all of which show linkage to *RBP3* (Simpson and Kidd, 1989a; Wu *et al.*, 1990).

To date all families that have been studied have, if informative for the markers used, shown linkage to chromosome 10. There is thus strong support for MEN 2A being a genetically homogeneous disease with one locus responsible for most, if not all, cases of MEN 2A. The total LOD score between the disease locus and *RBP3* from all of the published studies exceeds 35 at a recombination frequency of about 3%, averaging across all studies (Table III). This LOD score represents odds of $10^{35}{:}1$ favoring linkage at this average recombination frequency or a value close to it. However, while there is no question remaining about the existence of linkage and this the linkage is close, there is still considerable uncertainty about what the precise recombination frequency is. As discussed below, the uncertainty is highly relevant to the accuracy with which presymptomatic diagnoses can be made. To improve the estimates of the recombination fraction and to find other markers even closer for use in clinical applications, a genetic map of the larger region of chromosome 10 encompassing *RBP3* and

TABLE III
Summary of Published Linkage Studies of MEN2A and RBP3[a]

	Recombination frequency ($\theta_m = \theta_t$)				
Study	0	0.01	0.05	0.1	0.2
Nakamura *et al.* (1989)	6.8	17.8	17.7	16.1	11.8
Yamamoto *et al.* (1989)	5.2	5.1	4.7	4.1	3.0
Wu *et al.* (1990)	9.5	12.7	13.1	12.3	9.7
Totals	21.5	35.6	35.5	32.5	24.5

[a]Values are the LOD scores reported on the assumption of equal recombination frequencies in males and females. The three studies report on different sets of families, so the results can be combined; they also incorporate many results published earlier. Other recent publications (e.g., Narod *et al.*, 1989) report results that either do not allow combination with these data and/or that are partially included in one of the other summaries.

MEN2A is needed. This need spurred the development of additional markers and linkage maps of chromosome 10.

G. 1988–1989: MAPPING OF *MEN1* AND *MEN2B*

Recently, the *MEN1* locus was mapped to chromosome 11 (Larsson *et al.*, 1988; Nakamura *et al.*, 1989b; A. E. Bale *et al.*, 1989; S. J. Bale *et al.*, 1989). This unambiguously demonstrates that MEN 1 is not only a different disease clinically, but also that it has a fundamentally different etiology. In contrast, preliminary data on the *MEN2B* gene suggest that it is tightly linked to *D10Z1* (Jackson *et al.*, 1988; C. E. Jackson, personal communication). This raises two interesting possibilities: MEN 2B might be caused by a different mutation at the same locus as the abnormal allele causing MEN 2A, or there might be two distinct loci closely linked and closely related in function that possibly arose by duplication of an ancestral locus. Only very high-resolution genetic mapping of the region and the cloning of the gene(s) involved will be likely to resolve these possibilities.

V. Recent Refinements of the Position of *MEN2A* on Chromosome 10

A. BETTER GENETIC MAPS OF CHROMOSOME 10

In our initial paper demonstrating linkage to chromosome 10 (Simpson *et al.*, 1987), we used both *RBP3* (then known as *IRBP*) and *D10S5*. We showed that these two markers were linked to each other at approximately 9% recombination. While both were known to be near the centromere, the regional localizations of those two markers were overlapping in the proximal long arm. Consequently, it was impossible to give a clear orientation of the linkage map that we constructed:

$$MEN2A—7 \text{ cM}—RBP3—9 \text{ cM}—D10S5$$

MEN2A could have been anywhere from the proximal short arm to nearly the middle of the long arm, depending on the orientation of the two markers and the distribution of recombination events along the chromosome. The subsequent maps generated by Lathrop *et al.* (1988) and by our group (Farrer *et al.*, 1988) used largely different sets of markers, but clearly established that *MEN2A* was on the short-arm side of *RBP3*, with *D10S5* and several other markers extending down the long arm of chromosome 10. We shortly thereafter added two additional markers to our map (Miki *et al.*, 1988; Wu *et al.*, 1988a), and by May 1988 the two maps that had been generated were as shown in Fig. 5. Since then, extensive mapping work on chromosome 10 has proceeded (Nakamura *et al.*, 1988a, 1989a; Wu *et al.*, 1988a,b, 1990; Wu and Kidd, 1990a; White *et al.*, 1990). As a result chromosome 10 is now one of the best mapped of the human

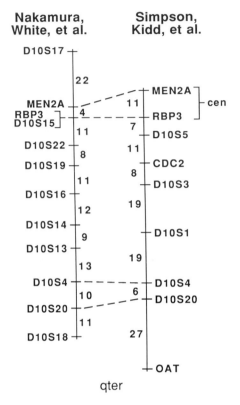

FIG. 5.   Two composite chromosome 10 maps based on work in White's laboratory (Lathrop *et al.*, 1988) and the Simpson and Kidd laboratories (see text) ($\theta_m = \theta_f$). Almost completely different sets of markers had been used, but there was close agreement—within statistically acceptable limits—for those markers in common. Both maps covered primarily the long arm.

chromosomes. Reviews of the maps that had been published (Smith and Simpson, 1989) and the map produced by the Centre d'Etude du Polymorphisme Humain (CEPH) consortium (White *et al.*, 1990) give a clear overview of virtually the entire chromosome. This basic human genetics work has significance far beyond MEN 2A, but in a real sense the rapid progress was a direct by-product of the search for the *MEN2A* gene.

B.   FLANKING MARKERS AND MORE ACCURATE LOCALIZATION OF *MEN2A*

Shortly after *MEN2A* was initially mapped, Nakamura *et al.* (1988a) showed that *D10S15* (probe pMCK2) was close to *RBP3*, thereby improving the informativeness of the proximal region of the long arm. Subsequent linkage studies have confirmed tight linkage between *RBP3* and *D10S15* (Wu *et al.*, 1990); physical–

molecular mapping studies indicate that they are within 200,000 bp of each other along the chromosome 10 DNA strand (N. Tanaka and T. Miki, personal communication). Nakamura *et al.* (1989a) have identified another marker, *D10S30* (probe TBQ16), that is just slightly distal to the *RBP3–D10S15* pair, possibly close to *D10S5*. Wu and Kidd (1990b) have also identified another marker, *D10S96* (probe KW31), that is just distal to *D10S5*, probably close to *D10S22* (probe pTB10.163). White *et al.* (1990) conclude that *D10S11* (probe CRI–L647) also belongs in the region, but could not precisely localize it. Thus, there are now several markers within about 15–20 cM on the long-arm side of *MEN2A*, but the *RBP3–D10S15* pair remains the closest long-arm marker to *MEN2A*.

In their first map Lathrop *et al.* (1988) had a short-arm marker, *D10S17*, that would almost certainly be on the opposite side of *MEN2A*, but it was so far away that it was not valuable. Wu *et al.* (1988b) mapped another marker, *D10S24*, in roughly the same place. The first evidence for a useful flanking marker came from Nakamura *et al.* (1989a), showing that *D10S34* (probe cTBQ14.34) was most likely on the short-arm side of *MEN2A*. This has been closely followed by studies showing that *FNRB*, the gene for the β subunit of fibronectin receptor and previously mapped to chromosome 10 (Zhang *et al.*, 1988; Goodfellow *et al.*, 1989), is definitely on the short-arm side of *MEN2A* and reasonably close (Wu *et al.*, 1989, 1990). Both *FNRB* and *D10S34* are now mapped to the proximal short arm (Smith and Simpson, 1989). The exact order of *FNRB* and *D10S34* is not yet known, but they should be close to each other. Thus, there are now two highly informative markers on the short-arm side of *MEN2A* within 5–6 cM.

More recently, Wu *et al.* (1990) showed that D10Z1, a highly polymorphic α-satellite DNA region at the centromere (Devilee *et al.*, 1988; Wu and Kidd, 1990a), is tightly linked to *MEN2A*. In the only published study using D10Z1 with *MEN2A* (Wu *et al.*, 1990) there were no cross-overs between the two. The several mapping studies reviewed above are all consistent with *MEN2A*'s being close to the centromere, but it is impossible to say whether *MEN2A* is in the short arm or the long arm. The several DNA markers known to be or might be useful in studying *MEN2A* are summarized in Table IV.

C.   THE SEX DIFFERENCE IN RECOMBINATION RATES

There is growing recognition that, in general and throughout the genome, the recombination frequency is different in male meiosis than in female meiosis (Kidd, 1987). The general tendency is for more recombination to occur in female meiosis (see, e.g., Donis-Keller *et al.*, 1986), but there are regions, especially near the telomeres, where recombination is more frequent in male meiosis (see, e.g., White *et al.*, 1985; Kramer *et al.*, 1977; O'Connell *et al.*, 1987; Reeders *et al.*, 1988; Nakamura *et al.*, 1988b,c). The early chromosome 10 maps indicated a slight overall excess of recombination in female meiosis. This has been confirmed by subsequent studies (see Simpson and Kidd, 1989b; Wu *et al.*, 1990).

TABLE IV
Chromosome 10 Pericentric DNA Markers and Their Polymorphisms[a]

Locus	Probe	Location	Restriction enzymes	Polymorphism information content
D10S24	p7A9	10p13–p12.1	MspI	0.55
			TaqI	
FNRB	pGEM-32	10p11.2	BanII	0.71
			HinfI	
			KpnI	
			BglII	
			SacI	
	pB/R2		MspI	
D10S34	cTBQ14–34	10p13–cen	TaqI	>.50
D10Z1	p10RP8	10cen	PstI	0.50
			EcoRV	
			HincII	
RBP3	H.4IRBP	10q11.2	BglII	0.67
			MspI	
	TBIRBP9	10q11.2	TaqI	
D10S15	pMCK2	10q11.2	PvuII	0.35
			RsaI	
D10S5	p9–12A	10q21.1	TaqI	0.49
			HincII	
			DraI	
D10S30	cTBQ16	10q11.2–q22	MspI	0.34
D10S22	pTB10.163	10q21.1	MspI	0.49
D10S96	KW31	10q21		
D10S11	CRI–L647	10q11.2	TaqI	0.48

[a]This summary is extracted from data included in the Human Gene Mapping Library computer database (see Kidd et al., 1989a, for the most recent printed summary). The polymorphism information content (Botstein et al., 1980) is a measure of how frequently the individual locus will be useful in mapping a disease locus such as MEN2A. Most of these loci will be useful individually more than half the time; some combination of loci will be useful in almost all families.

The CEPH Consortium map (White et al., 1990) finds that recombination rates are higher in female meiosis for at least 18 of the 27 intervals defined by 28 loci in the map. In the remaining nine intervals the difference was statistically significant for higher rates in male meiosis in four intervals, two of which are near the ends of the map. Our independent data give a similar picture overall (unpublished observations). However, we have found the magnitude of the sex difference in the region encompassing MEN2A to be surprisingly large.

Our study of the pericentromeric region (Wu et al., 1990) was the first to have a large enough sample size to show significant differences in male and female recombination frequencies in small regions. As shown in the summary in Fig. 6,

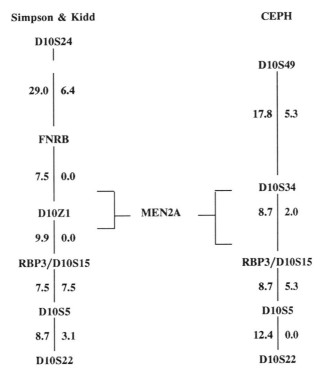

FIG. 6. Maps of the pericentromeric region of chromosome 10. The two maps are given in centimorgans, assuming Haldane's mapping function. The female map distances are on the left of each interval and the male distances are on the right. These two maps are based on independent sets of data and slightly different markers. The Simpson and Kidd map is based on data collected in 15 large kindreds, some with MEN 2A and some with other (or no) disorders (Wu *et al.*, 1990; unpublished observations). The CEPH map is based on the 40 nuclear families in the CEPH collaboration (White *et al.*, 1990).

there is no recombination detected in male meiosis from *FNRB* (in the proximal short arm) across the centromere (marked by *D10Z1*) to *RBP3* (in the proximal long arm). In contrast, each of the intervals on either side of the centromere shows about 8% recombination in female meiosis. The same is seen between *MEN2A* and each of the flanking markers, *FNRB* and *RBP3*, but the sample size (i.e., the number of meiotic products "assayed") is necessarily smaller for estimates involving *MEN2A* than for those involving just the markers. For example, the children can give information on recombination between markers in meiosis in the normal spouse as well as in the parent with MEN 2A, and families other than those with MEN 2 can be studied. As discussed in Section V, D, this sex difference in recombination frequencies has important clinical applications.

The difference might also be a major factor in the different estimates obtained by Ponder's group and ours for the distance from *RBP3* to *MEN2A* (see Nakamura *et al.*, 1989a).

D.   CLINICAL APPLICATIONS CURRENTLY POSSIBLE

Given the autosomal dominant inheritance pattern of MEN 2A, each child of an affected parent had a 50% risk of having inherited the abnormal allele at the *MEN2A* locus. The high risk and the fact that early surgery for MTC is curative justified screening programs, but half of those screened would never have the disease. Until a tumor developed or an at-risk family member remained disease free past early adulthood, there was little change from that 50:50 chance. Ponder *et al.* (1988) have given several examples of how age can be used to improve the risk estimates for unaffected individuals. Easton *et al.* (1989) have provided the first epidemiologically appropriate analysis to estimate the cumulative incidence distribution for MEN 2A. Unfortunately, there is a clear limit to the accuracy of risk estimates, even if the appropriate age-of-onset distribution is available. [For a discussion of the general problems of estimating age-of-onset distributions, see Heimbuch *et al.* (1980).] However, using DNA markers,highly accurate pre-symptomatic "diagnosis" is possible for a large percentage of families with MEN 2A. The diagnosis is based entirely on linkage and might be more accurately thought of as risk assessment. Using linkage, there is the possibility that an individual could be shown at an early age to have a specific risk for MEN 2A; this risk could be anything from virtually zero to virtually 100%, depending on the data and the amount of information on affected relatives.

In theory, it is possible with genetic linkage to know precisely who shares the identical relevant piece of DNA with an affected relative and who does not. In practice, what is known depends on several variables: how informative the nearby markers are, how close the markers are, and who else in the family can be studied. The best markers are those that allow the chromosome with the abnormal gene to be uniquely identified within the family. The five markers closest to *MEN2A* are all multiallelic, so there is a high probability for each one that an affected parent will have two different alleles, one on the chromosome with the abnormal *MEN2A* allele and a different one on the homolog with the normal allele. Sobol *et al.* (1989) discussed the use of *RBP3, D10S15* (probe pMCK2), and *D10S22* (probe pTB10.163) to improve risk assessment and concluded that even a set of markers on one side can significantly alter risks assigned for specific family members and can strongly reinforce the results of a screening test, especially if the test is borderline. They did not, however, consider sex-specific recombination frequencies in their calculations. Simpson and Kidd (1989b) have presented several examples of risk estimates, taking into account the sex of the parent with MEN 2A.

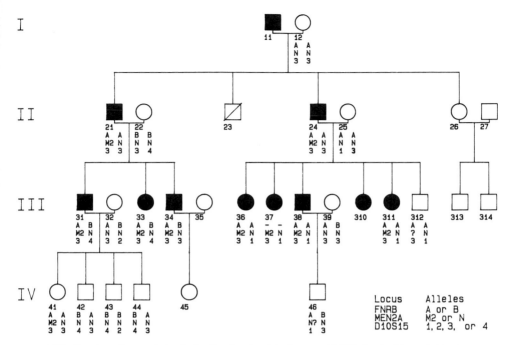

FIG. 7. A pedigree of the O family showing inheritance of MEN 2A (solid symbols), the observed marker alleles at two flanking loci, and the inferred genotypes at the *MEN2A* locus. The inferred chromosomes of each individual are represented by the two vertical columns of allele symbols. No obligate cross-overs are seen in this family. See text for a discussion of risk estimation.

Figure 7 shows four generations of a previously unpublished family in which several relevant points are illustrated. In the first generation the affected individual (#11) is dead, but his unaffected wife (#12) could be tested. In the second generation the two affected individuals (#21 and #24) both got the same alleles from their father, but since the unaffected sister (#26) was not studied, we do not know what the father's other chromosome was. Since the two brothers (#21 and #24) are homozygous for both flanking markers, we cannot use these markers to follow into their children the chromosome that had the abnormal *MEN2A* allele. Thus, we do not know whether the abnormal *MEN2A* allele was transmitted to the child (#312) that is still unaffected. However, in the first sibship in the third generation the affected children all got a different set of markers on the normal chromosome from their mother. As a result we know for certain that the affected son (#31), who himself has four young children, had the abnormal *MEN2A* allele (*M2*) on the chromosome flanked by the *A* allele at FNRB, and the *3* allele at *RBP3;* his other chromosome 10 has the normal allele at the *MEN2A* locus (*N*) flanked by the *B* allele at *FNRB* and the *4* allele at *RBP3*.

When we now look at his four young unaffected children, we see that three got his B4 chromosome and one (#41) got his A3 chromosome. Because the markers show very little recombination in male meiosis, the normal allele at the *MEN2A* locus is almost certainly still between the *B* and *4* alleles and the abnormal allele is still between the *A* and *3* alleles at these flanking loci. To be conservative, we could take 3% recombination on each side of *MEN2A* as the upper limit (remember, none has been observed in male meiosis). In order for the abnormal allele to be on the B4 chromosome, a cross-over would have to have occurred on each side of the *MEN2A* locus (a double cross-over) with a probability of $0.03 \times 0.03 = 0.0009$, or less than 1:1000. Thus, the maximum risk to these three children is still less than 0.001. Conversely, the abnormal allele is still present on the A3 chromosome, with a probability of 1:0.0009; the minimum risk for this child is greater than 0.999. These are numbers that are close to certainty and, if *D10Z1* were shown to be different on the two chromosomes and not to have recombined, the result would be indistinguishable from certainty. Just on available data the conclusion is that sons #42, #43, and #44 probably do not have the abnormal allele and that daughter #41 probably does. Rational patient management would mandate frequent screening of the daughter and suggest that the three sons have periodic check-ups to be on the safe side.

The caveat in such tests is always the possibility of laboratory error, which places a real practical limit on interpretation of results. However, the existence of multiple markers all showing the same pattern of inheritance in several family members provides a high level of confidence in results such as in this example.

Individual #312 presents a different problem, because the DNA marker data do not give any useful information on his genotype. For him we have only the age-of-onset distribution that, since he is still unaffected but over 35 years old, gives him a risk of less than 5% of having the abnormal (*M2*) allele. Additional markers need to be typed and can be combined with the age-dependent risk to refine, either lower or raise, our estimate of his risk.

Individual #46 represents a third situation. In his affected father (#38) the *FNRB* locus is homozygous, but the *D10S15* locus is heterozygous. Thus, we have useful marker information on only one side of the *MEN2A* locus. Individual #46 inherited from his father (#38) the *1* allele at the *D10S15* locus from his unaffected paternal grandmother (#25). If we take a conservative maximum estimate of recombination in his father (#38) of 3%, as above, there is a 97% chance that the normal allele (*N*) at the *MEN2A* locus was inherited with that grandmother's *1* allele. Conversely, the risk of having inherited the abnormal (*M2*) allele at the *MEN2A* locus is the probability that a cross-over took place: 3%. Individual #46 is too young for age to modify that risk and the clinical conclusion has to be that, while unlikely, he might have inherited the abnormal *MEN2A* allele and should be screened regularly. This is another case in which an additional marker closer to (e.g., *D10Z1*) or on the other side of (e.g., *D10S34*) the *MEN2A* locus should be tested to determine whether a cross-over did or did not occur. Such studies are under way to clarify this and the other residual uncertainties discussed above.

E.   STRATEGY TO FIND THE GENE

Available markers allow us to know who has the allele causing MEN 2A if we have sufficient appropriate family members to determine which marker alleles are being transmitted on the same chromosome as the abnormal allele. The markers are not a direct diagnosis. The objective now is to identify and clone the *MEN2A* gene itself. How do we go from the close linkage to cloning the gene? Unfortunately, there is no certain path, and some of what we know already indicates that there are particular problems.

One problem is that the size of the interval we must search is not known, but must be large on a molecular scale. *MEN2A* is 3–4 cM away from *RBP3* and about as much from *FNRB* or *D10S34* on the other side. We do not know how much DNA this is in kilobases because the relationship of linkage map distances in centimorgans to molecular length in kilobases) varies from place to place in the genome and also varies by sex. We can estimate that up to 8 million bp of DNA might separate each of these flanking markers from *MEN2A* in the middle. The α-satellite DNA itself is known to be, on average, 2 million bp long (Wevrick *et al.*, 1989). The distance is almost certainly too long to use molecular walking or jumping (as these were used to get to the *CF* gene) (Rommens *et al.*, 1989).

A second problem is the α-satellite DNA itself. By its nature it is repetitive and there is no way to walk out of it. Thus, though it is the closest marker we have and an obvious place to start from, we cannot apply standard molecular techniques. This is a unique problem faced in the cloning efforts on *MEN2A*, since no other disease gene has been mapped so close to a centromere. Any walking efforts must start from the single-copy markers on either side and move toward the centromere.

A third problem is that we do not know how we will recognize the *MEN2A* locus when we have cloned it. We do not know its function, even vaguely. We do not even know that it must be active in adult endocrine tissues. The hope is that other basic research on normal endocrine differentiation, development, and function will provide clues. Since it may take a few years to get molecularly close, the situation might improve.

Despite these problems, there is much that can be done. In the process ways to circumvent the problems might be found. The first requirement is many more clones from the area. While this might provide useful clones, simply pulling more clones at random from a chromosome 10 library will have a low specific yield, since the region between the flanking markers *FNRB* and *RBP3* is no more than about 5% of the total length of the chromosome. Strategies exist for making a library greatly enriched for the centromeric region of chromosome 10. These are being pursued to improve the chance of finding a random clone in the area. Interestingly, at this point the new clones do not need to identify polymorphisms to be useful, although they must be generally mapped to the region by some means.

From among the new clones some will identify polymorphisms and will be mapped closer to the *MEN2A* locus than the existing markers. To speed this process, it will be necessary to identify all MEN 2A families that have a cross-over between the *MEN2A* locus and the closest flanking markers, *FNRB* and *D10S34* on the short-arm side and *RBP3* and *D10S15* on the long-arm side. A multicenter collaboration to identify those rare parts of families was agreed to at the Third International Workshop on MEN 2A in Heidelberg in 1989. Currently, all groups are typing their families for all markers. There is even the hope that a cross-over with *D10Z1* will be found so that *MEN2A* can be mapped to either the short arm or the long arm. This work will provide tighter molecular bounds on the search for the *MEN2A* locus and will have the immediate clinical benefit of greater accuracy in risk estimation. The additional markers will also allow accurate risk estimates in even more families.

Having more molecular clones in the area will allow the molecular size of the region to be estimated more accurately using pulsed-field gel methods. It will also allow searches for microdeletions in patients and their tumors. While we are not optimistic that mechanisms exist for MEN 2A that are analogous to retinoblastoma and to Wilms' tumor, we cannot exclude these possibilities. While no deletion near the centromere of chromosome 10 has been seen at the cytological level, relevant deletions might be detectable at the molecular level, given the appropriate probes. Such a finding would open up many research strategies, such as the deletion mapping strategy used for molecular mapping of the Wilms' tumor gene (Gessler *et al.*, 1989).

Finally, there is the chance that linkage disequilibrium might help to identify the small molecular region containing the gene. Each of the original mutations occurred on a chromosome characterized by particular alleles at the markers on either side. Following just one of these mutants to its descendants several generations later, we can see that at marker loci that are far away, recombination will cause the mutation-bearing chromosomes to have all possible alleles. Although the marker loci are close (i.e., less than 1% recombination away from the *MEN2A* locus), most of the mutation-bearing chromosomes will still have the same alleles at these close marker loci even many generations later. If we can assemble large kindreds that might share a common abnormal *MEN2A* allele from 10 or more generations ago, we can use the linkage disequilibrium in this "population" to get even closer to the *MEN2A* locus.

Other molecular techniques are being used and/or developed. Zoo blots might help to identify functional genes by identifying sequences conserved in several different species. Yeast artificial chromosomes might help us to clone the large distance more quickly. New jumping procedures might give us many new nearby clones. These and other techniques will be used by the several research groups working on *MEN2A*. While no single approach is guaranteed to succeed, given current knowledge, the success with other disease genes and the rapid increase in knowledge should allow the gene itself to be identified in a few years.

VI. Speculations

A. "RECESSIVE" ONCOGENE HYPOTHESIS?

A major breakthrough in understanding the mechanisms of tumorigenesis was the demonstration by Cavanee *et al.* (1983) that retinoblastoma tumors were the result of loss of the normal allele for the *RB1* locus in the tumor cells, while normal cells retained the normal allele. Cavanee *et al.* (1985) provided beautiful documentation that this loss of the normal allele often occurred as the result of somatic recombination events. This and the earlier work on deletions (Sparkes *et al.*, 1980, 1983) provided a clear conceptual framework for understanding the autosomal dominant mode of inheritance in families, the variable age of onset, and the clonal origin of tumors. The autosomal dominant inheritance pattern is the result of either a nonfunctioning allele—a mutation rendering the locus inactive or the protein nonfunctional—or a small deletion removing the gene entirely from one chromosome. This single abnormal allele being transmitted through the family gives rise to a dominant mode of inheritance. However, the existence of a single normal allele on the other chromosome is sufficient for cells to show normal control of proliferation; a "second hit" that removes the normal allele is required for cells to proliferate, producing the tumor.

In retinoblastoma a common type of second hit is a mitotic error. Errors can be loss of an entire normal chromosome or misdivision such that one daughter cell gets two copies of the identical chromosome and none of its homolog. Other errors are the rare mitotic recombination events that produce daughter cells homozygous (strictly speaking, autozygous) for blocks of genes distal to the recombination event. This mechanism has greatly influenced the research on MEN 2A during the mid-1980s, but no evidence has been found that it is relevant to MEN 2A.

The evidence accumulated from numerous studies shows a few cases of allele loss for chromosome 10 markers, but no systematic pattern indicating anything other than these being consequences, not the cause of the transformation (Wurster-Hill *et al.*, 1986a; Tanaka *et al.*, 1987; Flejter *et al.*, 1988; Nelkin *et al.*, 1989b; Landsvater *et al.*, 1989). Other chromosomes have shown higher frequencies of allele loss than chromosome 10 (e.g., chromosome 1) (Mathew *et al.*, 1987). It is possible that these more frequently involved chromosomes indicate important secondary phenomena that must be considered in multistage development of the tumor. However, such studies are complicated by the fact that tumors frequently develop numerous chromosomal aberrations as a consequence of their altered growth and development.

B. A COMPLICATION RAISED BY THE CENTROMERIC LOCATION OF *MEN2A*

Does the negative evidence for loss of the normal allele on chromosome 10 argue that the primary mechanism in MEN 2A is really different from that in retinoblastoma? It is our opinion that this mechanism, in a general sense, is still a tenable hypothesis. In the case of MEN 2A, because the relevant locus is so close to the centromere, there is almost no room between the centromere and the *MEN2A* locus for somatic crossing-over to occur. Indeed, as we have demonstrated above, we have been unable to detect meiotic recombination between the centromere marker *D10Z1* and the *MEN2A* locus. The same argument can be made for deletions, including loss of the entire chromosome arm. For the cell to be viable, the centromere must be included in the daughter cell, and this leaves little molecular room for a breakpoint between *MEN2A* and the centromere.

The remaining major mechanism would be somatic mutation, occurring in the normal allele, at the locus itself, a mechanism which the molecular studies done to date could not detect. The high penetrance of MTC (generally believed to be essentially 100%, but see Easton *et al.*, 1989) in carriers of the abnormal *MEN2A* allele would indicate, if this were the mechanism, a high somatic mutation rate in the normal allele. A high rate would also be required by the multifocal origins of the tumors.

While no direct evidence supports the normal allele loss hypothesis, we feel the negative evidence—lack of allele loss for DNA markers on chromosome 10—is largely irrelevant, given the proximity of the locus to the centromere.

C. A DIFFERENT MECHANISM

In their excellent review of the topic, Nelkin *et al.* (1989a) concluded that the two-hit theory of Knudson (1971) might not be operative in familial MTC and polyposis coli if one limits that hypothesis to the two alleles at a single locus. However, Knudson did not so limit his initial general hypothesis, and Nelkin *et al.* (1989a) speculated on whether or not the second hit might involve other loci. The tumors in MEN 2A can have multiple origins, and there is even one report of two different types of tumor in one thyroid (Graham *et al.*, 1987). This suggests that different types of second hit might be possible, leading to different types of tumor. Nelkin *et al.* took as their primary focus the types of mechanisms that could/do cause the particular tumor type which sometimes is part of an inherited multitumor syndrome (MEN 2A or MEN 2B), sometimes an inherited pre-disposition to a single tumor type (e.g., MTCWP), sometimes as a sporadic tumor. Linkage data suggest that MTCWP is at the same locus; preliminary data suggest that MEN 2B is also at this locus. Each syndrome seems to be consistent within a family, which argues that it is the specific mutant (abnormal) allele in the germ line that determines the specific syndrome, not the type of second hit or the background genotype. Thus, the three syndromes seem likely to be allelic—caused by different abnormal forms of the same locus. (This is another argument against the recessive oncogene hypothesis.) All of this suggests that the *MEN2A* locus plays some fundamental role in the differentiation of endocrine tissues, which a dominant abnormal allele can disrupt in a manner specific to different abnormal alleles.

The abnormal proliferation of endocrine tissues is a fundamental characteristic of the MEN 2A syndrome. Nelkin *et al.* (1989a) note that hyperplasia of the target cell population is common for both MEN 2A (with the inherited chromosome 10 locus) and polyposis coli (determined by a chromosome 5 locus). Development of the precursor cells before the malignant tumors might be the phenotype of the heterozygote at the respective loci for these two different inherited cancers. The conversion of one of these cells to a tumor cell on a clonal basis might be the consequence of a second hit, possibly at another specific locus. Many different loci might be potential sites for such a second hit. For any of these hypothetical second-hit mechanisms, the inherited defect on chromosome 10 for MEN 2A would thus be necessary, but not sufficient, for development of endocrine tumors.

VII. Conclusions

The mapping of the *MEN2A* locus to chromosome 10 has been followed by refined localization of the gene to a region close to the centromere. Several close and flanking genetic markers are now available for clinical use. In most families with MEN 2A, these markers allow presymptomatic risk estimates that approach certainty—either the abnormal allele is most likely present or the abnormal allele is most likely absent. Additional markers will soon allow even more certain predictions, tantamount to diagnosis, to be made on an even higher proportion of families. Now the focus has shifted to work toward cloning the gene itself. How this work will progress is less clear. The uncertainty over the mechanism(s) producing the tumors in MEN 2A might not be resolved until the gene is cloned.

ACKNOWLEDGMENTS

The preparation of this paper and the research in our laboratories have been supported by National Institutes of Health Grant CA32066 (to K.K.K.) and by Grant MT 5783 (to N.E.S.) from the Medical Research Council of Canada. We want to thank our several colleagues and collaborators and especially, for their useful comments and assistance on this review, Dr. Myron Genel, Jingshi Wu, and

Judith R. Kidd. We also want to thank Dr. Andrew J. Pakstis, Dr. Claiborne Stevens, Mathew Hawley, Martin Mador, and Rowena Track for their help with the illustrations. Special thanks go to Rebecca Murray for typing the several drafts of this paper.

REFERENCES

Babu, V. R., Van Dyke, D. L., and Jackson, C. E. (1984). *Proc. Natl. Acad. Sci. U.S.A.* **81,** 2525–2528.

Babu, V. R., Van Dyke, D. ., Flejter, W. L., and Jackson, C. E. (1987). *Am. J. Med. Genet.* **27,** 739–748.

Bale, A. E., Friedman, E., Sakaguchi, K., Nakamura, Y., McBride, O. W., Spiegel, A. M., Aurbach, G. D., and Marx, S. J. (1989). *Cytogenet. Cell Genet.* **51,** 956.

Bale, S. J., Bale, A. E., Stewart, K., Dachowski, L., McBride, O. W., Glaser, T., Green, J. E., III, Mulvihill, J. J., Brandi, M. L., Sakaguchi, K., Aurbach, G. D., and Marx, S. J. (1989). *Genomics* **4,** 320–322.

Baylin, S. B., Gann, D. S., and Hsu, S. H. (1976). *Science* **193,** 321–323.

Baylin, S. B., Gann, D. S., Smallridge, R. C., and Wells, S. A. Jr., (1978). *Science* **199,** 429–431.

Birt, A. R., Hogg, G. R., and Dubé, W. J. (1977). *Arch. Dermatol.* **113,** 1674–1677.

Botstein, D., White, R. L., Skolnick, M., and Davis, R. W. (1980). *Am. J. Hum. Genet.* **32,** 314–331.

Butler, M. G., Kepaske, D. R., Joseph, G. M., and Phillips, J. A., III (1987a). *Cancer Genet. Cytogenet.* **24,** 129–135.

Butler, M. G., Rames, L. J., and Joseph, G. M. (1987b). *Cancer Genet. Cytogenet.* **28,** 253–260.

Carter, C., Easton, D. F., Mathew, C. G. P., Welander, G., Telenius, H., Telenius-Berg, M., and Ponder, B. A. J. (1987). *Cytogenet. Cell Genet.* **45,** 33–37.

Cavanee, W. K., Dryja, T. P., Phillips, R. A., Benedict, W. F., Godbout, R., Gallie, B. L., Murphree, A. L., Strong, L. C., and White, R. L. (1983). *Nature (London)* **305,** 779–784.

Cavanee, W. K., Hansen, M. F., Maumenee, I., Squire, J. A., Phillips, R. A., and Gallie, B. L., (1985). *Science* **228,** 501–503.

Cushman, P., Jr. (1962). *Am. J. Med.* **32,** 352–360.

Devilee, P., Kievits, T., Waye, J. S., Pearson, P. L., and Willard, H. F. (1988). *Genomics* **3,** 1–7.

Donis-Keller, H., Green, P., Helms, C., Cartinhour, S., Weiffenbach, B., Stephens, K., Keith, T. P., Bowden, D. W., Smith, D. R., Lander, E. S., Botstein, D., Akots, G., Rediker, K. S., Gravius, T., Brown, V. A., Rising, M. B., Parker, C., Powers, J. A., Watt, D. E., Kauffman, E. R., Bricker, A., Phipps, P., Muller-Kahle, H., Fulton, T. R., Ng, S., Schumm, J. W., Braman, J. C., Knowlton, R. G., Barker, D. F., Crooks, S. M., Lincoln, S. E., Daly, M. J., and Abrahamson, J. (1987). *Cell (Cambridge, Mass.)* **51,** 319–337.

Easton, D. F., Ponder, M. A., Cummings, T., Gagel, R. F., Hansen, H. H., Reichlin, S., Tashjian, A. H., Jr., Telenius-Berg, M., Ponder, B. A. J., and the Cancer Research Campaign Medullary Thyroid Group (1989). *Am. J. Hum. Genet.* **44,** 208–215.

Emmertsen, K. (1984). *Henry Ford Hosp. Med. J.* **32,** 238–243.

Emmertsen, K., Lamm, L. U., Rasmussen, K. Z., Elband, O., Hansen, H. H., Henningen, K., Jorgensen, J., and Peterson, G. B. (1983). *Cancer Genet. Cytogenet.* **9,** 251–259.

Farndon, J. R., Leight, G. S., Dilley, W. G., Baylin, S. B., Smallridge, R. C., Harrison, T. S., and Wells, S. A., Jr. (1986). *Br. J. Surg.* **73,** 278–281.

Farrer, L. A., Goodfellow, P. J., White, B. N., Holden, J. J. A., Kidd, J. R., Simpson, N. E., and Kidd, K. K. (1987a). *Cancer Genet. Cytogenet.* **27,** 327–334.

Farrer, L. A., Goodfellow, P. J., LaMarche, C. M., Franjkovic, I., Myers, S., White, B. N., Holden, J. J. A., Kidd, J. R., Simpson, N. E., and Kidd, K. K. (1987b). *Am. J. Hum. Genet.* **40,** 329–337.

Farrer, L. A., Castiglione, C. M., Kidd, J. R., Myers, S., Carson, N., Simpson, N. E., and Kidd, K. K. (1988). *Genomics* **3**, 72–77.

Ferrell, R. E., Saad, M. F., and Samaan, N. A. (1984). *Cancer Genet. Cytogenet.* **15**, 315–319.

Flejter, W. L., Babu, V. R., Van Dyke, D. L., and Jackson, C. E. (1988). *Cancer Genet. Cytogenet.* **32**, 301–303.

Gagel, R. F., Jackson, C. E., Block, M. A., Feldman, Z. T., Reichlin, S., Hamilton, B. P., and Tashjian, A. H., Jr. (1982). *J. Pediatr.* **101**, 941–946.

Gagel, R. F., Tashjian, A. H., Jr., Cummings, T., Papathanasopoulos, N., and Reichlin, S. (1987). *Henry Ford Hosp. Med. J.* **35**, 94–98.

Gagel, R. F., Tashjian, A. H., Jr., Cummings, T., Papathanasopoulos, N., Kaplan, M. M., DeLellis, R. A., Wolfe, H. J., and Reichlin, S. (1988). *N. Engl. J. Med.* **318**, 478–484.

Gessler, M., Thomas, G. H., Couillin, P., Junien, C., McGillivray, B. C., Hayden, M., Jaschek, G., and Bruns, G. A. P. (1989). *Hum. Genet.* **44**, 486–495.

Glowniak, J. V., Shapiro, B., Sisson, J. C., Thompson, N. W., Coran, A. G., Lloyd, R., Kelsch, R. C., and Beierwaltes, W. H. (1985). *Arch. Intern. Med.* **145**, 257–261.

Goldfarb, M., Shimizu, K., Perucho, M., and Wigler, M. (1982). *Nature (London)* **296**, 404–409.

Goodfellow, P. J., White, B. N., Holden, J. J. A., Duncan, A. M. V., Sears, E. V. P., Wang, H.-S., Berlin, L., Kidd, K. K., and Simpson, N. E. (1985). *Am. J. Hum. Genet.* **37**, 890–897.

Goodfellow, P. J., Duncan, A. M. V., Farrer, L. A., Holden, J. J. A., White, B. N., Kidd, J. R., Kidd, K. K., and Simpson, N. E. (1987). *Cytogenet. Cell Genet.* **44**, 112–117.

Goodfellow, P. J., Nevanlinna, H. A., Gorman, P., Sheer, D., Lam, G., and Goodfellow, P. N. (1989). *Ann. Hum. Genet.* **53**, 15–22.

Graham, S. M., Genel, M., Touloukian, R. J., Barwick, K. W., Gertner, J. M., and Torony, C. (1987). *J. Pediatr. Surg.* **22**, 501–503.

Graze, K., Spiler, I. J., Tashjian, A. H., Melvin, K. E. W., Cervi-Skinner, S., Gagel, R. F., Miller, H. H., Wolfe, H. J., DeLellis, R. A., Leape, L., Feldman, Z. T., and Reichlin, S. (1978). *N. Engl. J. Med.* **299**, 980–985.

Gusella, J. F., Wexler, N. S., Conneally, P. M., Naylor, S. L., Anderson, M. A., Tanzi, R. E., Watkins, P. C., Ottina, K., Wallace, M. R., Sakaguchi, A. Y., Young, A. B., Shoulson, I., Bonilla, E., and Martin, J. B. (1983). *Nature (London)* **306**, 234–238.

Gustavson, K. H., Jansson, R., and Öberg, K. (1983). *Clin. Genet.* **23**, 143–149.

Hamilton, B. P., Landberg, L., and Levine, R. J. (1978). *Am. J. Med.* **65**, 1027–1032.

Heimbuch, R. C., Matthysse, S., and Kidd, K. K. (1980). *Am. J. Hum. Genet.* **32**, 564–574.

Hodge, S. E., Morton, L. A., Tideman, S., Kidd, K. K., and Spence, M. A. (1979). *Am. J. Hum. Genet.* **31**, 761–762.

Hsu, T. C., Pathak, S., Samaan, N., and Hickey, R. C. (1981). *JAMA, J. Am. Med. Assoc.* **20**, 2046–2048.

Ikeuchi, T., Takai, S., Miki, T., Tateishi, H., Nishisho, I., and Kondo, I. (1987). *Cytogenet. Cell Genet.* **46**, 632.

Irvin, G. L., III, Fishman, L. M., and Sher, J. A. (1983). *Surgery* **96**, 938–940.

Jackson, C. E., Tashjian, A. H., Jr., and Block, M. A. (1973). *Ann. Intern. Med.* **78**, 845–852.

Jackson, C. E., Conneally, P. M., Sizemore, G. W., and Tashjian, A. H., Jr. (1976). *In* "Cancer and Genetics, Birth Defects: Original article series" (D. Bergsma, ed.), Vol. 12, pp. 159–164. Liss, New York.

Jackson, C. E., Norum, R. A., O'Neal, L. W., Nikolai, T. F., and Delaney, J. P. (1988). *Am. J. Hum. Genet.* **43**, A147.

Keiser, H. R., Beaven, M. A., Doppman, J., Wells, S., and Buja, L. M. (1973). *Ann. Intern. Med.* **78**, 561–579.

Kerem, B., Rommens, J. M., Buchanan, J. A., Markiewicz, D., Cox, T. K., Chakravarti, A., Buchwald, M., and Tsui, L. C. (1989). *Science* **245**, 1073–1080.

Kidd, K. K. (1987). *In* "Proceedings of the 7th International Congress of Human Genetics" (Vogel, F., Sperling, K. Eds.) pp. 99–106. Springer Verlag, New York.

Kidd, K. K., Kruger, S. D., Gerhard, D. S., Kidd, J. R., Housman, D., and Gertner, J. M. (1984). *Henry Ford Hosp. Med. J.* **32,** 262–265.

Kidd, K. K., Kidd, J. R., Castiglione, C. M., Genel, M., Darby, J., Cavalli-Sforza, L. L., and Gusella, J. F. (1986a). *Hum. Hered.* **36,** 243–249.

Kidd, K. K., Kidd, J. R., Castiglione, C. M., Pakstis, A. J., and Sparkes, R. S. (1986b). *Genet. Epidemiol.* **3,** 195–200.

Kidd, K. K., Bowcock, A. M., Schmidtke, J., Track, R. K., Ricciuti, F., Hutchings, G., Bale, A., Pearson, P., and Willard, H. F., with help from Gelernter, J., Giuffra, L., and Kubzdela, K. (1989a). *Cytogenet. Cell Genet.* **51,** 622–947.

Kidd, K. K., Klinger, H. P., and Ruddle, F. H. (1989b). *Cytogenet. Cell Genet.* **51,** 1–1147.

Knudson, A. G., Jr. (1971). *Proc. Natl. Acad. Sci. U.S.A.* **68,** 820–823.

Koufos, A., Hansen, M. F., Lampkin, B. C., Workman, M. L., Copeland, N. G., Jenkins, N. A., and Cavenee, W. K. (1984). *Nature (London)* **309,** 170–172.

Kramer, P. L., Farrer, L. A., Pakstis, A. J., and Kidd, K. K. (1986). *Genet. Epidemiol., Suppl.* **1,** 153–158.

Kruger, S. D., Gertner, J. M., Sparkes, R. S., Haedt, L. E., Crist, M., Sparkes, M. C., Genel, M., and Kidd, K. K. (1986). *Hum. Hered.* **36,** 6–11.

Landsvater, R. M., Mathew, C. G. P., Smith, B. A., Marcus, E. M., te Meerman, G. J., Lips, C. J. M., Geerdink, R. A., Nakamura, Y., Ponder, B. A. J., and Buys, C. H. C. M. (1989). *Genomics* **4,** 246–250.

Larsson, C., Skogseid, B., Öberg, K., Nakamura, Y., and Nordenskjöld, M. (1988). *Nature (London)* **332,** 85–87.

Lathrop, G. M., Lalouel, J.-M., Julier, C., and Ott, J. (1984). *Proc. Natl. Acad. Sci. U.S.A.* **81,** 3443–3446.

Lathrop, M., Nakamura, Y., Cartwright, P., O'Connell, P., Leppert, M., Jones, C., Tateishi, H., Bragg, T., Lalouel, J., and White, R. (1988). *Genomics* **2,** 157–164.

Lips, C. J. M., den Aantrekker, E., Jansen-Schillhorn van Veen, J. M., Geerdink, R. A., Griffioen, G., and van Slooten, E. A. (1984). *Henry Ford Hosp. Med. J.* **32,** 236–237.

Lulu, D. J., Corcoran, T. E., and Andre, M. (1968). *Am. J. Surg.* **115,** 695–701.

Mathew, C. B. P., Chin, K. S., Easton, D. F., Thorpe, K., Carter, C., Liou, G. I., Fong, S.-L., Bridges, C. D. B., Haak, H., Nieuwenhuijzen Kruseman, A. C., Schifter, S., Hansen, H. H., Telenius, H., Telenius-Berg, M., and Ponder, B. A. J. (1987). *Nature (London)* **328,** 527–528.

Maton, P. N., Norton, J. A., Nieman, L. K., Doppman, J. L., and Jensen, T. R. (1989). *JAMA, J. Am. Med. Assoc.* **262,** 535–537.

Miki, T., Nishisho, I., Tateishi, H., Chen, Y., Kidd, J. R., Wu, J., Pravtcheva, D., Pakstis, A. J., Takai, S., Ruddle, F. H., and Kidd, K. K. (1988). *Genomics* **3,** 78–81.

Morton, N. E. (1955). *Am. J. Hum. Genet.* **7,** 277–318.

Mulvihill, J. J. (1977). *In* "Genetics of Human Cancer" (J. J. Mulvihill, R. W. Miller, and J. F. Fraumeni, Jr., eds.), pp. 137–143. Raven, New York.

Mulvihill, J. J. (1984). *Henry Ford Hosp. Med. J.* **32,** 277–282.

Nakamura, Y., Lathrop, M., Bragg, T., Leppert, M., O'Connell, P., Jones, C., Lalouel, J. M., and White, R. (1988a). *Genomics* **3,** 389–392.

Nakamura, Y., Lathrop, M., O'Connell, P., Leppert, M., Barker, D., Wright, E., Skolnick, M., Kondoleon, S., Litt, M., Lalouel, J. M., and White, R. (1988b). *Genomics* **2,** 302–309.

Nakamura, Y., Lathrop, M., O'Connell, P., Leppert, M., Lalouel, J. M., and White, R. (1988c). *Genomics* **3,** 67–71.

Nakamura, Y., Mathew, C. G. P., Sobol, H., Easton, D. F., Telenius, H., Bragg, T., Chin, K.,

Clark, J., Jones, C., Lenoir, G. M., White, R., and Ponder, B. A. J. (1989a). *Genomics* **5,** 199–204.

Nakamura, Y., Larsson, C., Julier, C., Byström, Skogseid, B., Wells, S., Öberg, K., Carlson, M., Taggart, T., O'Connell, P., Leppert, M., Lalouel, J. M., Nordenskjöld, M., and White, R. (1989b). *Am. J. Hum. Genet.* **44,** 751–755.

Narod, S. A., Sobol, H., Nakamura, Y., Calmettes, C., Baullieu, J. L., Bigorgne, J. C., Chabrier, G., Couette, J., de Gennes, J. L., Duprey, J., Gardet, P., Guillausseau, P. J., Guilloteau, D., Houdent, C., Lefebvre, J., Modigliani, E., Parmentier, C., Pugeat, M., Siame, C., Tourniaire, J., Vandroux, J. C., Vinot, J. M., and Lenoir, G. M. (1989). *Hum. Genet.* **83,** 353–358.

Nelkin, B. D., de Bustros, A. C., Mabry, M., and Baylin, S. (1989a). *JAMA, J. Am. Med. Assoc.* **261,** 3130–3135.

Nelkin, B. D., Nakamura, Y., White, R. W., de Bustros, A. D., Herman, J., Wells, S. A., and Baylin, S. B. (1989b). *Cancer Res.* **49,** 4114–4119.

Noll, W. W., Maurer, L. H., Beisswenger, P. J., Quinn, B. M., Cate, C. C., Bassick, J. P., Clark, P. A., and Colacchio, T. A. (1984). *Henry Ford Hosp. Med. J.* **32,** 244–245.

Noll, W. W., Bowden, D. W., Maurer, L. H., Müller-Kahle, H., Gravius, T. C., Braeuler, C., Chamberlain, M., Knowlton, R. G., Memoli, V. A., Green, P., Colacchio, T. A., Brinck-Johnsen, T., Rediker, K., Powers, J., and Donis-Keller, H. (1988). *Am. J. Human Genet. Suppl.* **43,** abstr. 116.

O'Connell, P., Lathrop, G. M., Law, M., Leppert, M., Nakamura, Y., Hoff, M., Kumlin, E., Thomas, W., Elsner, T., Ballard, L., Goodman, P., Azen, E., Sadler, J. E., Cai, G. Y., Lalouel, J. M., and White, R. (1987). *Genomics* **1,** 93–102.

Orkin, S. H., Goldman, D. S., and Sallan, S. E. (1984). *Nature (London)* **309,** 172–174.

Ott, J. (1974). *Am. J. Hum. Genet.* **26,** 588–597.

Ott, J. (1985). *In* "Analysis of Human Genetic Linkage." The Johns Hopkins Univ. Press, Baltimore, Maryland.

Pakstis, A. J., Kidd, J. R., Castiglione, C. M., Pletcher, B. A., Murphy, P. D., Farrer, L. A., Genel, M., and Kidd, K. K. (1987). *Henry Ford Hosp. Med. J.* **35,** 164–167.

Partington, M. W., Ghent, W. R., Sears, E. V. P., and Simpson, N. E. (1981). *Can. Med. J.* **124,** 403–410.

Pearse, A. G. E. (1976). *Nature (London)* **262,** 92–94.

Pearson, P. L., Kidd, K. K., and Willard, H. F. (1987). *Cytogenet. Cell Genet.* **46,** 390–566.

Ponder, B. A. J. (1984). *Henry Ford Hosp. Med. J.* **32,** 233–235.

Ponder, B. A. J., Jeffreys, A. J., Hartley, N. E., Carter, C., Easton, D. F., Telenius, H., and Telenius-Berg, M. (1987). *Henry Ford Hosp. Med. J.* **35,** 161–163.

Ponder, B. A. J., Coffey, R., Gagel, R. F., Semple, P., Ponder, M. A., Pembrey, M. E., Telenius-Berg, M., and Easton, D. F. (1988). *Lancet* **1,** 397–400.

Reeders, S. T., Keith, T., Green, P., Germino, G. G., Barton, N. J., Lehmann, O. J., Brown, V. A., Phipps, P., Morgan, J., Bear, J. C., and Parfrey, P. (1988). *Genomics* **3,** 150–155.

Riordan, J. R., Rommens, J. M., Kerem, B., Alon, N., Rozmahel, R., Grzelczak, Z., Zielenski, J., Lok, S., Plavsic, N., Chou, J. L., Drumm, M. L., Iannuzzi, C., Collins, F. S., and Tsui, L. C. (1989). *Science* **245,** 1066–1073.

Rommens, J. M., Iannuzzi, M. C., Kerem, B., Drumm, M. L., Melmer, G., Dean, M., Rozmahel, R., Cole, J. L., Kennedy, D., Hidaka, N., Zsiga, M., Buchwald, M., Riordan, J. R., Tsui, L. C., and Collins, F. S. (1989). *Science* **245,** 1059–1065.

Saad, M. F., Ordonez, N. G., Rashid, R. K., Guido, J. J., Hill, C. S., Hickey, R. C., and Samaan, N. A. (1984). *Medicine* **63,** 319–342.

Schimke, R. N. (1986). *N. Engl. J. Med.* **314,** 1315–1316.

Shih, C., Padhy, L. C., Murray, M., and Weinberg, R. A. (1981). *Nature (London)* **290,** 261.

Simpson, N. E., and Falk, J. (1982). *Hum. Genet.* **60,** 157.

Simpson, N. E., and Kidd, K. K. (1987). *Henry Ford Hosp. Med. J.* **35,** 168–171.

Simpson, N. E., and Kidd, K. K. (1989a). *Henry Ford Hosp. Med. J.* **37,** 100–105.

Simpson, N. E., and Kidd, K. K. (1989b). *J. Horm. Metab. Res.* **21,** 5–9.

Simpson, N. E., Kidd, K. K., Goodfellow, P. J., McDermid, H., Myers, S., Kidd, J. R., Jackson, C. E., Duncan, A. M. V., Farrer, L. A., Brasch, K., Castiglione, C., Genel, M., Gertner, J., Greenberg, C. R., Gusella, J. F., Holden, J. J. A., and White, B. N. (1987). *Nature (London)* **328,** 528–530.

Sipple, J. H. (1961). *Am. J. Med.* **31,** 163–166.

Sipple, J. H. (1984). *Henry Ford Hosp. Med. J.* **32,** 219–222.

Sizemore, G. W., Heath, J., and Carney, J. A. (1980). *Clin. Endocrinol. Metab.* **9,** 299–315.

Smith, M., and Simpson, N. E. (1989). *Cytogenet. Cell Genet.* **51,** 202–225.

Sobol, H., Salvetti, A., Bonnardel, C., and Lenoir, G. (1988). *Lancet* **1,** 62.

Sobol, H., Narod, S. A., Nakamura, Y., Boneu, A., Calmettes, C., Chadenas, D., Charpentier, G., Chatal, J. R., Delepine, N., Delisle, M. J., Dupond, J. L., Gardet, P., Godefroy, H., Guillausseau, P. J., Guillausseau-Scholer, C., Houden, C., Lalau, J. D., Mace, G., Paramentier, C., Soubrier, F., Tourniaire, J., and Lenoir, G. M. (1989). *N. Engl. J. Med.* **321,** 996–1001.

Sparkes, R. S., Sparkes, M. C., Wilson, M. G., Towner, J. W., Benedict, W., Murphree, A. L., and Yunis, J. J. (1980). *Science* **208,** 1042–1044.

Sparkes, R. S., Murphree, A. L., Lingua, R. W., Field, L. L., Funderburk, S. J., and Benedict, W. F. (1983). *Science* **219,** 971–972.

Steiner, A. L., Goodman, A. D., and Powers, S. R. (1968). *Medicine* **47,** 371–409.

Takai, S., Miyauchi, A., Matsumoto, H., Ikeuchi, T., Miki, T., Kuma, K., and Kumahara, Y. (1984). *Henry Ford Hosp. Med. J.* **32,** 246–250.

Tanaka, K., Baylin, S. B., Nelkin, B. D., and Testa, J. R. (1987). *Cancer Genet. Cytogenet.* **25,** 27–35.

Tateishi, H., Takai, S., Nishisho, I., Miki, T., Motomura, K., Okazaki, M., Miyauchi, A., Ikeuchi, T., Yamamoto, K., Hattori, T., Kumahara, Y., Matsumoto, H., Honjo, T., and Mori, T. (1987). *Henry Ford Hosp. Med. J.* **35,** 157–163.

Telenius-Berg, M., Berg, B., Hamberger, B., Tibblin, S., Tisell, L., Ysander, L., and Welander, G. (1984). *Henry Ford Hosp. Med. J.* **32,** 225–232.

Thakker, R. V., Bouloux, P., Wooding, C., Chotai, K., Broad, P. M., Spurr, N. K., Besser, G. M., and O'Riordan, J. L. H. (1989). *N. Engl. J. Med.* **321,** 218–224.

Tsui, L. C., Buchwald, M., Barker, D., Braman, J. C., Knowlton, R., Schumm, J. W., Eiberg, H., Mohr, J., Kennedy, D., Plavsic, N., Zsiga, M., Markiewicz, D., Akots, G., Grown, V., Helms, C., Gravius, T., Parker, C., Rediker, K., and Donis-Keller, H. (1985). *Science* **230,** 1054–1057.

Van Dyke, D. L., Jackson, C. E., and Babu, V. R. (1981). *Am. J. Hum. Genet.* **33,** Suppl. 69a.

Van Dyke, D. L., Babu, V. R., and Jackson, C. E. (1984). *Henry Ford Hosp. Med. J.* **32,** 266–268.

Verdy, M. B., Cadotte, M., Schurch, W., Sturtridge, W. C., Cantin, J., Weber, A. M., Lacroix, A., and Forster-Gibson, C. (1984). *Henry Ford Hosp. Med. J.* **32,** 251–253.

Wells, S. A., Baylin, S. B., Linehan, W. M., Farrell, R. E., Cox, E. G., and Cooper, C. W. (1978). *Ann. Surg.* **188,** 139–141.

Wevrick, R., Bedford, H. M., and Williard, H. F. (1989). *Cytogenet. Cell Genet.* HGM10 51, 1107 [a2636].

White, R., Leppert, M., Bishop, D. T., Barker, D., Berkowitz, J., Brown, C., Callahan, P., Holm, T., and Jerominski, L. (1985). *Nature (London)* **313,** 101–105.

White, R., Lalouel, J. M., Nakamura, Y., Donis-Keller, H., Green, P., Bowden, D., Mathew, C., Easton, D. Robson, E., Morton, N., Gusella, J., Haines, J., Retief, A., Kidd, K. K., Murray, J., Lathrop, M., and Cann, H. (1990). *Genomics* **6,** 393–412.

Wu, J., and Kidd, K. K. (1990a). *Hum. Genet.* **84,** 279–282.

Wu, J., and Kidd, K. K. (1990b). *Nucleic Acids Res.* **13,** 1316.

Wu, J., Ramesh, V., Kidd, J. R., Castiglione, C. M., Myers, S., Carson, N., Anderson, L., Gusella, J. F., Simpson, N. E., and Kidd, K. K. (1988a). *Cytogenet. Cell Genet.* **48,** 126–127.

Wu, J., Cavanee, W. K., Miki, T., and Kidd, K. K. (1988b). *Cytogenet. Cell Genet.* **48,** 246–247.

Wu, J., Giuffra, L. A., Goodfellow, P. J., Myers, S., Carson, N. L., Anderson, L., Hoyle, L. S., Simpson, N. E., and Kidd, K. K. (1989). *Hum. Genet.* **83,** 383–390.

Wu, J., Carson, N. L., Myers, S., Pakstis, A. J., Kidd, J. R., Castiglione, C. M., Anderson, L., Hoyle, L. S., Genel, M., Simpson, N. E., and Kidd, K. K. (1990). *Am. J. Hum. Genet.* **46,** 624–630.

Wurster-Hill, D. H., Noll, W. N., Bircher, L. Y., Pettengill, O. S., and Grizzle, W. A. (1986a). *Cancer Genet. Cytogenet.* **20,** 247–253.

Wurster-Hill, D. H., Noll, W. W., Bircher, L. Y., Devlin, J., and Schultz, E. (1986b). *Cancer Res.* **46,** 2134–2138.

Yamamoto, M., Takai, S., Miki, T., Motomura, K., Okazaki, M., Nishisho, I., Tateishi, H., Honjo, T., Pakstis, A. J., and Mori, T. (1989). *Hum. Genet.* **82,** 287–288.

Zatterale, A., Stabile, M., Nunziata, V., DeGiovanni, G., Vecchione, R., and Ventruto, V. (1984). *J. Med. Genet.* **121,** 108–111.

Zhang, Y., Saison, M., Spaepen, M., De Strooper, B., Van Leuven, F., David, G., Van den Berghe, H., and Cassiman, J. J. (1988). *Somat. Cell Mol. Genet.* **14,** 99–104.

DISCUSSION

R.S. Swerdloff.   I believe there have been reports of a second chromosomal alteration in some of these families and of a two-hit hypothesis with regard to the manifestation of this disease. Can you bring us up to date on this?

K. K. Kidd.   There has been a lot of speculation on the two-hit hypothesis, but there is no consensus. Several people have examined tumor tissue from many different individuals, looking for loss of heterozygosity and for cytogenic anomalies in the tumor tissue that differ from those of the somatic tissue. Differences have been found on a large number of different chromosomes, but there is no single chromosome that stands out unequivocally. A few chromosomes, chromosome 1, for example, seem to show more frequent anomalies than any of the others, but a wide variety of chromosomes show anomalies. Almost all of these could be purely secondary phenomena. It is well known that cytogenic anomalies accumulate in tissue that has become malignant, and the lack of any consensus would tend to argue that these are just chance phenomena subsequent to the initial transformation and not part of the transformation. Alternatively, it could be that any of several different second hits might trigger the transformation and that some of these do represent different classes of second hits.

M. New.   I am just reeling from the idea that chromosome 10 is now a sex chromosome. Is it true that there are differences in the recombination ratios for other autosomes?

K. K. Kidd.   There is overall a very strong sex difference, the female showing something between one and a half to two times as much recombination as males through much of the human genome. In contrast, there tends to be an expansion of the genetic map near the telomeres in male meiosis. For example, at the tip of the short arm of chromosome 11 there is more recombination among loci in male meiosis than there is in female meiosis. This phenomenon also seems to be true at the tips of both the short and long arms of chromosome 10, and probably at the tips of the arms of several other chromosomes. The maps have only just begun to come together during the last year and a half, so it is very difficult to make generalizations. Though the linkage data are highly significant, from a statistical point of view, in terms of getting the correct order of loci in the maps, there are still huge confidence intervals on the actual distances between loci. Recombination frequency is inherently a statistical phenomenon; you are basically looking at the "dealing of cards or rolling of dice" as they occur in meiosis. Thus, there is no way of ignoring the statistics. Sample sizes for human maps are not quite large enough, in most cases, to give accurate estimates of sex differences. Our sample for the centromeric region of chromosome 10 is one of the largest samples, and it is the first time we have been able to show, for a single very small region, a very large sex effect with high statistical significance. In most other studies the statistical significance is based on larger regions because there are more events (meiotic products). To summarize, for most regions of the genome, the prior assumption has to be that there is a sex difference, and, in most cases, it favors more recombination in females than in males. But the consensus is growing that the telomeres show the opposite: more recombination in males.

G. B. Cutler.   Can anything be learned from the sporadic cases of these same tumors? Are they similar to the sporadic medullary thyroid cancer? Can they be searched for homozygosity or other abnormalities, deletions, etc., in this same area?

K. K. Kidd.   They certainly could be. Now that we are "honing" in on where the gene is, one of the important things to do is to study that region in sporadic tumors. The fact that we do not see much increase in homozygosity may be a function of where the gene is and the fact that the mechanisms that normally would generate homozygosity cannot. But, as we are now working to saturate the region with clones, we can look for microdeletions in that area. They may very well be important in sporadic tumors.

N. Josso.   Could the sex difference in recombination frequency be linked to the fact that in the female meiosis is a much more protracted procedure, since oocytes stay in the prophase of meiosis from fetal life to whenever ovulation occurs?

K. K. Kidd.   Yes, but I would phrase it in a different way. I think recombination events themselves probably take place prior to birth, and the protracted phase is subsequent to the actual recombination event. But I look at it in a broader framework: that male meiosis and female meiosis, though we have always thought of them as genetically identical, are physiologically and biologically completely different phenomena. Male meiosis does not even start until puberty, whereas in female meiosis the pairing and all the recombination events take place before birth and subsequent divisions do not take place until, one a month, each oocyte matures. In fact, the second meiotic division takes place only after the oocyte is fertilized by a sperm. If we can have duplicate genes that control salivary and pancreatic amylase (but one of many examples), we can certainly have duplicate genes or even different genes that control similar recombination functions, but under these very different cellular environments. Recombination is clearly, in the broadest sense, an enzymatically driven phenomenon; it is very precise at the molecular level, though it may be somewhat random in terms of where it occurs in any given cell. Thus, there is a very complicated mechanism involved and there may be—probably are—preferential recognition sequences where this complex attaches to the DNA, aligns the DNA, and causes this exchange of strands. If there are such recognition sequences, they may be very different for male meiosis and female meiosis. It may be differences in the numbers and distributions of these recognition sequences which result in the differences in male and female recombination rates. Many other hypotheses could explain the differences, but this hypothesis has emphasized to me that these are fundamentally different physiological processes.

G. B. Cutler.   One feature of the MEN disorder that intrigues me is that the thyroid gland disease virtually always progresses to malignancy, whereas the adrenal disease can either be benign or malignant and the parathyroid disease is virtually always benign. How does the same gene give rise to these clinically very different neoplastic processes?

K. K. Kidd.   I do not know, but that is what is so challenging and interesting about this disease. The tumors are different. They occur in different tissues and they have different age-of-onset spectrums and frequencies. Individuals in a family where PHEOs are common may have MTC and live a long time, but never develop pheochromocytoma. These are some of the intriguing aspects of this disease and of the underlying mechanism that must be involved.

G. B. Cutler. How do you calculate these LOD scores?

K. K. Kidd. The probability equations can be written out and the LOD scores calculated by hand. In almost all of these cases, however, a computer program is used. For example, my laboratory is one of the largest users of computers in the medical school; some of the analyses we have done have literally used a week of CPU time. On a time-sharing basis that may be 3 weeks from the "job in to the job out." These are the times on the largest available VAX computer. (I was very fortunate when I applied for a big computer. The reviewers' comments were "you didn't apply for a big enough one," and they actually overfunded me so I could get a bigger computer.) There are two commonly used statistical analysis programs distributed free of charge. One does marker-to-marker analyses, or marker-to-disease, just two loci at a time. The other does the multipoint analyses and will generate complex LOD score curves, using a much more elaborate computer algorithm. However, because it is more elaborate, it takes much longer to do the analysis. There are several other programs available. For some there is a charge; others are newer and are just being distributed. To do these types of analyses, very sophisticated computer programs and a lot of computer power are required.

INDEX